Advances in Ultrasound

Guest Editor

VIKRAM S. DOGRA, MD

ULTRASOUND CLINICS

www.ultrasound.theclinics.com

July 2009 • Volume 4 • Number 3

SAUNDERS an imprint of ELSEVIER, Inc.

W.B. SAUNDERS COMPANY
A Division of Elsevier Inc.

1600 John F. Kennedy Boulevard ● Suite 1800 ● Philadelphia, Pennsylvania 19103-2899

http://www.theclinics.com

ULTRASOUND CLINICS Volume 4, Number 3
July 2009 ISSN 1556-858X, ISBN-13: 978-1-4377-0553-9, ISBN-10: 1-4377-0553-7

Editor: Barton Dudlick
Developmental Editor: Theresa Collier

Ultrasound Clinics (ISSN 1556-858X) is published quarterly by W.B. Saunders, 360 Park Avenue South, New York, NY 10010-1710. Months of publication are January, April, July, and October. Business and editorial offices: 1600 John F. Kennedy Boulevard, Suite 1800, Philadelphia, Pennsylvania 19103-2899. Accounting and circulation offices: 6277 Sea Harbor Drive, Orlando, FL 32887-4800. Periodicals postage paid at New York, NY, and additional mailing offices. Subscription prices are $189 per year for (US individuals), $274 per year for (US institutions), $94 per year for (US students and residents), $215 per year for (Canadian individuals), $306 per year for (Canadian institutions), $229 per year for (international individuals), $306 per year for (international institutions), and $114 per year for (Canadian and foreign students/residents). To receive student/resident rate, orders must be accompanied by name of affiliated institution, date of term, and the signature of program/residency coordinator on institution letterhead. Orders will be billed at individual rate until proof of status is received. Foreign air speed delivery is included in all Clinics subscription prices. All prices are subject to change without notice. **POSTMASTER:** Send address changes to *Ultrasound Clinics,* Elsevier Health Sciences Division, Subscription Customer Service, 3251 Riverport Lane, Maryland Heights, MO 63043. **Customer Service (orders, claims, online, change of address): Telephone: 1-800-654-2452 (U.S. and Canada); 314-447-8871(outside U.S. and Canada). Fax: 314-447-8029. E-mail: journalscustomerservice-usa@elsevier.com (for print support); journalsonlinesupport-usa@elsevier.com (for online support).**

Reprints: For copies of 100 or more, of articles in this publication, please contact the Commercial Reprints Department, Elsevier Inc., 360 Park Avenue South, New York, NY 10010-1710. Tel.: (+1) 212-633-3812; Fax: (+1) 212-462-1935; E-mail: reprints@elsevier.com.

Contributors

GUEST EDITOR

VIKRAM S. DOGRA, MD
Professor of Radiology, Urology & Biomedical
Engineering, Department of Imaging Sciences,
University of Rochester Medical Center,
Rochester, New York

AUTHORS

MICHELE BERTOLOTTO, MD
Assistant Professor, Department of Radiology,
University of Trieste, Ospedale di Cattinara,
Trieste, Italy

SHWETA BHATT, MD
Department of Imaging Sciences, University
of Rochester, Rochester, New York

ORLANDO CATALANO, MD
Assistant, First Department of Radiology,
National Cancer Institute "Fondazione
G.Pascale", via M.Semmola, Naples, Italy

BHARGAVA K. CHINNI, MS
Department of Imaging Sciences, University
of Rochester, Rochester, New York

NIR VIKAR DAHIYA, MD
Assistant Professor of Radiology, Department
of Abdomen Imaging, Mallinckrodt Institute
of Radiology, Washington University School
of Medicine, Boulevard, St Louis, Missouri

VIKRAM S. DOGRA, MD
Professor of Radiology, Urology & Biomedical
Engineering, Department of Imaging Sciences,
University of Rochester Medical Center,
Rochester, New York

ALFONSO FAUSTO, MD
Consultant Radiologist, Department of
Diagnostic Imaging, San Giovanni di Dio
General Hospital, Gorizia, Italy

JASON GUTMAN, MD
Clinical Fellow, Division of Gastroenterology
and Hepatology, University of Rochester
Medical Center, Rochester, New York

JOSEPH J. JUNEWICK, MD
Assistant Clinical Professor, Michigan State
University, College of Human Medicine,
Helen DeVos Children's Hospital,
Michigan NE; Advanced Radiology Services,
PC, Grand Rapids, Michigan

NAVALGUND A. RAO, PhD
Center for Imaging Sciences, Rochester
Institute of Technology, Rochester, New York

GIORGIO RIZZATTO, MD
Director, Department of Diagnostic Imaging,
San Giovanni di Dio General Hospital, Gorizia,
Italy

A. THOMAS. STAVROS, MD, FACR
Radiologist, Sutter North Bay Women's Health
Center, Santa Rosa, California

KAI E. THOMENIUS, PhD, FAIUM
Chief Technologist, Ultrasound and Biomedical,
Imaging Technologies Organization, GE Global
Research, Niskayuna, New York

ASAD ULLAH, MD
Associate Professor of Medicine, Division of
Gastroenterology and Hepatology, University
of Rochester Medical Center, Rochester,
New York

KEERTHI S. VALLURU, MS
Department of Imaging Sciences, University of Rochester, Rochester, New York

TOMY VARGHESE
PhD, Associate Professor, Department of Medical Physics, The University of Wisconsin-Madison, Madison, Wisconsin

MARY C. WHITSETT, AS, BA, RT(R, T), RVT, RDMS
Clinical Ultrasound Specialist, St Luke's Hospital and Health Network, Ultrasound Department, Bethlehem, Pennsylvania

MAN ZHANG, MD, PhD
Department of Radiology, University of Michigan Health System, Ann Arbor, Michigan

Contents

radiological and cardiologic imaging. The commercialization of UCAs in different countries and the development of several scanning technologies have created a need for standardization of methodology and terminology. This article reviews the historical and physical basis of CEUS, illustrates the hepatic and extrahepatic applications, and discusses forthcoming developments.

Ultrasound Clinics

THE CLINICS ARE NOW AVAILABLE ONLINE!

Access your subscription at:
www.theclinics.com

GOAL STATEMENT

The goal of the *Ultrasound Clinics* is to keep practicing radiologists and radiology residents up to date with current clinical practice in ultrasound by providing timely articles reviewing the state of the art in patient care.

ACCREDITATION

The *Ultrasound Clinics* is planned and implemented in accordance with the Essential Areas and Policies of the Accreditation Council for Continuing Medical Education (ACCME) through the joint sponsorship of the University of Virginia School of Medicine and Elsevier. The University of Virginia School of Medicine is accredited by the ACCME to provide continuing medical education for physicians.

The University of Virginia School of Medicine designates this educational activity for a maximum of 15 *AMA PRA Category 1 Credits*™ for each issue, 60 credits per year. Physicians should only claim credit commensurate with the extent of their participation in the activity.

The American Medical Association has determined that physicians not licensed in the US who participate in this CME activity are eligible for a maximum of 15 *AMA PRA Category 1 Credits*™ for each issue, 60 credits per year.

Credit can be earned by reading the text material, taking the CME examination online at http://www.theclinics.com/home/cme, and completing the evaluation. After taking the test, you will be required to review any and all incorrect answers. Following completion of the test and evaluation, your credit will be awarded and you may print your certificate.

FACULTY DISCLOSURE/CONFLICT OF INTEREST

The University of Virginia School of Medicine, as an ACCME accredited provider, endorses and strives to comply with the Accreditation Council for Continuing Medical Education (ACCME) Standards of Commercial Support, Commonwealth of Virginia statutes, University of Virginia policies and procedures, and associated federal and private regulations and guidelines on the need for disclosure and monitoring of proprietary and financial interests that may affect the scientific integrity and balance of content delivered in continuing medical education activities under our auspices.

The University of Virginia School of Medicine requires that all CME activities accredited through this institution be developed independently and be scientifically rigorous, balanced and objective in the presentation/discussion of its content, theories and practices.

All authors/editors participating in an accredited CME activity are expected to disclose to the readers relevant financial relationships with commercial entities occurring within the past 12 months (such as grants or research support, employee, consultant, stock holder, member of speakers bureau, etc.). The University of Virginia School of Medicine will employ appropriate mechanisms to resolve potential conflicts of interest to maintain the standards of fair and balanced education to the reader. Questions about specific strategies can be directed to the Office of Continuing Medical Education, University of Virginia School of Medicine, Charlottesville, Virginia.

The faculty and staff of the University of Virginia Office of Continuing Medical Education have no financial affiliations to disclose.

The authors/editors listed below have identified no professional or financial affiliations for themselves or their spouse/partner:

Matthew J. Bassignani, MD (Test Author); Michele Bertolotto, MD; Shweta Bhatt, MD; Orlando Catalano, MD; Bhargava K. Chinni, MS; Nirvikar Dahiya, MD; Vikram S. Dogra, MD (Guest Editor); Barton Dudlick (Acquisitions Editor); Alfonso Fausto, MD; Jason Gutman, MD; Giorgio Rizzatto, MD; Kai E. Thomenius, PhD, FAIUM; Asad Ullah, MD; Keerthi S. Valluru, MS; Shahram Vaezy, PhD; Tomy Varghese, PhD; and, Man Zhang, MD, PhD.

The authors/editors listed below have identified the following professional or financial affiliations for themselves or their spouse/partner:
Joseph J. Junewick, MD serves on the Speakers' Bureau for General Electric.
Navalgund A. Rao, PhD is the Founder of AAIT, LLC.
A. Thomas Stavros, MD serves on the Speakers' Bureau for Medipattern and General Electric.
Mary C. Whitsett, AS, BA, RT(R,T), RVT, RDMS is employed by St. Luke's Hospital and Health Network, is employed by and is on the Advisory Committee/Board for Northampton Community College, and is an industry funded research/investigator for GE Medical.

Disclosure of Discussion of Non-FDA Approved Uses for Pharmaceutical Products and/or Medical Devices.
The University of Virginia School of Medicine, as an ACCME provider, requires that all faculty presenters identify and disclose any off-label uses for pharmaceutical and medical device products. The University of Virginia School of Medicine recommends that each physician fully review all the available data on new products or procedures prior to clinical use.

TO ENROLL

To enroll in the Ultrasound Clinics Continuing Medical Education program, call customer service at 1-800-654-2452 or visit us online at www.theclinics.com/home/cme. The CME program is available to subscribers for an additional fee of $205.00.

Preface

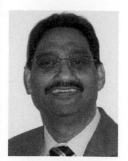

Vikram S. Dogra, MD
Guest Editor

This issue of *Ultrasound Clinics* takes a close look at the future of ultrasound and recent developments in the field. Ultrasound has evolved into a full modality and is the backbone of obstetrics and emergency radiology. Ultrasound equipment has become more compact and yet retains high-quality imaging capabilities. In this issue, we have tried to highlight current trends not only in ultrasound but also in related fields, such as elastography and photoacoustic imaging.

Elastography, photo acoustic imaging, and high-intensity focused ultrasound are evolving fields that will come to dominate the imaging world. Elastography provides a new method to image malignancy and is already proving very useful for detecting breast tumors. Photo acoustic imaging will open new doors to do functional imaging with prognostic and therapeutic capabilities. High-intensity focused ultrasound is already being used for the treatment of uterine fibroids. Other uses are being explored.

We assembled a group of leading radiologists and research scientists to provide information about the latest advances and new developments in ultrasound imaging. The information will be beneficial for general practitioners, for specialists, and for radiology residents and researchers in the field of imaging.

It is a privilege to be the guest editor for this issue of *Ultrasound Clinics*. I wish to thank Elsevier and, in particular, Barton Dudlick and our contributors for their outstanding work and cooperation.

Vikram S. Dogra, MD
Department of Imaging Sciences
University of Rochester Medical Center
601 Elmwood Avenue
Box 648, Rochester
NY 14642-8648, USA

E-mail address:
vikram_dogra@urmc.rochester.edu

Ultrasound Clin 4 (2009) xi
doi:10.1016/j.cult.2009.11.012
1556-858X/09/$ – see front matter

Acknowledgments

We are highly indebted to Patricia E. Miller for her secretarial assistance. Without her assistance, this task would not have been accomplished.

doi:10.1016/j.cult.2009.11.013

ultrasound.theclinics.com

Breast Imaging and Volume Navigation: MR imaging and Ultrasound Coregistration

Giorgio Rizzatto, MD*, Alfonso Fausto, MD

KEYWORDS

- Breast cancer • Ultrasound • MR imaging
- Elastography • Image registration • Fusion imaging

Increasing evidence suggests that for many women breast MR imaging provides the best possible accuracy, superior to both mammography and ultrasound (US). Additional cancers are identified independently of the mammographic breast density. MR imaging has the better accuracy in the evaluation of single or multifocal carcinoma and of the contralateral breast in women with recently diagnosed cancer. MR imaging is more accurate than mammography in detecting biologically aggressive ductal carcinoma in situ (DCIS). With this evidence in mind, Kuhl[1] elegantly notes that with an average lifetime risk as high as 12% to 14% in women, one could argue that "female gender" is already sufficient to call for screening methods that help compensate the limitations of mammography.

Breast MR imaging has a high sensitivity of 86% to 100%, but a variable specificity of 20% to 100% for the detection of breast cancer.[1–5] Even in expert hands there is still a high rate of suspicious MR imaging lesions that yield a benign diagnosis at pathology.[6]

There is a large overlap in the MR imaging findings of enhancing breast lesions, which often makes decisions regarding patient management difficult. All MR imaging lesions might be classified according to morphology, dynamics, and descriptors. If one considers drug intake, hormonal status,

previous therapy (surgery, radiation, and chemotherapy), and risk factors (familial or genetic predisposition to breast cancer), the same appearance might be differently classified.[7,8]

Tissue diagnosis is gaining popularity for lesions with suspicious or indeterminate features on MR imaging. MR imaging–guided biopsy has several disadvantages[4]: it is available only in selected centers, it is expensive, it requires trained personnel and scarce magnet time, it may not be tolerated by claustrophobic patients, and large patients may not be able to fit into the magnet. Unlike stereotactic and US-guided biopsies, MR imaging does not allow confirmation of lesion sampling. Vacuum-assisted biopsy with 9- or 11-gauge needles is preferred to automated core biopsy because a high proportion of MR imaging–detected lesions contain DCIS or atypical ductal hyperplasia; it may occur as a problem of progressively reducing conspicuity because of washout of contrast material; and localizing clips are better fitted for vacuum-assisted technology.[9] The mean time required to biopsy a single lesion varies from 35[9] to 70 minutes[10]; two lesions may require 90 minutes.[10] In expert hands this technique is highly successful, at around 98%[9,10]; complications are encountered in less than 5% of all patients. Many of the disadvantages of the MR imaging–guided biopsy are solved if it is

Department of Diagnostic Imaging, San Giovanni di Dio General Hospital, Viale Fatebenefratelli 34, 34170 Gorizia, Italy
* Corresponding author.
E-mail address: grizzatto@libero.it (G. Rizzatto).

Ultrasound Clin 4 (2009) 261–271
doi:10.1016/j.cult.2009.10.006
1556-858X/09/$ – see front matter © 2009 Elsevier Inc. All rights reserved.

possible to identify and biopsy the lesion with US. This is the reason why many centers try to target with a second-look US examination all the suspicious lesions that were previously seen only with MR imaging. The final solution should be a fully automatic integration of MR imaging and US to facilitate and reduce the costs of false-positive MR imaging diagnoses and to help in planning and performing therapies.

This article reviews the results of targeting conventional US to detect incidental enhancing, indeterminate, or suspicious MR imaging lesions. It adds information to ongoing research in the field of fusing MR imaging and US images; moreover, it presents the clinical possibilities offered by commercially available technologies with the addition of other US techniques, such as color Doppler and elastography.

CONVENTIONAL SONOGRAPHY AS SECOND-LOOK EXAMINATION FOR TARGETING LESIONS ON MR IMAGING

In many cases it is difficult to identify the lesion because the patient is positioned very differently from MR imaging. Comstock and Tartar[11] suggest not being rigid about lesion localization in the breast when looking for US correlates for breast MR imaging abnormalities. The mobility of breast tissue and positioning differences (prone versus supine or supine oblique positioning between MR imaging and US) introduce considerable variability in apparent position of corresponding lesions. They further suggest to examine with US at least a quadrant's worth of tissue on either side of the clock position of any concerning lesion identified on MR imaging. The distance from the nipple and the craniocaudal location with reference to the nipple are considered the most reliable data[4]; the MR imaging location near a distinct structure, such as a cyst, a fluid collection, or an implant, may provide further landmarks.

Correlating the imaging findings, the radiologist must be aware of the different descriptors related to US and MR imaging.[4] It has been suggested that having US performed by the same radiologist who interpreted the MR imaging study may increase the accuracy of targeted US.[4,12]

Second-look US may fail to identify a sonographic correlate in up to two thirds of MR imaging–detected lesions referred for biopsy.[13–15] In most of the cases the original lesion detected on MR imaging may not be confidently correlated or even not identified.

Different groups report variable sensitivity; in some cases sensitivity is quite higher, such as in the studies of Sim and colleagues[16] (67%) and

Beran and colleagues[17] (89%). Both studies are prospective, but quite small; they do not include comprehensive data to understand fully the correlation between imaging size and descriptors and the US false-negatives results.

In their recent study of 167 cases, DeMartini and colleagues[15] identified a US correlate in nearly half (46%) of MR imaging lesions overall. Sonographic detection was significantly more likely for MR imaging lesions characterized as masses (58%) than for findings described as foci (37%) or non-masslike enhancement (30%). LaTrenta and colleagues[13] found no significant difference in US detection based on lesion size.

These studies have some limitations, because both series are not very recent. To the authors' knowledge there is no published contribution with state-of-the-art technology comparing the overall sensitivity with the MR imaging and US descriptors, and with the type and the size of the gland.

It is common opinion that at least 50% of the MR imaging–detected lesions may have a clear correlate on second-look US. Second-look US is increasing in importance but the absence of a clear sonographic correlate may not spare the need for a biopsy under MR imaging guidance.

INTERMODALITY REGISTRATION

Intermodality registration involves the registration of breast images of the same patient obtained using diverse imaging modalities. The final goal is to assist clinicians in tracking normal and pathologic tissues across multiple imaging modalities. They can produce different measurements and images of the same disease; a coregistration algorithm helps to integrate the information from various sources into one image to combine analysis and synthesis. Complementary information can help to establish a diagnosis or assist the clinician for an optimal therapeutic approach.

The breasts are mostly composed of soft tissue; they easily deform and require nonrigid registration.[18,19] Many studies have been conducted to develop anatomically realistic sets of models of breast deformation under a variety of gravity loading conditions[19]; differences are not only related to breast position but also to morphology and the distribution of the different types of tissue within the breasts. Breast morphology varies with changing physiologic conditions and age of a woman and may be different for the two breasts. Breast morphology is also highly variable across individuals. This morphologic variation is also a result of the different stiffness of the breast tissues.[20,21]

The variation in mechanical properties of breast tissues across individuals is a major challenge in developing anatomically realistic individual models of the breast. One other major limitation, especially for non–real-time imaging, such as breast MR imaging, is the presence of motion artifacts caused by patient movement and breathing. Nonrigid registration needs to apply the best transformation algorithm that results in an alignment with the least error between two breast images. Finding the maximum of similarity measures is a multidimensional optimization problem.[18,19]

The registration process involves the deformation of one image (slave) so that it aligns with another image (target). No general method is able automatically to register any modality to any other modality.[18] Breast image coregistration methods are a compromise among accuracy; precision; reliability; robustness; and such issues as automation, interactivity, speed, and patient-friendliness.[18]

A wide variety of approaches have been proposed. On one extreme, patient position and algorithms have been developed to restrict the deformations induced by the mechanical behavior. This model restricts the deformations imposed on the slave to be physically realistic. An example is the hybrid biopsy system proposed by Causer and colleagues.[22] Both MR imaging and US are performed with the patient in the prone position using a redesigned bed and coil system. The location of the lesion is determined from its MR imaging coordinates relative to the fiducial markers and correlated to a dedicated US transducer stage. Remaining in the same position atop the redesigned bed, the patient is removed from the magnet room and taken to an adjoining room to undergo sonography. This system of

Causer and colleagues[22] has shown very accurate coregistration values in cases of masslike lesions, with plane errors of less than 2.5 mm.

At the other extreme, algorithms have been developed to model the deformations imposed on the images using simple functions. In this type of algorithm, landmarks are identified between the two images to be registered and a transformation is computed to coregister these landmarks. With regard to the breast, anatomic features can be either at the surface or internal. The former include skin boundary and the nipple, whereas the latter include the pectoral muscle, fibroglandular tissue, and vasculature (**Fig. 1**).[18]

MR IMAGING AND US REGISTRATION IN CLINICAL SETTING

For breast MR imaging and US imaging registration a commercially available US scanner with a magnetic tracking system and dedicated software for real-time volume navigation is used. The system is quite simple: a magnetic tracking system is used to determine the relative position of a pair of freehand sensors versus a fixed transmitter using a defined operating volume. In particular, an electromagnetic transmitter is positioned near the patient under examination and two light electromagnetic sensors are mounted on the conventional 6- to 15-MHz matrix array linear transducer bracket (**Fig. 2**). Transmitter and sensors are connected to a position-sensing unit embedded in the US scanner allowing one to track probe position and orientation within the electromagnetic field. Live US image is coregistered to a breast MR volume, previously acquired and loaded into the US system, by coupling at least three pairs of points. After US–MR imaging coregistration, the software reconstructs a real-time

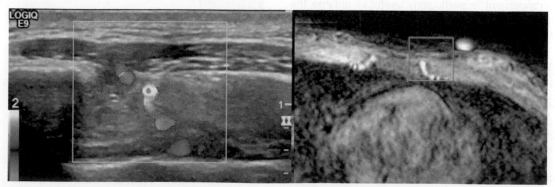

Fig. 1. Color Doppler imaging makes evident the correspondence of the position of the internal mammary artery and its perforating vessel in the side-by-side real-time US and MR imaging. Note the hyperintense oval shape of the vitamin E fiducial marker positioned on the skin during MR imaging supine scans. Internal mammary vessels may be used as additional fiducial markers to increase the accuracy of registration.

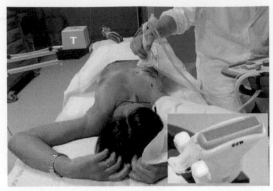

Fig. 2. The system is composed by a commercially available US scanner with a conventional 6- to 15-MHz matrix array transducer and a magnetic tracking system. The transmitter (T) is positioned near the patient. Two light sensors are mounted on a transducer bracket (close up).

multiplanar MR image of the corresponding live US image that is displayed side-by-side or in a blended overlaying format directly on the US scanner LCD monitor. Other commercially available technologies use slightly similar technologies; they may require a supplementary monitor or workstation.

The US platform and the transducer's geometry (both in conventional and in trapezoid imaging) allow one to visualize a wide field-of-view, still maintaining a high frame rate ($\geq$30 frames per second) and all the postprocessing capabilities. In addition to live B-mode and color Doppler images, it is possible to perform real-time US elastography. The elastographic color map is displayed in a blended overlaying B-mode format for a user-selected region of interest. The real-time volume navigation software makes it possible to visualize the real-time US scan in dual (with the corresponding MR image) or single mode: this last arrangement is particularly useful to enlarge the image of an already identified correlate when performing elastography.

TECHNIQUE AND ACCURACY OF MR IMAGING AND US COREGISTRATION

At the authors' institution diagnostic MR imaging examinations are performed on a 1.5-T MR imaging scanner in prone position using sensitivity encoding (SENSE) breast coil, seven elements. The protocol consists of a three-dimensional turbo field echo sequence with T1-weighted high-resolution isotropic voxel, 150 to 190 coronal 1-mm partitions with 120-second time resolution using a time interval depending on sequence acquisition time; dynamic evaluation is obtained with one

precontrast and four postcontrast phases, after automated intravenous administration (2 mL per second) of 0.05 mmol/kg of Gd-BOPTA followed by a flush of 20-mL saline solution using a cubital vein (30 mL if dorsal metacarpal vein is used).

To acquire the MR imaging volume for fusion imaging the authors perform a second MR imaging examination with the patient supine, after external positioning of three fiducial markers. Because of breast volume distortion, three softgel capsules of natural d-alpha tocopherol (vitamin E, 400 UI) are positioned over a corresponding black or blue surgical skin marker (**Fig. 3**). Each skin marker is drawn as large as capsule dimensions and subjectively positioned at 9-, 12-, and 3-o'clock radially to the nipple. Each capsule is fixed with a polyolefin single coated surgical tape during MR imaging examination and removed at the end. Skin markers are covered with a transparent dressing to prevent its alteration before US examination. MR imaging supine examination is performed on the 1.5-T MR imaging scanner with a three-dimensional turbo field echo sequence with T1-weighted high-resolution isotropic examination volume and spectral attenuated inversion recovery fat suppression, 200 axial 1-mm partitions (TR/TE = 4.7/2.3 milliseconds; flip angle = 10 degrees; field of view = 420 mm; matrix = 330 × 420 mm; time 8'30") with 120-second time resolution; one precontrast and three postcontrast phases, after automated intravenous administration (2 mL per second) of 0.05 mmol/kg of Gd-BOPTA followed by a flush of 20-mL saline solution using a cubital vein (30 mL if dorsal metacarpal vein was used). The patient is supine with upper extremities extended as for US examination. A double synergy body coil with SENSE covering both breasts is used. Breast compression is

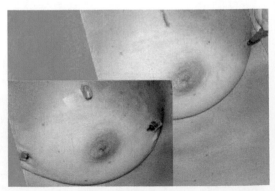

Fig. 3. Three vitamin E pills and their corresponding skin markers represent the fiducial markers used for the coregistration of MR imaging volume and US scan. Before the supine MR imaging examination a nurse prepares the patient.

minimized using a dedicated mattress and two straps. MR imaging examinations are uploaded on a dedicated postprocessing console for image evaluation. Native postcontrast sequence of the first or second dynamic phase with or without color-coded pixels describing wash-in and wash-out enhancement for fixed threshold are collected. Digital versatile disk rewritable or universal serial bus are used to store MR imaging volume data to be uploaded in the real-time volume navigation software.

US imaging is performed in supine position similar to that maintained during MR imaging examination (see **Fig. 2**). The US scanner system is configured with real-time volume navigation software and a high-frequency linear transducer is used after uploading MR imaging volume data and coupling the three fiducial points.

Two independent and experienced radiologists evaluated feasibility and accuracy.[23] They measured twice five point-to-probe distances in a series of healthy volunteers using a set of fiducial points (three external skin markers, nipple, and internal mammary artery). The real-time volume navigation coregistration was obtained in all the patients. Mean time to obtain real-time volume navigation was 9.5 minutes (5–13 minutes) without significant difference between the radiologists. Both the point-to-probe distances showed a good correlation: 6 ± 5 mm, 5 ± 3 mm, 6 ± 4 mm, and 4 ± 3 mm, respectively.

Good coregistration was confirmed in almost all the clinical cases (**Fig. 4**). It might be relatively important to obtain a perfect coregistration; with US the authors easily move in real-time and in all the planes, finding even lesions slightly apart. They have also found a good correspondence for the measurements obtained on both the side-by-side images (**Fig. 5**).

INTEGRATING COLOR DOPPLER AND ELASTOGRAPHY

Coregistration of MR imaging volumes and US imaging offers the unique capability to evaluate in real-time the US patterns of breast vascularity and elasticity. This integration may help to define correlated anatomic landmarks and pathologic features. These additional descriptors are not stand-alone; to enhance the diagnostic accuracy they must be integrated with the BI-RADS descriptors.

Color Doppler imaging is a valuable adjunct to conventional US in differentiating between malignant and benign breast lesions. The most specific descriptors for malignancy are the irregular morphology and the irregular velocities of the vessels inside a lesion. They predict the risk of malignancy (odds ratios of 5.8 and 3.2, respectively) according to the microvascular architecture of breast carcinomas.[24] At the same time color Doppler may help to assess benignity (ie, the nest morphology of the vessels of fibroadenomas and the regular morphology of the vessels within the hilum of lymph nodes) (**Fig. 6**).

Normal and pathologic breast tissues have different elastic modules[20,21] that can be defined with US; usually tumors are stiffer than benign lesions. Many commercially available scanners

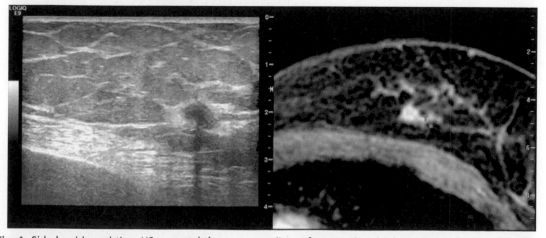

Fig. 4. Side-by-side real-time US scan and the corresponding reformatted multiplanar MR image during volume navigation (VNav). A GPS (global positioning system) marker (squared point and T) was positioned below the MR imaging lesion and automatically reproduced on the US scan. Shape and dimension of GPS marker change depending on lesion to probe distance allowing one to easily localize additional MR imaging detected findings. Distance discordance between GPS marker and the lesion represents the coregistration gap between the two volumes. In this a case the measurement error is less than 4 mm.

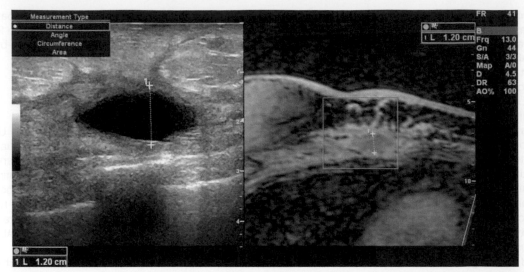

Fig. 5. VNav allows precise and comparable measurements. Patient with an inflammatory fluid collection of the left breast.

use strain-imaging methods, tracking tissue movement during compression to obtain an estimate of strain. This technique uses conventional signals from clinical scanners acquired before and after deformation is applied and derives relative hardness information (local strains) from a displacement function that is estimated by comparing the precompression and postcompression echo fields.[25] The final information is superimposed in real-time to the conventional image and is evaluated according to predefined patterns or scores.[26] Real-time elastography of the breast is accurate and reproducible, and may easily and quickly integrate conventional US and other breast imaging.[26–28] Elastography works better with small lesions, equal or less than 15 mm. Moreover, it is insensitive to the thickness and the echogenicity of the breast, and to the depth of the lesion. Elastographic scores are well reproducible. The indexes for intraobserver ($\kappa = 0.93$) and interobserver ($\kappa = 0.90$) agreement are very good.[28] This technique shows a very high

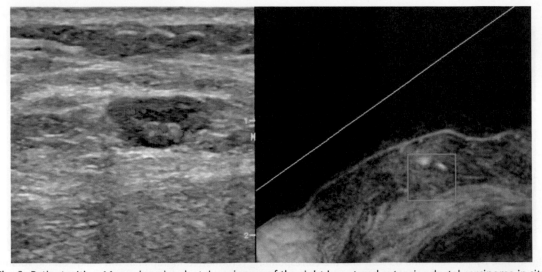

Fig. 6. Patient with a 14-mm invasive ductal carcinoma of the right breast and extensive ductal carcinoma in situ component. In the lower external quadrant of the left breast there is a second 9-mm contrast-enhanced lesion. VNav shows very well the correlate; color Doppler identifies the typical hilar vascularity of an intramammary lymph node. No further procedure was necessary. The patient was examined only in supine position because her size did not allow a prone study with the SENSE breast coil.

specificity in benign lesions, including BI-RADS for US category 3 lesions. With the best cutoff point between elasticity scores 3 and 4, the negative predictive value is around 98%.[28]

PRELIMINARY CLINICAL EXPERIENCE

From January to July 2009, the authors examined with real-time volume navigation software 41 patients (age range, 32–72 years; mean, 51 years) with MR imaging lesions. Only 20 lesions were first

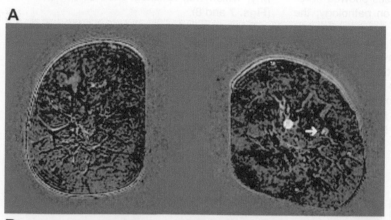

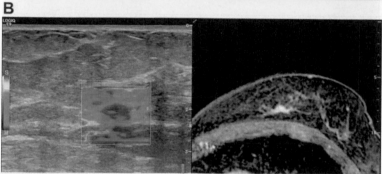

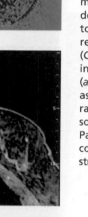

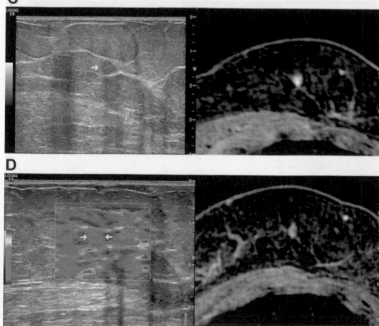

Fig. 7. (A) Coronal view of second postcontrast fast field echo T1-weighted subtracted sequence in prone position. A rounded 14-mm lesion is obvious in the nipple quadrant of the left breast. This is the index lesion of a trifocal invasive ductal carcinoma spreading at the upper inner quadrant. In the upper external quadrant of the same breast there is an inhomogeneous rounded lesion of 5 mm (arrow). (B) VNav correctly defines the index lesion; elastography shows a blue pattern, representative of a stiff lesion. (C) VNav also shows the lesion in the upper external quadrant (arrow). The lesion is classified as BI-RADS 3 for US; (D) elastography shows a pattern typical of soft, benign lesions (arrows). Pathology on US-guided 14-G core biopsy specimens demonstrated a fibroadenoma.

seen on MR imaging and were considered suspicious or indeterminate; the final prevalence of malignancy was 40%. In this group there was a good anatomic coregistration, but in three cases an abnormality on the US images could not be identified. These lesions underwent biopsy with MR imaging guidance. Two cases showed fibrocystic changes but no atypia on pathology; the third case was a 9-mm DCIS proved after MR imaging–guided biopsy. In all the other cases (85%) real-time volume navigation showed a good correlate. In four cases (two intramammary nodes and two fibroadenomas) the correlate was considered benign only based on the US descriptors. In the other 13 cases (six benign and seven malignant) an US-guided core biopsy was easily

performed directly with real-time volume navigation. Seven lesions showed an already suggestive US pattern, but it was decided to biopsy them all because the result might have changed the surgical approach. This event became more frequent when beginning to integrate elastography, which was routinely used since April 2005 (**Figs. 7** and **8**).

This series is too small to validate a statistical analysis on the accuracy of the method. During this period, the authors progressively refined the system settings and included new methods, such as elastography. Not all the cases are comparable. One must also consider that, although the method is simple, there is a learning curve; radiologists are not used to the MR images

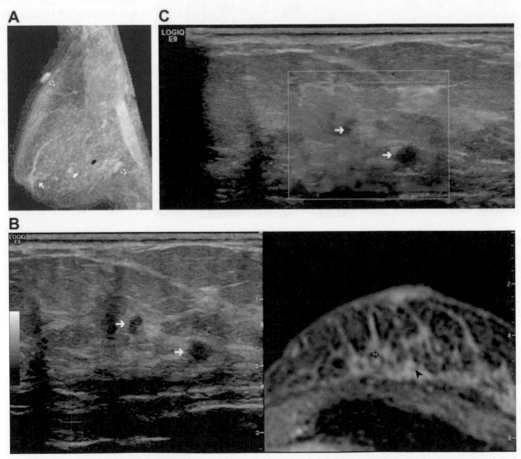

Fig. 8. (*A*) Left breast maximum intensity projection (MIP) of second postcontrast fast field echo T1-weighted subtracted sequence obtained in prone position. Two capsules of vitamin E are slightly visible (*open arrows*) because of a movement artifact. The superficial index lesion is spiculated and bilobulated (*arrow*); a second rounded, contrast-enhanced lesion is located deeper in the same quadrant (*white arrowhead*). (*B*) Being doubtful of a third focus near the pectoral muscle (*black arrowhead*) the radiologist decided to perform a VNav examination. Both the secondary foci (*white arrows*) are clearly demonstrated. The corresponding MR image of the deeper focus (*black arrowhead*) is confused within an area of enhancing fibroglandular tissue. (*C*) Both foci are stiff on elastography. Pathology on US-guided core biopsy confirmed the presence of invasive ductal carcinoma in both foci.

acquired in supine position and discover a very new correlative imaging in regard to both MR imaging and US.

SUGGESTED PROTOCOL FOR MR IMAGING AND US COREGISTRATION

Supine MR imaging is not generally recommended as a diagnostic technique; it gives less information compared with prone position. The coil is not specific for the breast and images may be slightly distorted by heart beating and respiration. There are, however, some advantages. With the SENSE body coil no compression is applied to the breast; moreover, the field of view is smaller than with axial sequence acquired in prone position. The time saved is used to increase time or spatial resolution without losing signal-to-noise ratio. The main disadvantage consists of breast dislocation along the chest wall in subjects with breast hypertrophy; the lesion position can be misleading.

Generally, the images obtained in prone position are used for diagnosis; they are brought into play every time further coregistration procedures are performed. If a lesion is found only in MR imaging that requires biopsy, first a second-look US

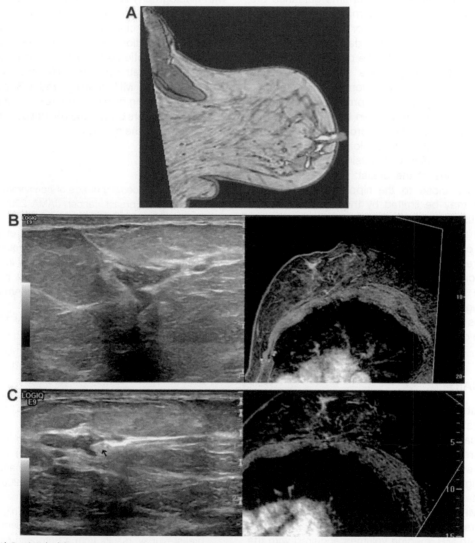

Fig. 9. (A) Sagittal oblique reconstructed second postcontrast fast field echo T1-weighted native image of the left breast acquired in prone position. A linear branched enhancing lesion of about 35 mm is shown in the nipple region. (B) Coregistration allowed tracing the dilated and filled ducts in their branching. (C) US real-time guidance allowed very precise positioning of the needle tip (*arrow*) and multiple specimens were collected along the major axis of some ducts. Pathology did not show significant atypias, but only "duct ectasia" and chronic inflammation.

examination is performed. The same radiologist who interpreted MR imaging usually performs US scan; in any case, this radiologist is present at the US examination. If a good correlate is not found, a new MR imaging examination in supine position and US real-time volume navigation is immediately proposed to the patient. The major advantage of studying the patient supine is the correspondence with standard sonographic and surgical positioning. A very good anatomic correlation is very helpful for both targeting and biopsy. Some studies have already pointed out the practical advantages of supine MR imaging as a guide for accurate breast-conserving surgery.[29,30] Anatomic landmarks and real-time guidance are both important when performing free-hand core biopsies. It is also easier for the radiologist to perform the biopsy in a standard setting; it is not so friendly to biopsy with the patient supine even with a dedicated guidance system. Lilienstein and colleagues[31] tried to correlate sonographic and MR imaging findings in prone position simply by scanning through an open MR imaging breast coil. They found relevant problems to evaluate lesions high in the axilla or close to the chest wall because the breast coil housing limits access to these portions of the breast; at the same time, for lesions close to the nipple, the transducer contact may be limited by the small amount of breast tissue located in that area. With real-time volume navigation there are no restrictions, the biopsy can be targeted in all directions, and it is very precise (**Fig. 9**). Moreover, the radiologist can decide to use the cheapest but best biopsy system according to the lesion type and the pathologist's needs; with MR imaging–guided biopsies guidelines are very strict in suggesting the use of vacuum systems.[32]

SUMMARY

Coregistration of MR imaging–US breast imaging and real-time volume navigation is becoming a clinical reality. Some commercially available scanners already have this capability. The positioning systems are quite simple and easy to use; they might not require adjunctive workstations or dedicated transducers. Most systems may integrate MR imaging volumes from different manufacturers. Coregistration is clinically acceptable even with MR imaging volumes acquired with the patient supine. Biopsies are very precise and cheaper than with MR imaging. The mean time that is required for a biopsy under real-time volume navigation guidance is 25 minutes, 10 to 45 minutes less than with MR imaging. In any case,

this results in relevant spare time for both radiologist and magnet.

The number of clear correlates is markedly increased. Still, conventional second-look US of all the incidental enhancing lesions first seen on MR imaging is the first procedure to reduce the number, the cost, and patients' discomfort of MR imaging–guided biopsy. Volume navigation is referred as a second-step procedure to identify patients who really need the procedure. There was a significant reduction of MR imaging–guided biopsies especially after the integration of volume navigation with elastography, which is known to increase the specificity for benignity. The interaction with elastography is promising; it is expected that one will be able to recognize the stiff pattern of some lobular carcinomas that do not show alteration on conventional B-mode. At the same time the future integration with contrast-enhanced analysis will help in better understanding the efficacy of the new drugs. MR imaging and US contrast-enhanced imaging give different results; unlike MR imaging enhancers US bubbles do not pass through the holes within the neoangiogenetic vessels.

REFERENCES

1. Kuhl CK. The coming of age of nonmammographic screening for breast cancer. JAMA 2008;299(18): 2203–5.
2. Sardanelli F, Giuseppetti GM, Panizza P, et al. Sensitivity of MRI versus mammography for detecting foci of multifocal, multicentric breast cancer in fatty and dense breasts using the whole-breast pathologic examination as a gold standard. AJR Am J Roentgenol 2004;183(4):1149–57.
3. Kuhl CK, Schrading S, Leutner CC, et al. Mammography, breast ultrasound, and magnetic resonance imaging for surveillance of women at high familial risk for breast cancer. J Clin Oncol 2005;23(33): 8469–76.
4. Erguvan-Dogan B, Whitman GJ. Breast ultrasound MR imaging correlation. Ultrasound Clin 2007;1: 593–601.
5. Sardanelli F, Podo F, D'Agnolo G, et al. Multicenter comparative multimodality surveillance of women at genetic-familial high risk for breast cancer (HIBCRIT study): interim results. Radiology 2007;242(3): 698–715.
6. Perlet C, Heywang-Kobrunner SH, Heinig A, et al. Magnetic resonance-guided, vacuum-assisted breast biopsy: results from a European multicenter study of 538 lesions. Cancer 2006;106(5):982–90.
7. Macura KJ, Ouwerkerk R, Jacobs MA, et al. Patterns of enhancement on breast MR images: interpretation and imaging pitfalls. Radiographics 2006;26(6): 1719–34.

8. Ojeda-Fournier H, Choe KA, Mahoney MC. Recognizing and interpreting artifacts and pitfalls in MR imaging of the breast. Radiographics 2007;27(Suppl 1):S147–64.

9. Liberman L. Percutaneous magnetic resonance imaging guided breast biopsy. In: Morris EA, Liberman L, editors. Breast MRI: diagnosis and intervention. New York: Springer; 2005. p. 297–316.

10. Perlet C, Heinig A, Prat X, et al. Multicenter study for the evaluation of a dedicated biopsy device for MR-guided vacuum biopsy of the breast. Eur Radiol 2002;12(6):1463–70.

11. Comstock CC, Tartar M. Detection of breast cancer: screening of asymptomatic patients. Case 12. In: Tartar M, Comstock CC, Kipper MS, editors. Breast cancer imaging. 1st edition. New York: Elsevier Health Sciences - Mosby; 2008. p. 26–8.

12. McMahon K, Medoro L, Kennedy D. Breast magnetic resonance imaging: an essential role in malignant axillary lymphadenopathy of unknown origin. Australas Radiol 2005;49(5):382–9.

13. LaTrenta LR, Menell JH, Morris EA, et al. Breast lesions detected with MR imaging: utility and histopathologic importance of identification with US. Radiology 2003;227(3):856–61.

14. Destounis S. The role of MRI and second-look ultrasound for evaluation of breast cancer. Appl Radiol 2006;35(10):10–20.

15. Demartini WB, Eby PR, Peacock S, et al. Utility of targeted sonography for breast lesions that were suspicious on MRI. AJR Am J Roentgenol 2009; 192(4):1128–34.

16. Sim LS, Hendriks JH, Bult P, et al. US correlation for MRI-detected breast lesions in women with familial risk of breast cancer. Clin Radiol 2005;60:801–6.

17. Beran L, Liang W, Nims T, et al. Correlation of targeted ultrasound with magnetic resonance imaging abnormalities of the breast. Am J Surg 2005;190(4): 592–4.

18. Guo Y, Sivaramakrishna R, Lu C, et al. Breast image registration techniques: a survey. Med Biol Eng Comput 2006;44(1–2):15–26.

19. Rajagopal V, Lee A, Chung JH, et al. Creating individual-specific biomechanical models of the breast for medical image analysis. Acad Radiol 2008; 15(11):1425–36.

20. Samani A, Zubovits J, Plewes D. Elastic moduli of normal and pathological human breast tissues: an inversion-technique-based investigation of 169 samples. Phys Med Biol 2007;52(6):1565–76.

21. Gefen A, Dilmoney B. Mechanics of the normal woman's breast. Technol Health Care 2007;15(4): 259–71.

22. Causer PA, Piron CA, Jong RA, et al. Preliminary in vivo validation of a dedicated breast MRI and sonographic coregistration imaging system. AJR Am J Roentgenol 2008;191(4):1203–7.

23. Fausto A, Preziosa A, Gruden M, et al. Advanced second-look ultrasound of MR detected lesions with fusion imaging. Eur Radiol, in press.

24. Less JR, Skalak TC, Sevick EM, et al. Microvascular architecture in a mammary carcinoma: branching patterns and vessel dimensions. Cancer Res 1991; 51(1):265–73.

25. Garra BS. Imaging and estimation of tissue elasticity by ultrasound. Ultrasound Q 2007;23(4):255–68.

26. Itoh A, Ueno E, Tohno E, et al. Breast disease: clinical application of US elastography for diagnosis. Radiology 2006;239(2):341–50.

27. Tardivon A, El Khoury C, Thibault F, et al. Elastography of the breast: a prospective study of 122 lesions. J Radiol 2007;88(5):657–62.

28. Rizzatto G. Ultrasound elastography. In: Programs and abstracts of Symposium Mammographicum 2008. Breast Cancer Res 2008; 10(Suppl 3):P4.

29. Tozaki M, Fukuda K. Supine MR mammography using VIBE with parallel acquisition technique for the planning of breast-conserving surgery: clinical feasibility. Breast 2006;15(1):137–40.

30. Ogawa T, Tozaki M, Yamashiro N, et al. New preoperative MRI marking technique for a patient with ductal carcinoma in situ. Breast Cancer 2008; 15(4):309–14.

31. Lilienstein J, Daniel BL, Ikeda DM. In vivo sonography through an open MRI breast coil to correlate sonographic and MRI findings. AJR Am J Roentgenol 2005;184(Suppl 3):S49–52.

32. Heywang-Köbrunner SH, Sinnatamby R, Lebeau A, et al. Interdisciplinary consensus on the uses and technique of MR-guided vacuum-assisted breast biopsy (VAB): results of a European consensus meeting. Eur J Radiol 2008, in press.

Decreasing Radiation Risks by Increasing Use of Ultrasound in Pediatric Imaging

Joseph J. Junewick, MD[a,b,]*

KEYWORDS

- Ultrasound • Ionizing radiation • Pediatric imaging

PRELUDE

The author was presenting a sonogram (**Fig. 1**) at a multidisciplinary conference and he paused for questions. The pediatric surgeon said, "I understand what I am seeing." The author was puzzled by the lack of sarcasm but the surgeon was quick to elaborate, "I see the anatomy; I know what to do."

INTRODUCTION

Ultrasonography has advanced to a new level. It is not just a screening tool or the gateway to computed tomography (CT) or magnetic resonance imaging (MRI). Transducer technology with new piezoelectric crystal design and higher frequencies has increased spatial resolution. Three-dimensional (3D) techniques including tomographic imaging, surface rendering, and volume assessment have increased accuracy and improved understanding of complex anatomy. Ultrasound images can be fused with digital imaging and communications in medicine (DICOM) data sets, allowing CT and MRI to guide ultrasound imaging with navigation technology. Indeed, it is an exciting time for ultrasonography.

However, ultrasonography needs to reassert itself, especially given the risks of radiation exposure. Any radiation exposure can increase the risk of cancer, and exposure when younger increases the lifetime risk of cancer. One needs to be judicious with radiation and creative about incorporating ultrasonography into imaging strategies.

Pediatric sonography in the United States is at the crossroads, presenting the following opportunities: ultrasonography is increasingly accepted and understood by clinicians; technological advancements are helping to increase one's diagnostic confidence and accuracy, and the risk of ionizing radiation is real. One needs to capitalize on these opportunities and reshape imaging paradigms.

The purpose of this article is to review some clinical scenarios where ultrasonography can substitute for ionizing radiation in pediatric imaging. For each scenario, the author briefly discusses the opportunity for dose reduction, the imaging technique/protocol that is used at his institution, and the pathophysiology ultrasonographic features of various disease entities.

RIGHT LOWER QUADRANT PAIN

Suspected appendicitis is the most common reason for abdominal surgery in children.[1] The classic presentation of anorexia, nausea, and right lower quadrant pain with fever and rebound tenderness poses no clinical dilemma. However, the signs and symptoms in children with appendicitis are often vague and require imaging for verification. Initially, ultrasonography was the modality

[a] Michigan State University, College of Human Medicine, Helen DeVos Children's Hospital, 100 Michigan NE, Grand Rapids, MI 49503, USA
[b] Advanced Radiology Services, PC, 3264 North Evergreen Drive NE, Grand Rapids, MI 49525, USA
* Michigan State University, College of Human Medicine, Helen DeVos Children's Hospital, 100 Michigan NE, Grand Rapids, MI 49030.
E-mail address: jjunewick@advancedrad.com

Ultrasound Clin 4 (2009) 273–284
doi:10.1016/j.cult.2009.10.007

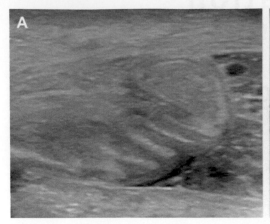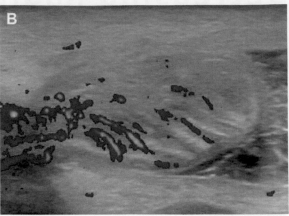

Fig. 1. (*A, B*) 6-week-old former 29-week gestation infant with nonreducible scrotal mass. Ultrasound scan demonstrates small bowel traversing the inguinal canal into the scrotum with thickened and hyperechoic valvulae (*A*) with hyperemia on color Doppler (*B*), indicating necrotizing enteritis. Strangulated hernia was found at surgery.

of choice, although more recently, CT has supplanted its use.[2] This trend can only be reversed by increasing one's experience and consequently one's accuracy in performing and interpreting appendix ultrasonography.

Graded compression sonography of the right lower quadrant is performed from the cecum, along the iliac vessels to the bladder base, and documented with static and cinegraphic images. Additional static images of the gall bladder, right kidney, and urinary bladder are obtained; ovarian anatomy is also imaged in females.

The basic pathophysiology of appendicitis is related to luminal obstruction, usually enteric contents (fecalith) or lymphoid hyperplasia. Because the mucosa of the appendix is secretory, the appendix becomes progressively dilated with obstruction of the lumen. Appendiceal dilation results in lymphatic and venous obstruction and subsequently, mural edema. As mural edema increases, perfusion becomes compromised and ischemia, necrosis, and ulceration occur.

Generally, less abdominal fat, smaller patient size, and smaller field of view (FOV) optimize pediatric imaging; lack of patient cooperation, pain, bowel gas, and appendix location may work against a successful examination.[3,4] The normal appendix is seen in up to 82% of pediatric patients (although the author's experience is less).[5] The normal appendix is to 6 mm or less in diameter, although it can be larger and still normal in patients with chronic constipation (eg, cystic fibrosis).[3,5] A central uninterrupted echogenic stripe representing the coapted mucosa is surrounded by the hypoechoic muscularis propria. Occasionally, the serosa is seen as a thin echogenic layer peripheral to the muscularis propria. Intraluminal gas or

enteric contents may be present[5]; intraluminal appendiceal fluid is seen in about 5% of normal patients but should measure less than 2.6 mm.[6]

The sensitivity of CT for the diagnosis of acute appendicitis is greater than ultrasonography, although when considering radiation safety, the 2 modalities are fairly equivalent. Any portion of the appendix that measures more than 6 mm in diameter and is noncompressible usually secures the diagnosis of appendicitis. Visualization of the entire appendix with normal dimension and compressibility excludes appendicitis.

Occasionally, the examination is not clearly normal or abnormal, but many other sonographic findings can be used to increase the confidence in the diagnosis of appendicitis. Loss of the echogenic mucosal stripe (**Fig. 2**) reflects ischemic ulceration. Appendicoliths (**Fig. 3**) are associated with a higher rate of perforation. Loculated

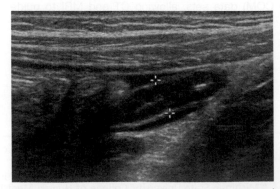

Fig. 2. Interrupted central stripe indicating mucosal necrosis and ulceration. Also, the appendix was noncompressible, measured 7 mm in diameter, and was associated with periappendiceal fluid.

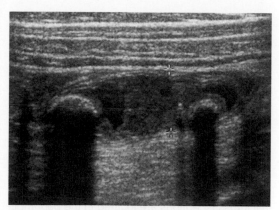

Fig. 3. Appendicitis with 3 appendicoliths. The appendix is distended with fluid and echogenic debris; note the mural thinning.

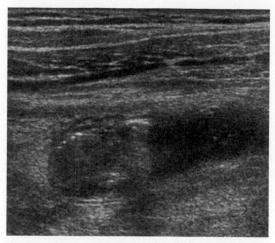

Fig. 5. Dilated appendix with mural thinning and pneumatosis, representing gangrenous appendicitis.

periappendiceal fluid is virtually diagnostic of perforated appendicitis. Mural hyperemia (Fig. 4) on color Doppler image indicates inflammation. Mural pneumatosis (Fig. 5) and lack of color Doppler flow are seen with gangrenous appendicitis. Close attention to the periappendiceal region can also improve the accuracy of appendicitis diagnosis. Increased periappendiceal and pericecal echogenicity (Fig. 6) is related to mesenteric or omental inflammation. Periappendiceal fluid, mesenteric adenopathy (Fig. 7), and adynamic small bowel are less specific sonographic findings, but with other sonographic signs, can increase the certainty of diagnosis.

INTUSSUSCEPTION

Patients with colicky abdominal pain, vomiting, lethargy, and "currant jelly" stool usually proceed to fluoroscopy and enema.[7,8] Some of these patients may have hemolytic uremic syndrome, volvulus, gastroenteritis, or Henoch-Schönlein purpura, rather than intussusception. Many infants with even just one of these findings may also end up in fluoroscopy because of the gravity of non-diagnosis of intussusception. Ultrasonography can reliably exclude intussusception and differentiate between ileoileal and ileocolic intussusception, and therefore, can replace diagnostic fluoroscopic enemas and prevent unnecessary radiation exposure.[7–11]

Graded compression of all 4 quadrants is performed with a linear 15 MHz transducer, carefully searching the periphery of the abdomen for the target or pseudokidney sign representing intussusception. Mural thickness, peristalsis, and caliber of bowel should be assessed. If intussusception is found, color Doppler should be applied.

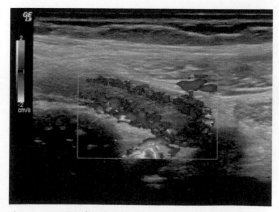

Fig. 4. Longitudinal section of an inflamed appendix with mural hyperemia on Doppler interrogation.

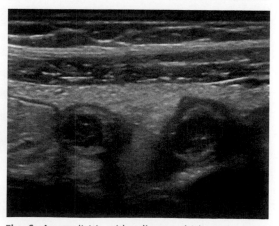

Fig. 6. Appendicitis with adjacent thickened mesentery/omentum. The lumen is distended by fluid and associated with submucosal edema giving rise to the so-called target sign.

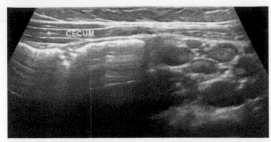

Fig. 7. Primary mesenteric adenitis may be a cause of right lower quadrant pain but approximately half the patients with appendicitis have secondarily enlarged mesenteric lymph nodes.

Intussusception (**Fig. 8**) is the result of the bowel invaginating into itself and can be asymptomatic or symptomatic. Asymptomatic intussusception typically involves a short segment of small bowel and is transient and incidental. Symptomatic intussusception typically involves a long segment of small bowel and colon (ileocolic) and requires urgent attention. Most symptomatic intussusceptions occur between 2 months and 3 years of age and are related to disordered bowel peristalsis or a "lead point." Most often the lead point is hypertrophied intestinal lymphoid tissue (Peyer patches). If intussusception is encountered outside of this age range, an underlying abnormality of the bowel, such as Meckel diverticulum, polyp, appendicitis (**Fig. 9**), celiac disease, Kawasaki disease, lymphoma (**Fig. 10**), bleeding diathesis (**Fig. 11**), or polyarteritis nodosum could be considered.[7]

Differentiating symptomatic ileocolic (see **Fig. 8A, B**) from asymptomatic ileoileal (see **Fig. 8C**) intussusception is fairly easy. Most ileoileal intussusceptions are located in the periumbilical region or right lower quadrant and measure less than 1.4 cm in diameter, and the outer bowel wall thickness is less than 3 mm. Most ileocolic intussusceptions are located in the upper quadrants or left lower quadrant and measure more than 2.5 cm in diameter, and the outer bowel wall thickness is greater than 5 mm.[9,10]

Several other signs may be helpful in the sonographic evaluation of intussusception. The presence of lymph nodes in the intussusceptum

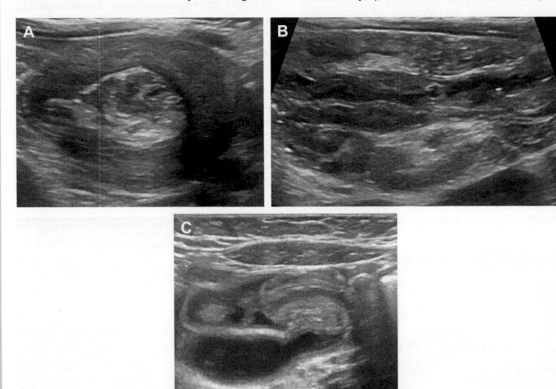

Fig. 8. Transverse (*A*) and longitudinal (*B*) images in a 7-month-old male with irritability and vomiting, demonstrating ileocolic intussusception in the right upper quadrant measuring 2.9 cm in diameter. The patient returned 5 days after successful hydrostatic reduction with vomiting, with longitudinal (*C*) image demonstrating incidental ileoileal intussusception in the periumbilical region measuring 0.9 cm in diameter.

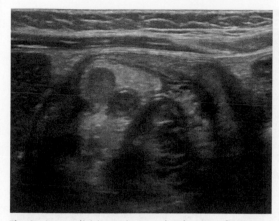

Fig. 9. Appendicitis serving as a lead point of an intussusception. The intussusceptum contains dilated fluid-filled appendix, small bowel, and lymph nodes.

(Fig. 12) is pathognomonic of ileocolic intussusception. The presence of free fluid or dilated proximal small bowel and the absence of color flow[11] of the intussusceptum are poor predictors of hydrostatic reduction, probably reflecting prolonged obstruction.

ABDOMINAL TRAUMA

CT is the primary modality for evaluating major trauma.[12] The role of ultrasonography in trauma has been limited to FAST (focused assessment with sonography for trauma) scanning in the trauma bay.[13–16] However, ultrasonography could replace CT in the setting of subacute trauma, minor trauma, single organ queries, and in the follow-up of known visceral injuries. Working with

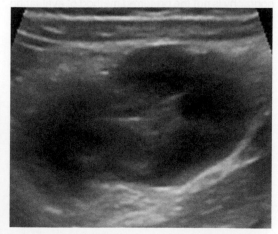

Fig. 10. Pseudokidney appearance of intussusception in 5–year-old female with chronic recurrent abdominal pain. Note the nodular thickening of the outer rim of bowel. Biopsy revealed Burkitt lymphoma.

the trauma surgeons, emergency physicians, and pediatricians to convert imaging preference to sonography could have an enormous impact on dose reduction.

The sonographic detection of hemoperitoneum and visceral injury varies depending on the technique. The FAST technique is a means to rapidly triage trauma patients. The bilateral subphrenic spaces, the hepatorenal space, the perisplenic space, the pelvic peritoneum (retrovesical space), and the pericardium are observed in 2 planes. Otherwise, directed organ examination or abdominal survey examination with color and power Doppler is performed.

FAST has a favorable sensitivity and specificity and an accuracy for injuries requiring surgery, but false-negative examinations were encountered with liver and spleen injuries without hemoperitoneum. Those clinically unstable patients with sonographic evidence of hemoperitoneum or visceral injury are usually taken directly to the operating room; those who are stable are examined with CT or observed.[13–16]

A subset of patients may benefit from ultrasonography as the only diagnostic imaging test. Patients with minor trauma or subacute injury who do not demonstrate peritoneal signs or abnormal laboratory studies (eg, amylase and hepatic enzymes) may allow more thorough scrutiny with conventional ultrasound imaging and Doppler (**Fig. 13**).

Serial CT imaging of the abdomen is often used, especially in patients with nonoperative management of trauma, to evaluate for infection/abscess; progression of hemoperitoneum or visceral hematoma; development of vascular injuries (pseudoaneurysms, dissection, and thrombosis); and evaluation of occult visceral injury.[12,17] Sonographic survey or directed examination could easily supplant CT in these cases, with the added benefit of lower cost and portability. Newer sonographic techniques such as 3D imaging with reconstruction and navigation sonography (fusing previously obtained CT to guide real-time sonography) allow confident and accurate assessment (**Fig. 14**).

VOMITING INFANT

Ultrasonography and barium upper gastrointestinal examinations are the predominant means to evaluate a vomiting infant. Both examinations are successful in the diagnosis of pyloric stenosis, gastroesophageal reflux, and volvulus. The clinical overlap of these diagnoses may make the fluoroscopic option preferable to some, but the

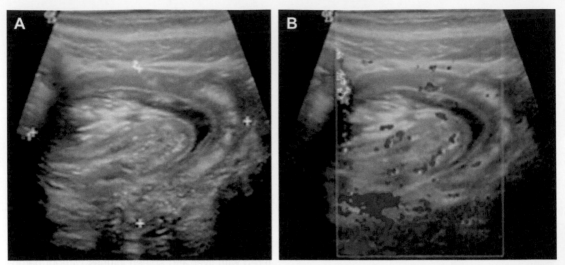

Fig. 11. A 1-year-old male with cramping abdominal pain and vomiting and recently diagnosed with Henoch-Schönlein purpura. (*A*) The hyperechoic regions in the thickened outer rim of bowel represent intramural hemorrhage. (*B*) Color Doppler flow in the mesentery, intussuscipiens, and intussusceptum predicts high likelihood of successful hydrostatic reduction.

sonographic examination can easily answer both clinical questions.

Static high-resolution transverse and longitudinal images of the pylorus and cinegraphic clips of gastric peristalsis and the pyloric channel are obtained. If pyloric stenosis is not demonstrated, (1) the relationship of the superior mesenteric artery and vein is documented with gray-scale and color Doppler, (2) a single image of each kidney is obtained to exclude renal or retroperitoneal cause of vomiting, and (3) the gastroesophageal junction is evaluated.

Elongation and thickening of the pylorus eventually results in gastric outlet obstruction. The incidence of pyloric stenosis is 2 to 3.5 cases per 1000 live births. Pyloric stenosis is more common in males and firstborns; there may also be a familial or genetic predisposition. The typical age at onset

is between 3 and 5 weeks, and is very rare after 12 weeks. Sonographic findings of pyloric stenosis (**Figs. 15** and **16**) include thickened pyloric mucosa, thickened pyloric muscularis, elongated pyloric channel, pyloric mass effect on the antrum and duodenal bulb, and altered gastric peristalsis (either vigorous or absent).[18,19]

Volvulus is related to abnormal bowel rotation, which gives rise to a narrow retroperitoneal attachment of the bowel and susceptibility to torsion. Initially there is venous and lymphatic obstruction, followed by arterial compromise and eventually, bowel ischemia. Most patients with malrotation present in the first month of life. Although ultrasonography is not the preferred method of evaluating malrotation/volvulus, it may be helpful in situations

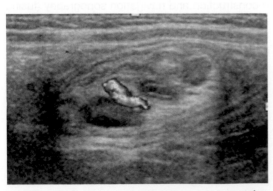

Fig. 12. Lymph nodes in the intussusceptum is pathognomonic of ileocolic intussusception.

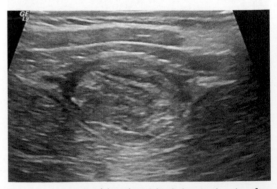

Fig. 13. A 2-year-old male with abdominal pain after fall. Ultrasonography demonstrates deep abdominal-wall hematoma. No visceral injury or hemoperitoneum was seen and confirmed with CT.

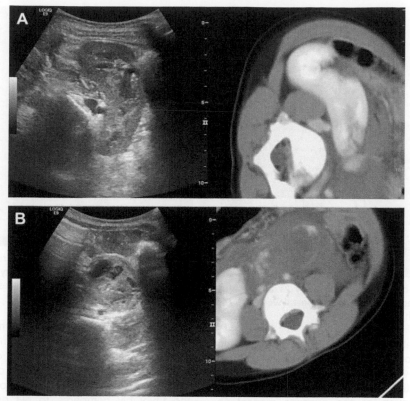

Fig. 14. A 7-year-old female with a horseshoe kidney who was kicked in the abdomen by a horse. The renal laceration/contusion (*A, B*) and perinephric hematoma (*B*) was followed up by navigation ultrasonography; the DICOM data from the initial CT examination was used to guide the ultrasonography, allowing accurate follow-up assessment of the post-traumatic findings.

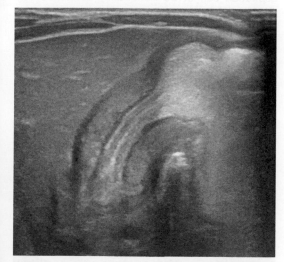

Fig. 15. 5-week-old female with projectile vomiting. The pyloric muscle measures 4 mm and the pyloric channel measures 20 mm. Note the marked mucosal hyperplasia.

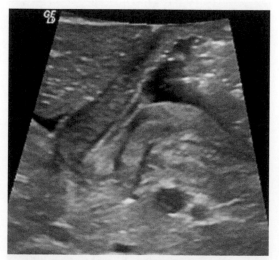

Fig. 16. 6-week-old male with pyloric stenosis. Note the normal superior mesenteric artery and vein relationship.

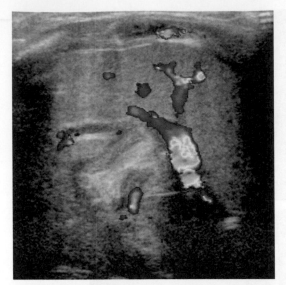

Fig. 17. 1-day-old male with trisomy 21 and bilious emesis showing a preduodenal portal vein that is associated with malrotation.

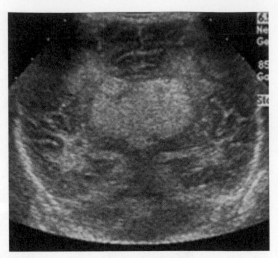

Fig. 19. Newborn with neonatal depression demonstrating gangliothalamic echodensity and diffuse cerebral white matter edema representing status marmoratus.

where the pretest probability is low. Sonographic findings of volvulus include superior mesenteric artery and vein inversion ("whirlpool" sign), duodenal dilation with distal tapering, fixed midline bowel, truncation of the superior mesenteric artery, and dilation of the superior mesenteric vein (Fig. 17).[20,21]

Gastroesophageal reflux (Fig. 18) is a common malady in infants; so common, that some view it as a normal event. Ultrasonography can easily demonstrate the gastroesophageal junction and hiatus. The patient is imaged supine with a linear

high frequency transducer, using the liver as an acoustic window . The patient can ingest any fluid meal (formula, dextrose solution, or electrolyte solution). Sonography accurately quantifies the number of episodes of gastroesophageal reflux and favorably compares to pH probe assessment.[22] A short intraabdominal segment of the esophagus, rounded gastroesophageal angle, and a "beak" at the gastroesophageal junction are associated with gastroesophageal reflux.[22] Ultrasonography can also diagnose hiatus hernia.[22] Swallowing function, inflammatory changes of the esophagus, and endotracheal aspiration cannot be adequately evaluated with sonography.

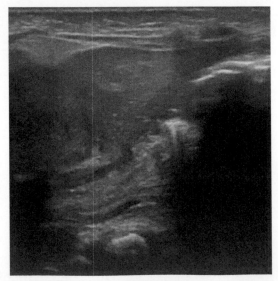

Fig. 18. Infant with vomiting shown to have gastroesophageal reflux.

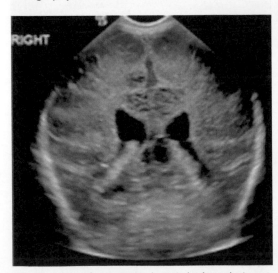

Fig. 20. Bilateral parasagittal cystic leukomalacia representing maturing watershed ischemia.

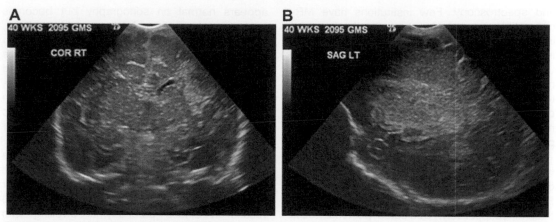

Fig. 21. Coronal (A) and sagittal (B) images from a screening neurosonogram of a 1-week-old former 40-week gestation infant, with congenital diaphragmatic hernia on extracorporeal membrane oxygenation therapy demonstrating echodense ischemic change in the left-middle cerebral artery distribution.

Other causes of vomiting in infancy are unusual, but they may be evident on sonography of the upper abdomen, including duodenal duplication cyst, choledochal cyst, hydronephrosis, neuroblastoma, meconium pseudocyst, intussusception, and bowel hematoma.

NEONATAL SEIZURE OR DEPRESSION

Neonatal seizure or depression is most often due to a hypoxic-ischemic event or intracranial hemorrhage. Probably the best single examination for the evaluation is MRI with diffusion-weighted imaging

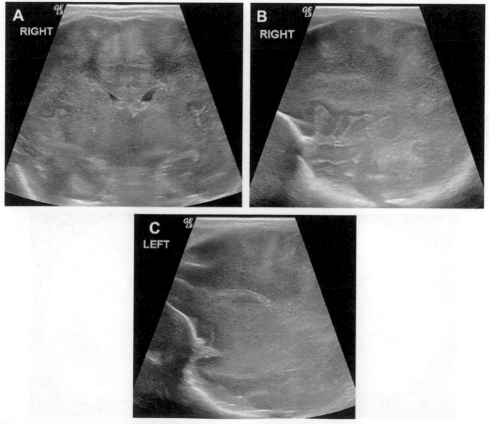

Fig. 22. Newborn former 35-week-gestation infant with perinatal distress. Coronal (A), right parasagittal (B) and left parasagittal (C) images demonstrate diffuse cerebral edema, loss of gray-white distinction, and effacement of the cerebrospinal fluid-containing spaces.

and spectroscopy. Few institutions have MR-compatible incubator systems or the neonatal intensive care support to safely image these fragile infants, and consequently, MR is usually not used. CT is quick and often used as the alternative means of imaging. It may not seem intuitive, but ultrasonography is superior to CT in the evaluation of hypoxic-ischemic injury, very good in the diagnosis of intracranial hemorrhage, and able to triage patients for MR imaging.

Sagittal and coronal imaging is performed through the anterior fontanelle using a curved 8MHz and a linear 15 MHz transducer with the FOV set to the foramen magnum and inferior thalami, respectively. Dedicated posterior fossa imaging is performed through the posterolateral fontanelle using the curved 8 MHz transducer with the FOV set to the contralateral sigmoid sinus. Spectral Doppler tracing of the anterior cerebral artery with resistive index calculation is also obtained.

In the newborn, several patterns of hypoxic-ischemic injury may be evident.[23,24] Selective neuronal injury of the striatum (**Fig. 19**) initially appears normal on sonography but becomes hyperechoic over several days, related to edema, gliosis, or calcification. Parasagittal watershed ischemia (**Fig. 20**) occurs along the intersections of the anterior and middle and the middle and posterior cerebral arteries, related to hypoperfusion or hypoxia; parasagittal ischemia is often associated with selective neuronal injury. Ischemic perinatal stroke (**Fig. 21**) is related to arterial or venous thrombosis. Initially, small discreet echogenic foci are evident, which show progressive distortion of the gray-white matter junction and sulci and eventual hyperemia on color Doppler imaging. Diffuse hypoxic-ischemic injury (**Fig. 22**) results in diffuse parenchymal swelling with effacement of the ventricles and sulci and loss of gray-white matter differentiation.

Doppler assessment of the intracranial arteries can reveal perfusion disturbance and predict hypoxic-ischemic injury before there are gray-scale changes.[25,26] A normal Doppler image of the anterior or middle cerebral arteries in a term infant should demonstrate uniform systolic and diastolic velocities and a resistive index between

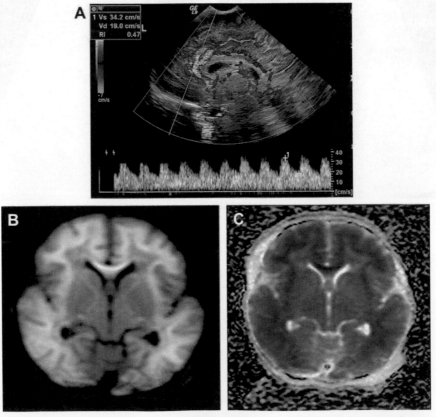

Fig. 23. Newborn with seizure. Spectral Doppler imaging (*A*) demonstrates elevated diastolic flow in the anterior cerebral artery. Diffusion-weighted (*B*) and apparent diffusion coefficient map (*C*) confirm extensive cytotoxic edema.

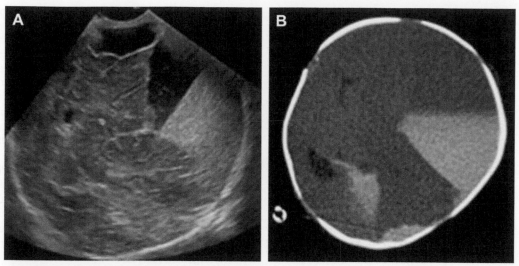

Fig. 24. (*A, B*). A 2-day-old infant born at home with a history of delayed administration of vitamin K, now with seizures. Large extra-axial hemorrhage on the left with effacement of the left lateral ventricle and rightward shift of the midline are demonstrated. The ultrasound image (*A*) was reconstructed from a 3D acquisition, at the workstation to correspond to the follow-up CT (*B*) to allow accurate comparison.

0.6 and 0.8. Low resistive index (increased diastolic velocity) reflects cerebral hyperemia from vasodilation after a hypoxic-ischemic event (**Fig. 23**). Nonuniform systolic or diastolic velocities may indicate loss of autoregulation.

Intracranial hemorrhage in the newborn may be related to birth trauma (dystocia or precipitous delivery), coagulopathy, vascular malformation, hypertension, or ischemia.[27,28] Hemorrhage may be intra-axial, extra-axial (**Fig. 24**), solitary, or multifocal. Intra-axial hyperacute and nonclotted blood tends to be cystic or hypoechoic; otherwise, hemorrhage is hyperechoic relative to the parenchyma. Detectability of extra-axial hemorrhage by ultrasonography can be difficult, but thorough evaluation to include cinegraphic imaging and tilt views and the use of multiple acoustic windows can help.

SUMMARY

Five clinical scenarios where ultrasonography could be used instead of ionizing radiation were reviewed. Numerous additional clinical opportunities for radiation reduction using ultrasonography exist and have been variably supported in the literature, including pyelonephritis diagnosis, tumor surveillance, hydrocephalus follow-up, gall bladder ejection fraction assessment, diagnosis of vesicoureteral reflux, musculoskeletal injury evaluation, and others. Whenever possible one needs to be creative and have an open mind when pursuing nonradiation imaging alternatives to answer the clinical question.

Significant recent advances in sonographic technology will help us to be more confident in sonographic diagnosis and should translate into less reliance on imaging with ionizing radiation. This is especially important in children, because they are at the greatest risk of developing radiation-induced cancer.

By becoming more confident in sonographic diagnosis and using ultrasonography as an alternative to imaging with ionizing radiation, one will make an impact and reshape imaging paradigms.

REFERENCES

1. Doria AS. Optimizing the role of imaging in appendicitis. Pediatr Radiol 2009;39:144–8.
2. Sivit CJ. Contemporary imaging in abdominal emergencies. Pediatr Radiol 2008;38(Suppl 4):S675–8.
3. Holscher HC, Heij HA. Imaging of acute appendicitis in children: EU versus US...or US versus CT? A European perspective. Pediatr Radiol 2009;39: 497–9.
4. Frush DP, Frush KS, Oldham KT. Imaging of acute appendicitis in children: EU versus US...or US versus CT? A North American perspective. Pediatr Radiol 2009;39:500–5.
5. Wiersma F, Sramek A, Holscher HC. US features of the normal appendix and surrounding area in children. Radiology 2005;235:1018–22.
6. Moteki T, Horikoshi H. New CT criterion for acute appendicitis: maximum depth of intraluminal appendiceal fluid. AJR Am J Roentgenol 2007;188:1313–9.
7. Applegate KE. Intussusception in children: evidence-based diagnosis and treatment. Pediatr Radiol 2009;39(Suppl 2):140–3.

8. Ko HS, Schenk JP, Troger J, et al. Current radiologic management of intussusception in children. Eur J Radiol 2007;17:2411.

9. Wiersma F, Allema JH, Holscher HC. Ileoileal intussusception in children: ultrasonic differentiation from ileocolic intussusception. Pediatr Radiol 2006; 36:1177–81.

10. Park NH, Park SI, Park CS, et al. Ultrasonographic findings of small bowel intussusception, focusing on differentiation from ileocolic intussusception. Br J Radiol 2007;80:798–802.

11. Lim HK, Bae SH, Lee KH, et al. Assessment of reducibility of ileocolic intussusception in children: usefulness of color doppler sonography. Radiology 1994;191:781–5.

12. Sivit CJ. Imaging children with abdominal trauma. AJR Am J Roentgenol 2009;192:1179–89.

13. Luks FI, Lemire A, Saint-Vil D, et al. Blunt abdominal trauma in children: the practical value of ultrasonography. J Trauma 1993;34(5):607–11.

14. Richards JR, Knopf NA, Wang L, et al. Blunt abdominal trauma in children: evaluation with emergency ultrasound. Radiology 2002;222:749–54.

15. Marco G, Diego S, Giulio A, et al. Screening US and CT for blunt abdominal trauma: a retrospective study. Eur J Radiology 2005;56(1):97–101.

16. Browning JG, Wilkinson AG, Beattie T. Imaging paediatric blunt abdominal trauma in the emergency department: ultrasound versus computed tomography. Emerg Med J 2008;25(10):645–8.

17. Eeg K, Khoury A, Halachim S, et al. Single center experience with application of the ALARA concept to serial imaging studies after blunt renal trauma in children – is ultrasound enough? J Urol 2009; 181(4):1834–40.

18. Hernanz-Schulman M. Infantile pyloric stenosis. Radiology 2003;227(2):319–31.

19. Hernanz-Schulman M. Pyloric stenosis: the role of imaging. Pediatr Radiol 2009;39:134–9.

20. Chao HC, Kong MS, Chen SJ, et al. Sonographic features related to volvulus in neonatal malrotation. J Ultrasound Med 2000;19(6):371–6.

21. Sze RW, Guillerman RP, Krauter D, et al. A possible new ancillary sign for diagnosing midgut volvulus: the truncated superior mesenteric artery. J Ultrasound Med 2002;21(4):477–80.

22. Westra SJ, Wolf BH, Staalman CR. Ultrasound diagnosis of gastroesophageal reflux and hiatal hernia in infants and young children. J Clin Ultrasound 2005; 18(6):477–85.

23. Heinz ER, Provenzale JM. Imaging findings in neonatal hypoxia: a practical review. AJR Am J Roentgenol 2009;192:41–7.

24. Chao CP, Zaleski CG, Patton AC. Neonatal hypoxic-ischemic encephalopathy: multimodality imaging findings. Radiographics 2006;26:S159–72.

25. Stark JE, Siebert JJ. Cerebral artery doppler ultrasonography for prediction of outcome after perinatal ischemia. J Ultrasound Med 1994;13:595–600.

26. Blankenburg FG, Loh NN, Norbash AM, et al. Impaired cerebrovascular autoregulation after hypoxic ischemic injury in extremely low birth weight neonates: detection with power and pulsed wave doppler US. Radiology 1997;205(2):562–8.

27. Ykilmaz A, Taylor GA. Cranial sonography in term and near-term infants. Pediatr Radiol 2008;38: 605–16.

28. Daneman A, Epelman M, Blaser S, et al. Imaging of the brain in full-term neonates: does sonography still play a role. Pediatr Radiol 2006;36:636–46.

New Advances in Breast Ultrasound: Computer-Aided Detection

A. Thomas Stavros, MD, FACR

KEYWORDS

- Computer-aided technologies for breast ultrasound screening
- Radiology breast imaging reporting and data system ultrasound lexicon
- Characterizing solid nodules
- Computer-aided diagnosis for breast ultrasound

To fully take advantage of ultrasound's ability to make a more specific diagnosis than that which can be made with clinical findings and mammography alone, efficacious sonographic characterization of solid breast nodules is essential. One specific goal of diagnostic breast ultrasound is to minimize the number of biopsies that prove benign while maximizing identification of lesions that prove malignant on biopsy. In characterizing a breast nodule, a single or feature can be useful as a starting point. However, sensitivity can be improved greatly by analyzing multiple features and applying a strict algorithmic approach.[1]

CHARACTERIZING SOLID NODULES

The American College of Radiology Breast Imaging Reporting and Data System (BI-RADS) was developed to help standardize findings, terminology, and management of breast lesions. This was first developed for mammography, then later for ultrasound and magnetic resonance imaging. The BI-RADS Ultrasound Lexicon is currently undergoing revision and soon version 2 will be released. The system describes and illustrates features that can be used to characterize solid nodules.[2] It further defines with feature analysis the risk and categories that

should be used in characterizing solid breast nodules. To generate a BI-RADS category and its corresponding recommendation, clinicians must identify multiple features per lesion and assess the relative importance of each feature. These tasks can be can be time-consuming and tedious (**Box 1, Table 1**).

COMPUTER-AIDED DIAGNOSIS; COMPUTER-AIDED DETECTION

Computer technology should be useful for both diagnosis and detection. Thus, the terms *computer-aided diagnosis* and *computer-aided detection* have been coined, both with the acronym CAD. However, regulatory nuances within the United States have muddied the distinction between computer-aided detection and computer-aided diagnosis. Computer-aided detection is what has been used in mammography to aid in discovering lesions. Computer-aided diagnosis is what is used in diagnostic ultrasound to aid in lesion characterization after the lesion has been found. However, the term *computer-aided diagnosis* tends to be avoided in favor of *computer-aided detection* because United States regulatory authorities have approved computer-aided detection but not computer-aided diagnosis.

Sutter North Bay Women's Health Center, 625 Steele Lane Santa Rosa, CA 95403, USA
E-mail address: tstavros@riaco.com

Ultrasound Clin 4 (2009) 285–290
doi:10.1016/j.cult.2009.10.010

Box 1
BI-RADS features

Shape
- Oval
- Round
- Irregular

Margin
- Circumscribed
- Not circumscribed
  - Indistinct
  - Angular
  - Microlobulated
  - Spiculated

Lesion boundary
- Abrupt
- Echogenic halo

Orientation
- Parallel
- Not parallel

Posterior features
- No posterior features
- Enhancement
- Shadowing
- Combined pattern

Echo pattern
- Anechoic
- Hyperechoic
- Hypoechoic
- Isoechoic
- Complex echogenicity

Calcifications
- Macrocalcifications
- Microcalcifications out of mass
- Microcalcification in mass

Surrounding tissue
- Duct change
- Cooper ligament
- Edema
- Architectural distortion
- Skin thickening
- Skin retraction

Vascularity
- None
- In lesion

- Adjacent to lesion
- Diffuse

Special cases
- Clustered microcysts
- Complicated cysts
- Mass in or on skin
- Foreign body
- Intramammary lymph nodes

Thus, the term *CAD for breast ultrasound* is inaccurately considered computer-aided detection, when more precisely it is a technique for diagnosis. CAD for breast ultrasound applies ultrasound CAD algorithms to find the edge of a solid nodule and then characterize it. The algorithm assesses individual BI-RADS features and suggests a BI-RADS category. CAD feature analysis and BI-RADS classification are always suggestions that can be overridden by the reader if appropriate. As noted in the term *computer-assisted*, CAD exists to aid the reader, not to replace the reader.

ADVANTAGES AND DRAWBACKS OF COMPUTER-ASSISTED DIAGNOSIS
Advantages

Computers and well-written software not only can help make feature analysis less cumbersome and more consistent, but can also facilitate proper use of each feature within a strict algorithm. Properly written CAD software should impose strict adherence to the BI-RADS Lexicon, decrease interobserver variability, and may even improve assignment of BI-RADS categories (at least for less experienced breast sonologists). Furthermore, by strictly adhering to the BI-RADS Ultrasound Lexicon, a well-written CAD program can facilitate structured reporting, which in turn can generate concise and accurate printed reports, automatically fax or e-mail reports, triage urgent reports, and minimize transcription costs and errors.

Finally, each BI-RADS–compliant entry, including indication, history, risk factors, clinical findings, sonographic findings, BI-RADS category, and management recommendation, can be assigned to a field in a database. From the database generated by using CAD software, regular turnkey weekly, monthly, quarterly, and annual reports can be generated, which are essential for continuous quality improvement and accreditation processes. Such databases could also be invaluable for

Table 1
BI-RADS ultrasound categories

Category	Finding
0	Incomplete: Additional imaging evaluation needed before final assessment
1	Negative: No lesion found; routine follow-up
2	Benign finding(s): No malignant features (eg, cyst); routine follow-up for age; clinical management
3	Probably benign finding: Malignancy is highly unlikely (eg, fibroadenoma); initial short-interval follow-up
4 (4a, 4b, 4c)	Suspicious abnormality: Low to moderate probability of cancer; biopsy should be considered
5	Highly suggestive of malignancy: Almost certainly cancer; appropriate action should be taken
6	Known cancer: Biopsy proven malignancy before institution of therapy

research. It is always interesting and educational to be able to assess individual findings and BI-RADS categories for any specific indication, BI-RADS category, or histologic diagnosis. Data could be used, for example, (1) to assess the false-negative rate for second-look ultrasound after contrast enhanced magnetic resonance imaging, (2) to assess the percentage of malignant lesions within the BI-RADS 3 category for a radiology group or an individual radiologist, or (3) to assess the sonographic findings in micropapillary carcinoma in situ. Since the database would be standardized, it would greatly enhance ability to perform multicenter studies.

Because the risk of malignancy within the BI-RADS 4 category is so large (3%–94%), version 1 of the BI-RADS Ultrasound Lexicon allows for voluntary subdivision of the BI-RADS 4 category into 4a, 4b, and 4c categories. However, no specific percentages of malignancy were defined for each subcategory and no rules for placement in each of the subcategories were defined. A database that strictly adhered to the BI-RADS Lexicon and that could be generated from multiple facilities might form a foundation for developing rules for BI-RADS 4 subcategorization.

Drawbacks

The main drawback of CAD is possible inaccuracy of CAD-assessed features and CAD-determined BI-RADS risk categories. Because accuracy may vary from one software package to another, each CAD software package must prove itself scientifically. The only other major drawback, at least as far as the regulatory agencies within the United States are concerned, is that the reader will rely entirely upon CAD and will not assess the images

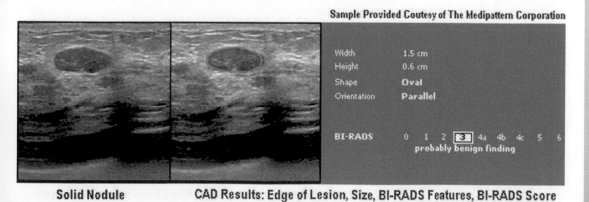

Sample Provided Coutesy of The Medipattern Corporation

Width	1.5 cm
Height	0.6 cm
Shape	**Oval**
Orientation	**Parallel**

BI-RADS   0   1   2   **3**   4a   4b   4c   5   6
probably benign finding

Solid Nodule   CAD Results: Edge of Lesion, Size, BI-RADS Features, BI-RADS Score

Fig. 1. Nodule proven through histology to be fibroadenomas and correctly characterized as BI-RADS 3. (*Left*) Original image. (*Right*) CAD results. Edges of nodule traced in green. Suggested BI-RADS features and BI-RADS score shown to the right of the CAD image.

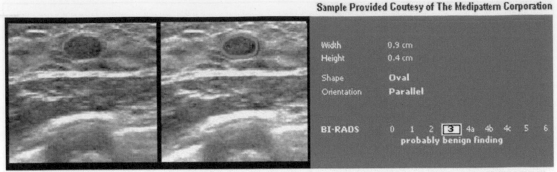

Width	0.9 cm
Height	0.4 cm
Shape	**Oval**
Orientation	**Parallel**
BI-RADS	0 1 2 **3** 4a 4b 4c 5 6
	probably benign finding

Solid Nodule   **CAD Results: Edge of Lesion, Size, BI-RADS Features, BI-RADS Score**

Fig. 2. Nodule proven through histology to be fibroadenomas and correctly characterized as BI-RADS 3. (*Left*) Original image. (*Right*) CAD results. Edges of nodule traced in green. Suggested BI-RADS features and BI-RADS score shown to the right of the CAD image.

at all. Such use of CAD is, indeed, inappropriate and should never be condoned. However, as noted above, CAD is meant to assist the reader, not to replace the reader.

EXAMPLES OF COMPUTER-AIDED DIAGNOSIS FOR BREAST ULTRASOUND IN PRACTICE

Solid nodules characterized as BI-RADS 3 are considered probably benign. Nodules characterized into BI-RADS 4a, 4b, 4c, and 5 categories are considered positive for purposes of correlation with histology. In practice, the most challenging determination is between subgroup BI-RADS 3 and the BI-RADS 4a subgroup. This forms the testing ground for determining how well CAD adheres to the strict algorithm that we use to interpret solid nodules. Each of the cases in this section shows CAD results from these two subgroups.

The original image is displayed on the left in **Figs. 1–5**. The CAD results are displayed on the

right. The CAD algorithm finds the edge of the nodule and automatically traces the outline of the lesion in green directly on the image shown in the right panel. The suggested BI-RADS features and BI-RADS score are shown to the right of the image with CAD. All three of these elements—lesion segmentation, features, and score—comprise the CAD results.

Figs. 1 and **2** show solid nodules proven through histology to be fibroadenomas and correctly characterized as BI-RADS 3, in which case 6-month follow up can be offered as an alternative to biopsy. The CAD algorithm automatically finds BI-RADS features that correspond to benign findings and correctly suggests that the nodule is likely benign. **Figs. 3–5** are solid nodules proven to be malignant. The CAD algorithm correctly finds BI-RADS features that are suspicious for malignancy and then suggests a BI-RADS classification appropriate for the suspicious findings and also concordant with the malignant histology in all three cases.

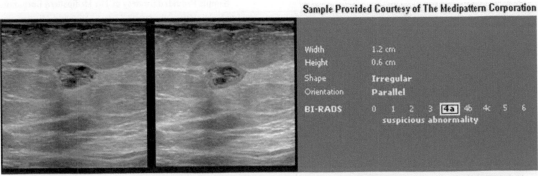

Width	1.2 cm
Height	0.6 cm
Shape	**Irregular**
Orientation	**Parallel**
BI-RADS	0 1 2 3 **4a** 4b 4c 5 6
	suspicious abnormality

Solid Nodule   **CAD Results: Edge of Lesion, Size, BI-RADS Features, BI-RADS Score**

Fig. 3. Histologically proven ductal carcinoma in situ (BI-RADS 4a). (*Left*) Original image. (*Right*) CAD results. Edges of nodule traced in green. Suggested BI-RADS features and BI-RADS score shown to the right of the CAD image.

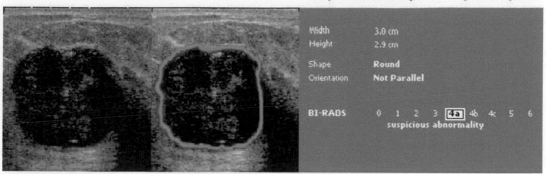

Fig. 4. Histologically proven invasive ductal carcinoma (BI-RADS 4a). (*Left*) Original image. (*Right*) CAD results. Edges of nodule traced in green. Suggested BI-RADS features and BI-RADS score shown to the right of the CAD image.

SCREENING BREAST ULTRASOUND: THE NEED FOR COMPUTER-AIDED DETECTION

Originally, one of the expected uses for breast ultrasound was as a screening tool as an adjunct to screening mammography. The recent ACRIN (American College of Radiology Imaging Network) 6666 Trial results[3] indicate that handheld whole-breast ultrasound used in addition to screening mammography increases the sensitivity for cancer over mammography alone in women who are at high risk of breast cancer and who have dense breast tissue on mammography.[4] However, at least in the United States, not enough qualified breast radiologists or sonographers are available to perform handheld screening breast ultrasound, which is much more tedious and time-consuming than is targeted diagnostic breast ultrasound. Thus, there has been renewed interest in automated

screening breast ultrasound. Several companies have accepted the challenge and are building automated breast ultrasound scanners. These machines generate numerous images that vary from machine to machine, with breast size, and in some cases, with the percentage of the breast that is comprised of breast tissue. The number of images needing to be analyzed ranges from a few hundred to 5000. The main problems for the reader are fatigue and brief attention lapses. In some cases, viewing 5000 images at 10 frames per second requires 10 minutes. Maintaining concentration and focus for that long is exceedingly difficult. Even a brief attention lapse of 5 seconds could mean 50 missed images. Some small carcinomas may be seen only on 5 or even fewer images. Computer-aided detection could be invaluable in such cases, especially if there were auditory as well as visual cues to the abnormalities detected. However, we must

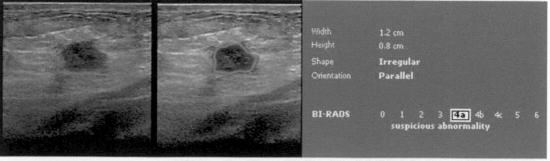

Fig. 5. Histologically proven invasive ductal carcinoma (BI-RADS 4a). (*Left*) Original image. (*Right*) CAD results. Edges of nodule traced in green. Suggested BI-RADS features and BI-RADS score shown to the right of the CAD image.

remember that screening is not diagnosis. In screening studies, computer-aided diagnosis would be less important than computer-assisted detection. Also, an abnormal screening study should instigate a formal diagnostic ultrasound, at which time computer-assisted diagnosis would be needed.

SUMMARY

In 1995 we published a prospective study showing that, by using multiple sonographic findings in a strictly followed algorithm, we could identify a group of solid breast nodules that had less than a 2% risk of being malignant while still characterizing more than 98% of malignant lesions as suspicious or malignant. Since then, the role of diagnostic breast ultrasound progressively expanded well beyond merely distinguishing cyst from solid. The volume of breast ultrasound and the number of images per study have increased dramatically. CAD could serve a very useful role in assisting the breast-imaging physician. Just as a pilot's checklist ensures that the pilot checks all of the indicators before landing, CAD can ensure each sonographic finding is sought, noted, and appropriately reported. This can be helpful in many ways. It may improve performance amongst less experienced readers, decrease interobserver variability, generate concise and accurate reports, save transcription costs, and create an invaluable database useful for accreditation, continuous quality improvement, and research. CAD will likely eventually be invaluable in breast ultrasound screening. Unfortunately, no single CAD program achieves all these goals yet and only limited

versions of CAD are approved for use within the United States. Far more robust versions have been approved for use virtually everywhere outside the United States. To fulfill its promise, CAD will have to evolve to remain compliant with version 2 of the BI-RADS Ultrasound Lexicon, detection must be added to aid us in screening, a database function with turnkey reports will need to be added, and CAD will have to overcome United States regulatory hurdles that prevent American clinicians now from having the full-featured CAD programs available to clinicians outside the United States. Finally, breast imagers can never forget that CAD is meant to aide, not replace, the breast imager.

REFERENCES

1. Stavros AT. Ultrasound of solid breast nodules: distinguishing benign from malignant. In: Stavros AT, editor. Breast ultrasound. Philadelphia: Lippincott Williams & Wilkins; 2004. p. 445–527.
2. American College of Radiology (ACR), Breast Imaging Reporting And Data System Atlas (BI-RADS Atlas). 1st edition. Reston (VA): American College of Radiology; 2003.
3. Berg WA, Blume JD, Cormack JB, et al. Combined screening with ultrasound and mammography vs mammography alone in women at an elevated risk of breast cancer. JAMA 2008;299:2151–63.
4. Kelly KM, Dean J, Comuldada WS, et al. Breast cancer detection using automated whole breast ultrasound and mammography in radiographically dense breasts. Eur Radiol 2009. [Epub ahead of print].

Three-Dimensional Ultrasound: Technique and Applications Revisited

Nirvikar Dahiya, MD

KEYWORDS

- Three-dimensional ultrasound • Volume acquisition
- Ultrasound applications
- Postprocessing of volume datasets

Three-dimensional ultrasound (3DUS) has been around long enough to warrant a comprehensive discussion of its capabilities. From the infamy of "baby faces" for entertainment value, no less served by the highly publicized story of a celebrity buying the equipment to look at his unborn child, to the real diagnostic capabilities that include volume acquisition and multiplanar imaging, 3DUS has seen it all.

For several years now, 3DUS seems to have been hanging between "promise" and "delivery." However, faster computing platforms and improved software have recently enabled much better postprocessing techniques. A change in the mindset of the user has shifted attention from the surface-rendering abilities of 3DUS (as used for "baby faces") to its "volume" capabilities.

Volume acquisition is the new paradigm where the ability to do multiplanar reconstruction has given 3DUS enhanced diagnostic value and widened its acceptance. A frequent complaint against general ultrasound has been its "operator dependence." 3DUS offers the promise of leveling the playing field between computed tomography, magnetic resonance imaging, and ultrasound by enabling multiplanar imaging and decreasing the dependence on the operator. Regardless, a skilled sonologist is still required as good three-dimensional (3D) acquisition depends on a good two-dimensional (2D) orientation. Comprehensive volume acquisition by 3DUS should enable the development and use of standardized scanning protocols, which should reduce dependence on the operator.

This article provides an overview of the technology and explains the features available in current state-of-the-art ultrasound imaging equipment. Some of the main clinical applications are listed.

ACQUISITION OF VOLUME

There are three basic ways of acquiring a 3D volume dataset: freehand technique, automatic acquisition, and automatic acquisition with matrix transducers.[1–3]

> Freehand technique: With the freehand technique, volume is acquired with a conventional 2D transducer. This requires a fair bit of skill in moving the transducer in a manner that limits artifacts. This method does not have volumetric accuracy and can be done with or without a position-sensing device. If volume is acquired without a position-sensing device, the geometric accuracy of the resulting images cannot be relied on for measurements.

Department of Abdomen Imaging, Mallinckrodt Institute of Radiology, Washington University School of Medicine, 510 S. Kingshighway Boulevard, St Louis, MO 63108, USA
E-mail address: dahiyan@mir.wustl.edu

Ultrasound Clin 4 (2009) 291–306
doi:10.1016/j.cult.2009.10.004
1556-858X/09/$ – see front matter © 2009 Elsevier Inc. All rights reserved.

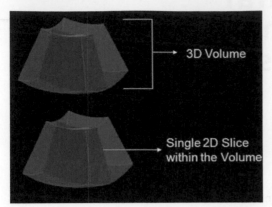

Fig. 1. Three-dimensional volume. (*Top*) The general shape of an acquired 3D volume. This volume contains multiple contiguous 2D planes. (*Bottom*) A single 2D slice.

Automatic acquisition: Automatic acquisition employs a dedicated mechanical volume transducer to help in acquisition of volume. Here, a 2D transducer is housed in a casing with position-sensing device. With the aid of a motor, the transducer sweeps at a pre-defined angle for acquiring volume. A real-time 3D acquisition and display is also known as four-dimensional (4D) (the fourth dimension being time) ultrasound.

Automatic acquisition with matrix trans-ducers: Matrix transducers use arrays of active elements that acquire large volume datasets and reduce the artifacts related to respiration. These were initially used in cardiac applications and have slowly grav-itated to general ultrasound.

Once a volume dataset has been acquired, it is important to understand that the volume is in the shape of a trapezoid and is essentially made up of multiple 2D slices (**Fig. 1**). The quantity or width of the volume depends on the sweep angle selected before acquiring the volume. Larger sweep angles will result in longer acquisition times and more chances of artifacts if the patient is not able to hold breath for that duration. After an auto-matic transducer acquires the volume, it retains all the geometric information needed to create the orthogonal planes. Knobs provided on the equip-ment or on the workstations help rotate the 2D planes within the volume to obtain other sections (**Fig. 2**). The volume dataset can be postprocessed in multiple ways to obtain relevant diagnostic information.

POSTPROCESSING OF VOLUME DATASET

The two postprocessing tools most often used on a volume dataset are those for rendering and for sectional anatomy.

Rendering in a Volume Dataset

Rendering of a volume demonstrates information stored within the entire volume by selecting display modes that preferentially enhance certain aspects of the anatomy. Surface rendering exploits the interface between two structures. If fluid surrounds the surface, the surface rendering is easily identifiable, as is the case with the fetal face, which is surrounded by amniotic fluid (**Fig. 3**). Gallbladder mucosa is similarly rendered because the lumen has fluid (bile) (**Fig. 4**). If the surface rendering is performed through the solid

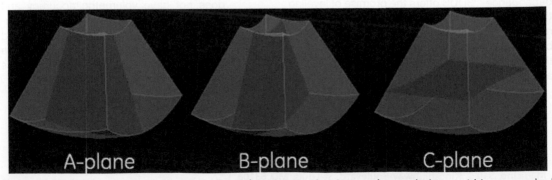

Fig. 2. Multiplanar imaging. A, B, and C planes demonstrate the three orthogonal planes within an acquired volume. One of these planes is the primary plane of acquisition while the other two planes are reconstructed from the volume dataset.

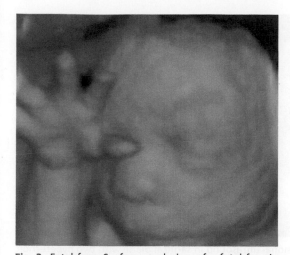

Fig. 3. Fetal face. Surface rendering of a fetal face in the second trimester.

portion of an organ, the displayed anatomy behaves like a thick slice of the volume. Depending upon the direction from where the rendering is done, the final rendered image is a display of the sum of voxels in a selected area (**Fig. 5**).

Vendors have made available various modes for rendering acquired volume. These include the surface-rendering mode, the maximum-transparency mode, the gradient-light mode and others. A mix of two different rendering modes is possible and the best sonographic results are obtained by learning to experiment with different mix selections.

The earliest 3DUS machines were somewhat limited in their rendering capabilities. The frame rates were slow and volumes acquired per second were small, resulting in a significant lag between acquisition and display of information. Over time,

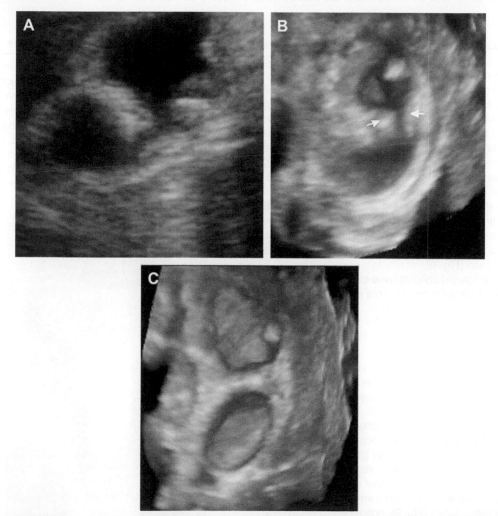

Fig. 4. Gallbladder rendering. (*A*) Two-dimensional image of a case of adenomyomatosis of the gallbladder with midbody constriction and a calculus lodged in the fundus. (*B*) Rendered image in the same plane with rendering of the mucosa and calculus. Arrows point to mid body constriction. (*C*) A section through the constriction band that divides the gallbladder lumen into two. The "threshold" in C was increased to better evaluate the mucosa.

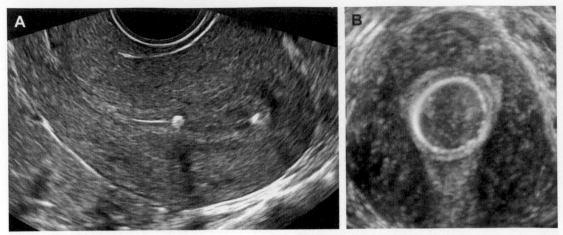

Fig. 5. Intrauterine contraceptive device. (*A*) Two-dimensional ultrasound in sagittal plane with two hyperechoic foci in the endometrium. (*B*) Coronal reconstruction of the rendered plane through the endometrium. The two-echogenic foci seen on the 2D image are part of intrauterine ring contraceptive device.

significant software and hardware improvements have contributed to an expansion of 3DUS rendering applications.

One of the most significant improvements in the rendering mode is the ability to curve the rendering line. This enables the operator to follow the physiologic curve of an anatomic structure so that the structure could be laid out in its entirety in the rendered image. The technique for rendering the uterine endometrial stripe is a perfect example. Earlier it was difficult to reconstruct a coronal plane that showed the endometrium as a continuous line. It had to be imaged separately in the uterine body and in cervical segments. With the curved rendering, the entire endometrium can be easily seen (**Fig. 6**).

The rendering abilities have expanded to include the color Doppler mode. This enables the use of a pseudoangiographic mode, where the vascularity of a volume dataset can be visualized in an enhanced manner by subduing the gray voxels (**Fig. 7**).

Another rendering addition has been the introduction of the inversion mode.[4,5] This technique involves an algorithm that inverts the dark/black voxels into bright/white voxels. Thus, the anechoic (dark/black) fluid-filled structures appear echogenic (bright/white) and echogenic structures appear dark. Additionally the gray-scale voxels of the volume dataset are removed. The final rendered image shows white casts of fluid-filled cavities (**Fig. 8**). This mode can be used to investigate dilated tubes (**Fig. 9**), hollow viscous cavities, or even vascular channels. The threshold and levels of transparency can be changed to fine tune the appearance of the final rendered image.

Sectional Anatomy in a Volume Dataset

The second most often used option to evaluate a volume dataset is that for reviewing sectional anatomy. Sectional anatomy in a given volume can be reviewed simultaneously in all three orthogonal planes. As in computed tomography and magnetic resonance imaging, this enables multiplanar evaluation. With mechanical transducers, the primary plane of acquisition has the best resolution. The other two orthogonal planes are

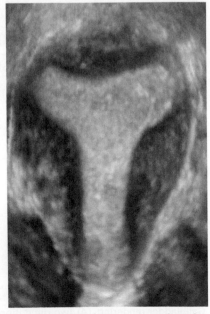

Fig. 6. Coronal plane of uterus. Curved rendered line enables continuous display of the entire endometrial stripe.

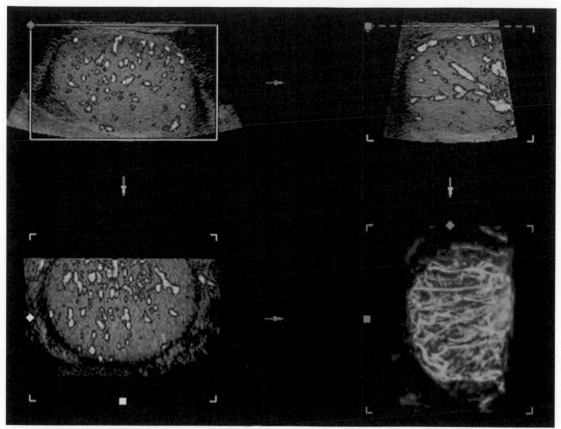

Fig. 7. Pseudoangiographic mode of 3DUS. Multiplanar display of the testes is shown with the final rendered image of color voxels at the bottom right. The rendered image shows the sum of vascularity in the entire testicular volume.

reconstructed from the volume dataset and therefore have a lower resolution (**Fig. 10**). For this purpose, it makes sense to acquire the volume in the plane most pertinent to the diagnosis. It is believed that matrix probes in the future will be able to circumvent this issue and provide isotropic resolution in all planes.

Ultrasound tomography is an offshoot of multiplanar imaging. Here information is displayed as multiple parallel slices. Similar to a computed tomography scanogram, a primary reference plane is chosen and then multiple parallel slices are re-created in an orthogonal plane for display of information (**Fig. 11**).

Taking postprocessing of the volume dataset a notch higher are algorithms that allow for visualization of parts of the volume in a high-contrast manner. This technology is known as volume contrast imaging (GE Healthcare, Milwaukee, WI).[6] This is essentially real-time volume acquisition

with a very small elevation sweep angle. A combination of surface and maximum gradient rendering is used to deliver improved contrast to the ultrasound image (**Fig. 12**).

Another algorithm enables capture of multiple volumes and synchronizes them based on a calculated heart rate. This is known as spatiotemporal image correlation (STIC) and has been extensively used to study the fetal heart.[7]

MEASUREMENTS ON THE VOLUME DATASET

The acquisition of a volume dataset enables clinicians to take measurements remotely. The measurement of a relevant organ or lesion is easy since all the planes needed for measurement are available in the dataset. Additionally, the ability to calculate an accurate volume of the lesion or the organ is possible, irrespective of the contour. This

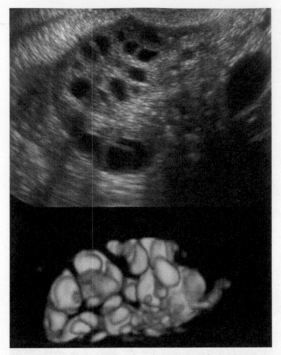

Fig. 8. Inversion mode. (*Top*) Large polycystic ovary with multiple follicles on 2D ultrasound rendered using the inversion mode. (*Bottom*) The anechoic follicles represented by the white casts of their volume.

technique has been described as virtual organ computer-aided analysis.

This semiautomated technique uses a complex mathematical formula to calculate volume. It enables the user to outline the contour of a lesion serially through different planes, as the volume is rotated 180° about a central axis. Measurement accuracy is excellent when a small rotation step is used as this generates multiple planes for the user to measure and integrate for each single volume calculation (**Fig. 13**). An enhancement of the above technique is SonoAVC (GE Medical Systems, Zipf, Austria), which has been very successful in automatically calculating volumes of individual ovarian follicles in work-up and treatment of infertility.[8,9]

CLINICAL APPLICATIONS

Many clinical studies have looked at 3DUS applications in obstetric ultrasound mainly because the fetus, surrounded by amniotic fluid, lends itself to volume imaging and rendering. With the exception of applications involving the uterus and the adnexa in gynecologic examinations, nonobstetric areas have rarely been addressed in 3DUS studies.

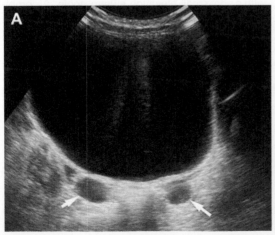
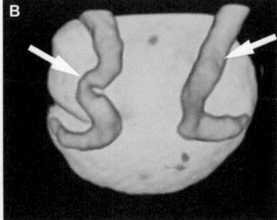

Fig. 9. Inversion mode. (*A*) Two-dimensional image of a urinary bladder with two anechoic well-defined areas (*arrows*) posterior to the bladder representing the dilated ureters in a case of posterior urethral valve. (*B*) Inversion mode–rendered image rotated 180° to demonstrate the dilated ureters (*arrows*) posterior to the urinary bladder.

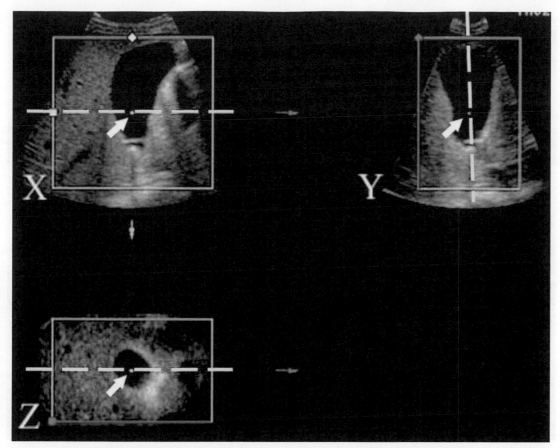

Fig. 10. Multiplanar display. The three orthogonal planes have been demonstrated. The yellow dotted line represents the central axis in the volume and are the X, Y, and Z coordinates of the dataset. In the center of the image slice is a small dot that represents the point of intersection of the three coordinates. This point can be moved by the operator to evaluate different sections of anatomy.

A review of all the clinical applications is beyond the scope of this article. Some of the more widely used applications are mentioned.

Obstetric Three-dimensional Ultrasound

Many studies have compared the performance of 3DUS and 2D ultrasound (2DUS) in detecting fetal anomalies.[10–16] The major applications have centered on surveys of the fetal anatomy in the first trimester using a dedicated volume transvaginal transducer and of the fetal anatomy in the second trimester using a curvilinear transducer.

First trimester three-dimensional ultrasound
The transvaginal transducer enables a wide angle of volume acquisition. The entire fetus is acquired in one volume sweep and this makes it easier to manipulate the postacquisition volume for diagnostic information. This technique has been used to locate ectopic pregnancies, especially cornual and cervical pregnancies (**Fig. 14**); to conduct biometric and anatomic surveys; and to measure nuchal translucency. Nuchal translucency thickness (NTT) has been measured in multiple studies by many investigators. Paul and colleagues[17] reported a high visualization rate of the NTT if the primary plane of acquisition is in a sagittal plane. They reported a clear visualization of NTT in 38 of 40 cases using the above technique. This was more significant when compared with the low rate of visualization they had with respect to measurement of NTT in volumes captured using a different primary plane of acquisition.

Fetal abnormalities detected by 3DUS in the first trimester include anomalies of the central nervous

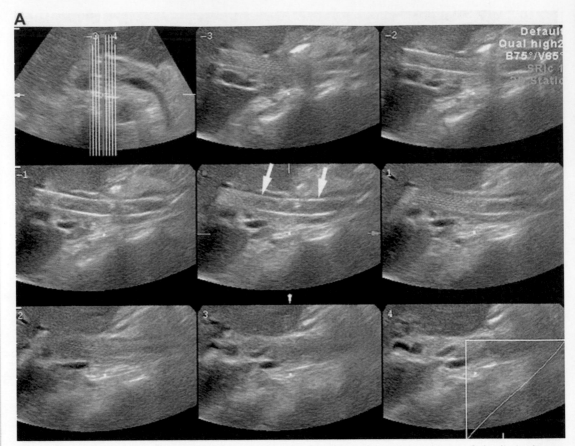

Fig. 11. Tomographic sonography. (*A*) Multiple tomographic planes through the hilum of the liver, demonstrating a biliary stent (*arrows*). The top left image is a transverse image of the distal bile duct at the head of the pancreas. This image was used as a reference to re-create the sagittal tomographic planes. (*B*) Multiple contiguous axial reconstructions through the female urethra (*arrows*) with a urethral diverticulum (*arrowheads*). The top left reference image is a sagittal image of the urethra.

system, the skeletal system, and heart. Volume measurements of normal gestation sac and yolk sac have been reported.

Second and third trimester three-dimensional ultrasound

The fetal face was one of the first structures to be rendered by 3DUS. Multiple studies have reported that 3DUS of the fetal face is complementary to 2DUS. It is possible to reconstruct the true midline sagittal plane and thus evaluate the fetal face profile for nasal bone or mandible anomalies (**Fig. 15**). The surface-rendered frontal view helps in diagnosing cleft lip and palate, midfacial, and orbital abnormalities.[18–24]

With greater focus on multiplanar aspects of 3DUS, internal bony and soft tissue evaluations of the skull have become more common. Mueller and colleagues[25] and Wang and colleagues[26] have focused on comparing the 3D and 2D central nervous system anomalies. 3DUS has been very successful in reconstructing the axial planes of the brain. This has improved visualization of the ventricles, corpus callosum, and cerebellum.

The fetal thorax has been evaluated for congenital thoracic (**Fig. 16**) and heart anomalies. Measurements of normal fetal lung volumes have been published.[27–30] Significantly lower lung volume is associated with congenital diaphragmatic hernia. STIC is frequently used for

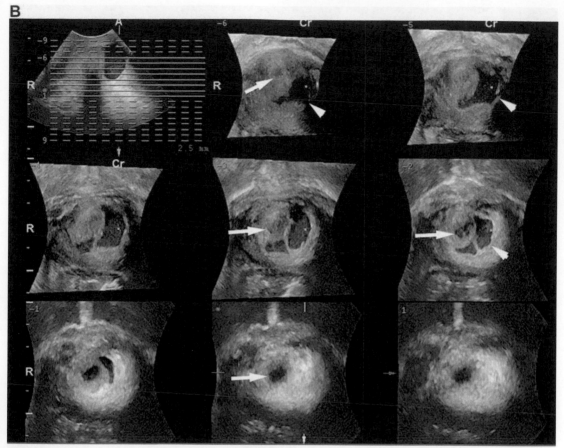

Fig. 11. (*continued*)

real-time evaluation of the fetal heart. Multiple congenital anomalies are readily visualized.

Clinicians conducting evaluations of the fetal skeletal have commonly used the maximum intensity mode so that the bony structures stand out. Developmental skeletal anomalies, such as skeletal dysplasias and bony deformities, have been reliably diagnosed.[31] The fetal spinal deformities have been extensively reported upon.[25,32–34] The surface rendering ability has helped in extremity evaluations and real-time 3DUS can be used to assess motor functions of hands and feet.

Three-dimensional volume acquisition with color Doppler enables imaging of fetal abdominal vasculature. A recent study was able to identify with consistency all the abdominal arteries and veins in the fetal abdomen.[35]

Non-obstetric Three-dimensional Ultrasound

Clinicians have been slow to develop 3DUS applications for the abdomen. The most widely accepted nonobstetric application for 3DUS is gynecologic evaluation. The coronal plane reconstruction provides an entirely new plane of interrogation on ultrasound, which is valuable for assessing congenital uterine anomalies. The ability to reconstruct the coronal plane gives clinicians a frontal-plane view like that from a magnetic resonance image. This helps in evaluating the uterine fundal contour (**Fig. 17**). Ghate and colleagues[36] showed in their study that 3D reformations improve visualization of the fundal contour deformity during 3D sonohysterography. However, they did not see benefit by 3DUS in detecting endometrial abnormalities. Still, 3DUS is a valuable

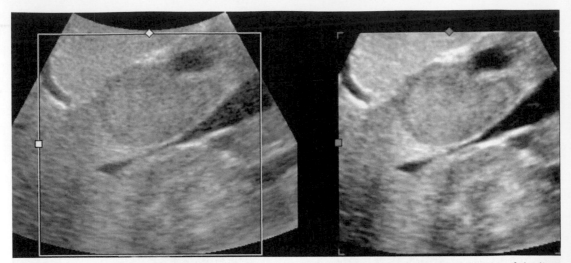

Fig. 12. Volume contrast imaging. (*Left*) Two-dimensional image shows a lesion in the caudate lobe of the liver. (*Right*) Volume contrast imaging rendering mode enhances the contrast and enables better appreciation of the margins of the lesion.

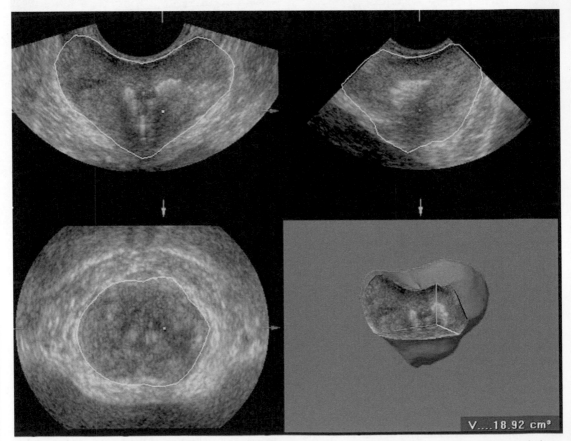

Fig. 13. Volume calculation by virtual organ computer-aided analysis. The three representative orthogonal planes are visualized with a final volume-rendered image (*Bottom right*) that shows a calculated prostate volume. The calculation itself is done on one plane but incremental rotations of that plane enable contour changes in other planes to be factored in.

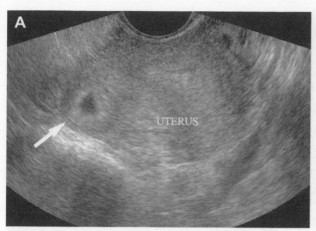

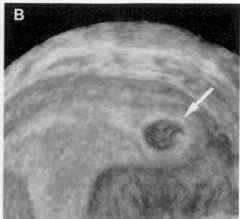

Fig. 14. Uterine 3DUS. (*A*) Two-dimensional ultrasound showing an eccentrically located gestation sac (*arrow*), raising concern about a possible cornual pregnancy. (*B*) Three-dimensional ultrasound enabled multiplanar evaluation of the gestation sac, which was found to be within the endometrium.

problem-solving tool for endometrial abnormalities, often helping to differentiate between a polyp and a submucosal fibroid.

Nongynecologic applications of 3DUS have included evaluations of liver, gallbladder, kidney, urinary bladder, small parts (eg, thyroid), scrotum, and the musculoskeletal system.[37–46] Such

structures as the gallbladder and the urinary bladder contain fluid and thus can be rendered using the fluid interface (**Fig. 18**).

Vascular evaluations have included studies of the abdominal aorta for aneurysms and even calculation of plaque volume in carotid arteries as an indicator for treatment response. Volume calculations of organs and lesions using virtual organ computer-aided analysis have been more precise and have been used for follow-up of cancers after therapy.[47–49]

Multiplanar reconstruction has played a greater role in abdominal imaging than rendering alone (**Fig. 19**). Nevertheless, a combination of the two provides the spatial information needed in different planes. The ability to reimage in multiple planes after the patient has left the examination room enhances the role of 3DUS as a problem-solving tool that complements 2DUS.

THREE-DIMENSIONAL ULTRASOUND AND WORKFLOW

With 3DUS, acquired volume can be stored for diagnostic interpretation later. This capability opens up the possibility of remote interpretation of the volume data. Nelson and colleagues[50] investigated this ability of 3DUS and found that off-line review of 3DUS data generally was able to comply with the American Institute of Ultrasound in Medicine and American College of Radiology guidelines to produce a diagnostically adequate study. An offshoot of this ability is the

Fig. 15. Micrognathia. Three-dimensional ultrasound rendering of the fetal face showing micrognathia.

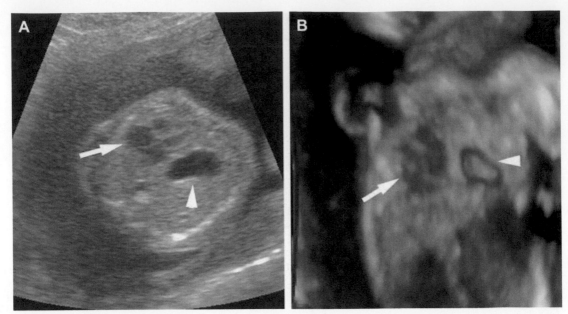

Fig. 16. Congenital diaphragmatic hernia. (*A*) Axial 2D plane showing a cystic structure (*arrowhead*) in close proximity to the heart (*arrow*). (*B*) Coronal 3D rendering showed the cystic structure (*arrowhead*) to be the herniated stomach in the thorax. Arrow indicates heart.

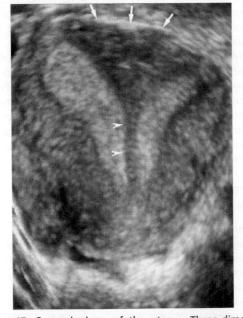

Fig. 17. Coronal plane of the uterus. Three-dimensional reconstruction of the coronal plane shows an intact fundal myometrium (*arrows*) with a thin uterine septum (*arrowheads*).

capability to dedicate a 3D workstation for review of volume data and reconstruction of relevant planes for measurements. This can tremendously improve the efficiency of an ultrasound department.

Bromley and colleagues[51–53] have documented in their study that the standard fetal anatomic survey of a fetus between 17 and 21 weeks' gestation can be performed and interpreted with 3DUS in a much shorter time than is possible with standard 2DUS. The same group in an earlier paper showed how 3DUS could provide a rapid, efficient, and accurate way to perform transvaginal gynecologic scans. Their results proved that four volume acquisitions encompassing the uterus and ovaries reduce significantly the actual time patients spend in an examination room, thus improving turnover times of ultrasound examinations.

Hagel and colleagues[54] have also shown that implementing 3DUS volume protocols in a community hospital setting can significantly save time. They specifically tested 3DUS for nonobstetric applications, such as pelvic, small parts, renal, and shoulder scans. Wilson and colleagues[55] in a recent study in the *American Journal of Roentgenology* scanned 200 consecutive patients using mechanical volumetric acquisitions of each

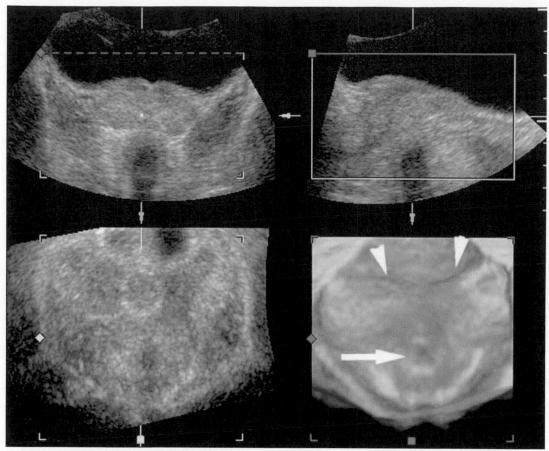

Fig. 18. Three-dimensional rendering of the urinary bladder. A multiplanar view of the urinary bladder with the bottom right image showing the rendering of the bladder base (trigone). The distal ureteral ridges (*arrowheads*) and the urethral opening (*arrows*) are shown.

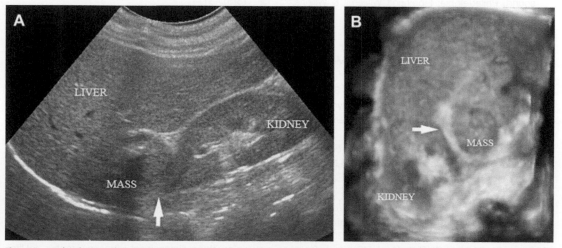

Fig. 19. Multiplanar abdomen sections. (*A*) Two-dimensional coronal image of the right kidney with a mass (*arrow*) between the upper pole of the kidney and the inferior edge of the liver. Clinicians were concerned about the possibility of an exophytic renal mass or a suprarenal mass. (*B*) Three-dimensional reconstruction in an oblique axial plane showed a distinct interface (*arrow*) between the kidney and the suprarenal mass.

abdominal organ, including the liver, gallbladder, pancreas, kidneys, spleen, bowel, and aorta. They reported that the technique was most successful for imaging the right kidney, followed by the left kidney, gallbladder, and liver. The technique was least successful for imaging the spleen. Poor resolution in the reconstructed planes was identified as a technical limitation. This may be a less cumbersome issue with the introduction of matrix transducers that will provide isotropic resolution in all planes.

FUTURE DIRECTIONS

Multiple developments have kept 3DUS on a steady path toward wider recognition and acceptance. Advancements in technology, the development of standards in volume acquisition techniques, and improvements in postprocessing will dictate future developments in 3DUS. Optimization of volume displays and intervendor compatibility for picture archiving and communication systems will play a significant role in adaptation and propagation of 3DUS.

REFERENCES

1. Pretorius DH, Borok NN, Coffler MS, et al. Three-dimensional ultrasound in obstetrics and gynecology. Radiol Clin North Am 2001;39:499–521.
2. Timor-Tritsch IE, Platt LD. Three-dimensional ultrasound experience in obstetrics. Curr Opin Obstet Gynecol 2002;14:569–75.
3. Nelson TR, Downey DB, Pretorius D, et al. Acquisition methods. In: Nelson TR, Downey DB, Pretorius D, et al, editors. Three-dimensional ultrasound. Philadelphia: Lippincott Williams & Wilkins; 1999. p. 11–32.
4. Lee W, Goncalves LF, Espinoza J, et al. Inversion mode: a new volume analysis tool for 3-dimensional ultrasonography. J Ultrasound Med 2005; 24:201–7.
5. Benacerraf BR. Inversion mode display of 3D sonography: applications in obstetric and gynecologic imaging [review]. AJR Am J Roentgenol 2006; 187(4):965–71.
6. Available at: http://www.gehealthcare.com/euen/ ultrasound/docs/education/whitepapers/Ultrasound TechnologyUpdate-STIC.pdf. Accessed September 21, 2009.
7. Available at: http://www.gemed.com.ar/usen/ultra sound/education/docs/UltrasoundTechnologyUp date-VCI.pdf. Accessed September 21, 2009.
8. Rizzo G, Capponi A, Pietrolucci ME, et al. Sonographic automated volume count (SonoAVC) in volume measurement of fetal fluid-filled structures: comparison with virtual organ computer-aided analysis (VOCAL). Ultrasound Obstet Gynecol 2008;32(1):111–2.
9. Raine-Fenning N, Jayaprakasan K, Clewes J, et al. SonoAVC: a novel method of automatic volume calculation. Ultrasound Obstet Gynecol 2008;31(6): 691–6.
10. Merz E, Bahlmann F, Weber G, et al. Three-dimensional ultrasonography in prenatal diagnosis. J Perinat Med 1995;23:213–22.
11. Platt LD, Santulli T Jr, Carlson DE, et al. Three-dimensional ultrasonography in obstetrics and gynecology: preliminary experience. Am J Obstet Gynecol 1998;178:1199–206.
12. Baba K, Okai T, Kozuma S, et al. Fetal abnormalities: evaluation with real-time-processible three-dimensional US—preliminary report. Radiology 1999;211: 441–6.
13. Dyson RL, Pretorius DH, Budorick NE, et al. Three-dimensional ultrasound in the evaluation of fetal anomalies. Ultrasound Obstet Gynecol 2000;16: 321–8.
14. Scharf A, Ghazwiny MF, Steinborn A, et al. Evaluation of two-dimensional versus three-dimensional ultrasound in obstetric diagnostics: a prospective study. Fetal Diagn Ther 2001;16:333–41.
15. Xu HX, Zhang QP, Lu MD, et al. Comparison of two-dimensional and three-dimensional sonography in evaluating fetal malformations. J Clin Ultrasound 2002;30:515–25.
16. Merz E, Welter C. 2D and 3D ultrasound in the evaluation of normal and abnormal fetal anatomy in the second and third trimesters in a level III center. Ultraschall Med 2005;26:9–16.
17. Paul C, Krampl E, Skentou C, et al. Measurement of fetal nuchal translucency thickness by three-dimensional ultrasound. Ultrasound Obstet Gynecol 2001; 18(5):481–4.
18. Kozuma S, Baba K, Okai T, et al. Dynamic observation of the fetal face by three-dimensional ultrasound. Ultrasound Obstet Gynecol 1999;13: 283–4.
19. Kuno A, Akiyama M, Yamashiro C, et al. Three-dimensional sonographic assessment of fetal behavior in the early second trimester of pregnancy. J Ultrasound Med 2001;20:1271–5.
20. Campbell S. 4D, or not 4D: that is the question. Ultrasound Obstet Gynecol 2002;19:1–4.
21. Merz E, Weber G, Bahlmann F, et al. Application of transvaginal and abdominal threedimensional ultrasound for the detection or exclusion of malformations of the fetal face. Ultrasound Obstet Gynecol 1997;9:237–43.
22. Pretorius DH, Nelson TR. Fetal face visualization using three-dimensional ultrasonography. J Ultrasound Med 1995;14:349–56.
23. Lee W, Kirk JS, Shaheen KW, et al. Fetal cleft lip and palate detection by three-dimensional

ultrasonography. Ultrasound Obstet Gynecol 2000; 16:314–20.

24. Kuo HC, Chang FM, Wu CH, et al. The primary application of three-dimensional ultrasonography in obstetrics. Am J Obstet Gynecol 1992;166: 880–6.

25. Mueller GM, Weiner CP, Yankowitz J. Three-dimensional ultrasound in the evaluation of fetal head and spine anomalies. Obstet Gynecol 1996;88: 372–8.

26. Wang PH, Ying TH, Wang PC, et al. Obstetrical three-dimensional ultrasound in the visualization of the intracranial midline and corpus callosum of fetuses with cephalic position. Prenat Diagn 2000; 20:518–20.

27. Ruano R, Benachi A, Joubin L, et al. Three-dimensional ultrasonographic assessment of fetal lung volume as prognostic factor in isolated congenital diaphragmatic hernia. BJOG 2004; 111:423–9.

28. Moeglin D, Talmant C, Duyme M, et al. Fetal lung volumetry using two- and three-dimensional ultrasound. Ultrasound Obstet Gynecol 2005;25: 119–27.

29. Chang CH, Yu CH, Chang FM, et al. Volumetric assessment of normal fetal lungs using three-dimensional ultrasound. Ultrasound Med Biol 2003;29: 935–42.

30. Sabogal JC, Becker E, Bega G, et al. Reproducibility of fetal lung volume measurements with 3-dimensional ultrasonography. J Ultrasound Med 2004;23: 347–52.

31. Krakow D, Williams J III, Poehl M, et al. Use of three-dimensional ultrasound imaging in the diagnosis of prenatal-onset skeletal dysplasias. Ultrasound Obstet Gynecol 2003;21:467–72.

32. Johnson DD, Pretorius DH, Riccabona M, et al. Three-dimensional ultrasound of the fetal spine. Obstet Gynecol 1997;89:434–8.

33. Lee W, Chaiworapongsa T, Romero R, et al. A diagnostic approach for the evaluation of spina bifida by three-dimensional ultrasonography. J Ultrasound Med 2002;21:619–26.

34. Bonilla-Musoles F, Machado LE, Osborne NG, et al. Two- and three-dimensional ultrasound in malformations of the medullary canal: report of four cases. Prenat Diagn 2001;21:622.

35. Gindes L, Pretorius DH, Romine LE, et al. Three-dimensional ultrasonographic depiction of fetal abdominal blood vessels. J Ultrasound Med 2009; 28(8):977–88.

36. Ghate SV, Crockett MM, Boyd BK, et al. Sonohysterography: do 3D reconstructed images provide additional value? AJR Am J Roentgenol 2008;190: W227–33.

37. Campani R, Bottinelli O, Calliada F, et al. The latest in ultrasound: three-dimensional imaging.

Part II [review]. Eur J Radiol 1998;27(Suppl 2): S183–7.

38. Yoon HJ, Kim PN, Kim AY, et al. Three-dimensional sonographic evaluation of gallbladder contractility: comparison with cholescintigraphy. J Clin Ultrasound 2006;34(3):123–7.

39. Badea R, Socaciu M, Lupşor M, et al. Evaluating the liver tumors using three-dimensional ultrasonography. A pictorial essay [review]. J Gastrointestin Liver Dis 2007;16(1):85–92.

40. Riccabona M, Fritz GA, Schöllnast H, et al. Hydronephrotic kidney: pediatric three-dimensional US for relative renal size assessment–initial experience. Radiology 2005;236(1):276–83.

41. Fernandez LJ, Aguilar A, Pardi S. Three-dimensional ultrasound in small parts: Is it just a nice picture? Ultrasound Q 2004;20(3):119–25.

42. Lyshchik A, Drozd V, Reiners C. Accuracy of three-dimensional ultrasound for thyroid volume measurement in children and adolescents. Thyroid 2004; 14(2):113–20.

43. Elwagdy S, Razmy S, Ghoneim S, et al. Diagnostic performance of three-dimensional ultrasound extended imaging at scrotal mass lesions. Int J Urol 2007;14(11):1025–33.

44. Elwagdy S, Ghoneim S, Moussa S, et al. Three-dimensional ultrasound (3D US) methods in the evaluation of calcular and non-calcular ureteric obstructive uropathy. World J Urol 2008;26(3): 263–74.

45. Hünerbein M, Raschke M, Khodadadyan C, et al. Three-dimensional ultrasonography of bone and soft tissue lesions. Eur J Ultrasound 2001;13(1): 17–23.

46. Wallny TA, Theuerkauf I, Schild RL, et al. The three-dimensional ultrasound evaluation of the rotator cuff–an experimental study. Eur J Ultrasound 2000; 11(2):135–41.

47. Riccabona M, Nelson TR, Pretorius DH, et al. In vivo three-dimensional sonographic measurement of organ volume: validation in the urinary bladder. J Ultrasound Med 1996;15:627–32.

48. Riccabona M, Nelson TR, Pretorius DH. Three-dimensional ultrasound: accuracy of distance and volume measurements. Ultrasound Obstet Gynecol 1996;7:429–34.

49. Suwanrath C, Suntharasaj T, Sirapatanapipat H, et al. Three-dimensional ultrasonographic bladder volume measurement: reliability of the virtual organ computer-aided analysis technique using different rotation steps. J Ultrasound Med 2009;28(7): 847–54.

50. Nelson TR, Pretorius DH, Lev-Toaff A, et al. Feasibility of performing a virtual patient examination using three-dimensional ultrasonographic data acquired at remote locations. J Ultrasound Med 2001;20(9):941–52.

51. Bromley B, Shipp TD, Benacerraf B. Assessment of the third-trimester fetus using 3-dimensional volumes: a pilot study. J Clin Ultrasound 2007; 35(5):231–7.

52. Benacerraf BR, Shipp TD, Bromley B. Three-dimensional US of the fetus: volume imaging. Radiology 2006;238(3):988–96.

53. Benacerraf BR, Shipp TD, Bromley B. Improving the efficiency of gynecologic sonography with 3-dimensional volumes: a pilot study. J Ultrasound Med 2006;25(2):165–71.

54. Hagel J, Bicknell SG. Impact of 3D sonography on workroom time efficiency. AJR Am J Roentgenol 2007;188(4):966–9.

55. Wilson SR, Gupta C, Eliasziw M, et al. Volume imaging in the abdomen with ultrasound: How we do it. AJR Am J Roentgenol 2009;193(1): 79–85.

High-Intensity Focused Ultrasound (HIFU) Therapy Applications

Vikram S. Dogra, MD[a],*, Man Zhang, MD, PhD[b], Shweta Bhatt, MD[a]

KEYWORDS

- High-intensity focused ultrasound • Therapy • HIFU
- Ultrasound • Tumor

The development of the modern ultrasound transducer dates back to 1880, when Jacques and Pierre Curie discovered the piezoelectric effect. In the early 1900s, Paul Langevin and colleagues used the piezoelectric properties of quartz crystal to build the first ultrasound transducer as submarine sonar. Several years later, Wood and Loomis reported the biologic effects of high-intensity ultrasound, leading to the exploration of therapeutic ultrasound. Those early studies on the use of ultrasound in medicine were summarized.[1,2]

The initial applications of high-intensity focused ultrasound (HIFU) on biologic tissues were proposed.[3] From the 1950s to 1970s, HIFU was used as a therapeutic modality to treat the diseases of the central nervous system.[4–18] In particular, Fry[19] designed and tested the first HIFU system for the treatment of neurologic disorders including Parkinson's disease. Although some progress had been achieved by optimizing the parameters of the ultrasound source, it was still difficult to achieve a precise tissue ablation in Parkinson's disease.

In 1956, Burov[20] suggested using high-intensity ultrasound to treat malignant tumors, and the bioeffects and specific properties of focused ultrasound on tissues were investigated in further studies.[21–25] Researchers also applied HIFU to treat tumors in animals and further improved the capability of HIFU to ablate tumors.[26,27] These experiments successfully demonstrated complete tumor destruction and shrinkage in the size of tumor.

Another early application was for the treatment of ocular diseases. As early as 1938, Zeiss[28] demonstrated that in vitro cataracts could be induced by ultrasound. Lavine and colleagues[29] described focused ultrasound beams that might induce cataract. Studies using focused ultrasound to treat the retina, ciliary body, crystalline lens, and choroid plexus followed. In 1958, Baum and colleagues[30] showed that an ultrasound beam can disperse the ocular blood. During the 1960s and 1970s, Purnell and colleagues[31–33] established early HIFU results for both cataract development and potential chorioretinal lesion treatment. Coleman and colleagues[34–36] produced cataracts in rabbit lenses, showing the consistency of their sizes and shapes and a thermal mechanism. They also obtained the first threshold curves for chorioretinal lesions in albino rabbit eyes in vivo for the retinal detachment treatment. In the 1980s, a series of animal experiments were performed to explore the treatment of simulated ocular disorders, and a device was set up for the treatment of glaucoma and ocular tumors.[37–40] They set up a device for

[a] Department of Imaging Sciences, University of Rochester Medical Center, 601 Elmwood Avenue, PO Box 648, Rochester, NY 14692, USA
[b] Department of Radiology, University of Michigan Health System, 3232 Medical Sciences Building I, 1301 Catherine Street, Ann Arbor, MI 48109, USA
* Corresponding author.
E-mail address: vikram_dogra@urmc.rochester

Ultrasound Clin 4 (2009) 307–321
doi:10.1016/j.cult.2009.10.005
1556-858X/09/$ – see front matter © 2009 Elsevier Inc. All rights reserved.

the treatment of glaucoma and ocular tumors. The clinical trials found that an efficiency rate of 79.3% was achieved for the treatment of glaucoma with ultrasound at 1-year follow-up. The successful large-scale clinical studies (>1000 patients involved) led to approval by the Food and Drug Administration (FDA) of the first HIFU clinical system: Sonocare CST-100 by Sonocare Inc.

Although the earlier results of HIFU studies were promising, its potential for clinical use had not been established until a recent development in advanced medical imaging technology. In the past 2 decades, applications of HIFU have been widely investigated, in both research and clinical practice, for the treatment of benign and malignant tumors, hemostasis, uterine fibroids, wound healing, and so forth.

PRINCIPLE OF HIGH-INTENSITY FOCUSED ULTRASOUND
What is High-Intensity Focused Ultrasound?

HIFU refers to a technique wherein HIFU beams are emitted from a high-powered transducer that can noninvasively target a tissue volume inside the body without affecting the intervening and surrounding tissue. HIFU causes an increased temperature within the focal volume, resulting in tissue coagulative necrosis.

Mechanism of Action

Two principle mechanisms, hyperthermia and acoustic cavitation, are responsible for the tissue destruction. Because human tissues have viscoelastic characteristics, the acoustic energy is lost and converted to heat. As a result, tissue temperature increases rapidly above 80°C in the focal region, resulting in the protein denaturization (>43°C) and the formation of a necrotic lesion with a sharp demarcation. Compared with hyperthermia, acoustic cavitation is more complex and unpredictable. It appears to cause cell necrosis via nonlinear high-amplitude pressure oscillations by which gas bubbles are generated and oscillate or collapse rapidly, resulting in tissue destruction and localized heat. However, recent studies show the attractive prospect of using acoustic cavitation to enhance the level of HIFU ablation and reduce its exposure times. If the cavitation process can be controlled, it could feasibly avoid any problems occurring with near-field heating.[41]

Advantages and Limitations of High-Intensity Focused Ultrasound

HIFU treatment has some distinct advantages over other thermal ablation techniques such as cryotherapy, laser ablation, microwave coagulation, and radiofrequency (RF) ablation. It is noninvasive and nonionizing, which means it can be repeated as desired because it has no long-term cumulative effects. It increases tissue temperature in the focal area up to 60°C and as high as 100°C in seconds, which is sufficient to induce thermal coagulation while minimizing blood perfusion effects. The energy can also be focused precisely on tissue volumes as small as 20 mm^3 without damaging the intervening or surrounding tissue. The desired size and shape of a larger HIFU target can be achieved by multiple sonications combining individual lesions in a matrix format.

However, potential limitations to the clinical application of HIFU still exist. Currently, HIFU is conducted under anesthesia, which may be hazardous to some patients with serious conditions. Another disadvantage is the long treatment time, mostly because of the large volume of a tumor. But with improvement in HIFU techniques, the time will possibly be shortened to satisfy the desired value. In some cases, patients complain about local pain after HIFU therapy, although this is not very common. Finally, owing to the restrictions of ultrasound interacting with human tissues such as lung and bone, HIFU cannot be clinically implemented in these areas in the body.

SET-UP OF HIGH-INTENSITY FOCUSED ULTRASOUND TREATMENT
High-Intensity Focused Ultrasound Parameters and Applications

A typical HIFU system consists of a signal generator, a power amplifier, a 3-dimensional positioning system, and a therapeutic transducer (**Fig. 1**). The signal generator controls the frequency and initial amplitude of the input signal, which is amplified using the power amplifier. The amplified signals are transmitted to the HIFU transducer to generate the desired ultrasound beam. HIFU transducers can be spherical-shaped transducers or phased arrays. They are constructed to converge ultrasound beams and deposit maximum acoustic energy into the focal millimeter-sized volume. HIFU systems commonly operate in the frequency range of 1 to 5 MHz, generating focal intensities in the range of 1000 to 10,000 W/cm^2. Such rapid (<3 seconds) and high-level intensities can result in cell destruction, protein denaturization, and coagulation necrosis. Under the parameters mentioned previously, individual necrotic lesions, developed in the direction of the ultrasound beam, are ellipsoidal in shape with an extension about three-fourths in front of

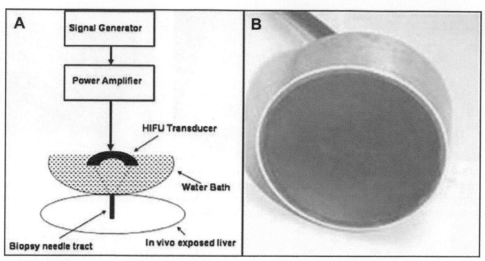

Fig. 1. (A) Schematic diagram depicting the HIFU experimental setup for the hemostasis study. (B) The HIFU transducer has a focal length of 5 cm, a diameter of 42 mm, an F number of 1.2 (focal length/diameter), and a center of frequency of 4.23 MHz. HIFU pulses of 10- to 75-second duration were generated in the experiment. (*From* Deng CX, Dogra V, Exner AA, et al. A feasibility study of high intensity focused ultrasound for liver biopsy hemostasis. Ultrasound Med Biol 2004;30:1531–37.)

the focus and one-fourth behind. Focal dimensions are determined by the geometry of the transducer (aperture and focal length) and its operating frequency, and are somewhat dependent on the tissue type and local structures. For the treatment of large volumes, multiple exposures with repositioning of the HIFU transducer are required to cover the whole region. Between each successive exposure, an interval of 30 to 60 seconds is necessary to avoid overdose damage to normal tissues. Further studies on treatment plans and dosimetry to optimize HIFU therapy are ongoing.

Imaging Modalities for High-Intensity Focused Ultrasound Guidance and Monitoring

In recent years, the potential of HIFU for clinical use has been enhanced greatly by combining HIFU treatment with advanced imaging modalities. Imaging guidance allows accurate HIFU dose delivery to the target tissue with minimal damage to the surrounding normal tissue, while monitoring evaluates the tissue response to the HIFU dose to determine the need for follow-up or further treatment. Methods in current clinical use and under investigation include magnetic resonance imaging (MRI), ultrasound, and elasticity imaging. The excellent soft-tissue resolution afforded by MRI enables accurate planning of the tissue to be targeted. MRI parameters have an intrinsic sensitivity

to temperature change and therefore can be adapted to provide accurate, near real-time thermometry, and thermal damage caused by focused ultrasound therapy and can be assessed immediately using MRI.[42] MRI provides better tissue discrimination and image quality, but is expensive and patient selective. The MRI-guided focused ultrasound therapy system ExAblate 2000 (InSightec) fully integrates with a 1.5-T MRI system (Signa, GE Health care) to enable focused ultrasound therapy to be planned directly with MR images and to give real-time MR thermometry feedback of each sonication.

Ultrasound imaging has also been implemented to guide and monitor the treatment. In clinical practice, the therapeutic system is integrated with the imaging system so that the target region can always be visualized on the diagnostic image.[43–45] Ultrasound imaging can be real-time when it is synchronized with bursts of HIFU. The advantage is lower cost and shorter treatment duration, but the image quality is not as good as that of MRI. Because tissue elasticity provides additional diagnostic information to conventional ultrasound imaging, elasticity imaging has undergone significant development for monitoring HIFU treatment. New elastography techniques (**Figs. 2 and 3**) include real-time sonoelastography imaging developed,[46] elastographic visualization of HIFU lesions proposed by Ophir's group,[47–49]

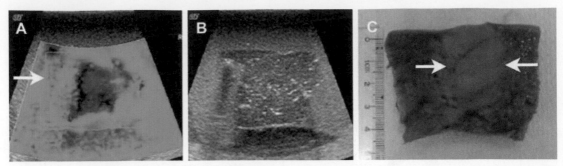

Fig. 2. (*A*) Sonoelastography and (*B*) B-scan images of an HIFU lesion verified by (*C*) gross pathology (*arrows*). The yellow outline (*arrows*) on the sonoelastography image is the profile of the liver sample obtained from the B-mode ultrasound image. The HIFU lesion is isoechoic in the B-Scan image, but the pathology result validates the lesion that is clearly demarcated by sonoelastography imaging.

acoustic radiation force monitoring,[50] and supersonic shear imaging.[51]

INVESTIGATIONS AND CLINICAL APPLICATIONS OF HIGH-INTENSITY FOCUSED ULTRASOUND
Tumor Treatment

HIFU has been promoted as a noninvasive method of treating benign and malignant tumors in human tissues such as liver, prostate, breast, kidney, and so forth. In these applications, focal high intensities are used to generate tumor tissue necrosis.

Liver
Each year, more than 2 million cases of primary and secondary liver cancer are diagnosed in the world. Only a few of them can be removed surgically. Even after surgery, the 5-year survival rates are fairly low. For this reason, HIFU is increasingly under investigation as an alternate to surgical treatment. Early studies in the 1980s established the essential HIFU exposure parameters for liver tissue destruction.[27] A number of liver tumor models were then used to explore the HIFU effects on liver cancer before human clinical trials.[52–56] Recently, Wu and colleagues[57] reported that a total of 474 patients with hepatocellular carcinoma (HCC) were treated with ultrasound-guided HIFU ablation. The tumor size ranged from 4 to 14 cm in diameter. Histologic changes, such as homogeneous coagulative necrosis in the treated region and a sharp margin between the destructed tissue and viable tissue were found 1 to 2 weeks after the HIFU treatment. Severe destruction of tumor blood vessels was observed using follow-up Doppler ultrasound and single-photon emission computed tomography (SPECT). MRI results at 1 to 2 weeks post-HIFU showed a reduction in contrast uptake in HIFU-treated regions whose volume shrank by 20% to 50% at 6 to 12 months.

More recently, in another HIFU study of HCC, 50 patients were treated, 26 with transarterial chemoembolization (TACE) alone (Group 1) and 24 with

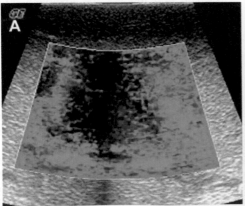
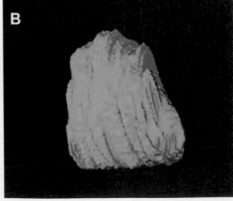

Fig. 3. (*A*) Two-dimensional sono image of a compound HIFU lesion. (*B*) Three-dimensional lesion reconstruction.

Table 1
Results of a HIFU study of HCC, 50 patients were treated, 26 with transarterial chemoembolisation (TACE) alone (Group 1) and 24 with TACE and HIFU (Group 2)[58]

Tumor Reduction After Treatment	1 mo %	3 mo %	6 mo %	12 mo %
Group 1	4.8	7.7	10	0 (<.01)
Group 2	28.6	35	50	50

TACE and HIFU (Group 2).[58] **Table 1** shows the results indicating that the combination of HIFU ablation and TACE is a promising approach in patients with advanced-stage HCC, but large-scale randomized clinical trials are necessary for confirmation. In this clinical trial, investigators used an ultrasound-guided HIFU therapeutic system designed by Chongqing Haifu (HIFU) Tech Co, Ltd, China. This device uses a 12-cm diameter piezoelectric ceramic transducer PZT-4 with a focal length of 9 to 16 cm and an operating frequency of 0.8 to 3.2 MHz. It also has a built-in 3.5- to 5.0-MHz diagnostic scanner for guidance and monitoring. In China, it has been used for HIFU treatment of liver cancer, breast cancer, osteosarcoma, and other solid malignancies.[57,59] In Oxford, United Kingdom, the same HIFU system has been investigated in clinical trials since November 2002.[60–62] Currently, phase I clinical trials of HIFU treatment of liver cancer have been completed at the Royal Marsden Hospital, England, and phase II trials are in process.

Prostate
Since the 1990s, HIFU has been investigated to treat benign prostate hyperplasia (BPH) and prostate cancer. Several groups have conducted the early feasibility studies on HIFU ablation of prostate tissue. In those studies, they used either a transrectal probe with dual capability of imaging and therapy[63,64] or a HIFU transducer combined with ultrasound scanner.[65] Subsequently, clinical phase I/II trials with a large number of BPH patients were accomplished in multiple sites, most of which used the commercial Sonablate HIFU device. The common findings include an increase of maximum urinary flow rate (Q_{max}), a drop of International Prostate Symptom Scores (IPSS), an improvement in quality of life (QOL), and prostate shrinkage in the year following HIFU treatment, although these changes were moderate.[66–72] One long-term study[73] indicated that 43.8% of patients underwent transurethral resection of the prostate (TURP) within a 4-year follow-up, and HIFU would not be considered an alternative to TURP until further assessment.[74,75]

A review of HIFU in the treatment of BPH was also provided by Hegarty and Fitzpatrick.[76]

In 1992, preliminary results of in vivo effects of HIFU on prostate carcinoma in rats were published, which suggested the use of HIFU for the treatment of small localized prostate malignant tumors.[77] Later on, Madersbacher and colleagues[78] first investigated the potential of HIFU therapy on prostate cancer. Several phase I/II clinical trials along with follow-up results were reported thereafter.[79–92] Two transrectal devices, HIFU Sonablate 500 (Focal Surgery, Milpitas, CA) and Ablatherm HIFU (Technomed International, Lyon, France), were used in most of the aforementioned studies.

The probes of HIFU Sonablate 500 have focal lengths varying from 2.5 to 4.5 cm, operating at 4 MHz for both imaging and therapy. This device produces multiple slices of prostate for treatment planning slice by slice, and images are shown before and during treatment, monitored by a doctor. It has been approved for prostate cancer treatment in Canada, Europe, and Mexico. Sanghvi[69] reviewed the 5-year experience of the treatment of prostate cancer by using the Sonoblate 500 in global multi-center study. Based on the clinical study inclusion criteria of (1) stage T1-2N0M0, (2) prostate volume less than 50 mL, (3) no large calcification in the prostate, and (4) no anal stricture, a total of 302 patients were enrolled in the study from January 1999 to April 2004. The relationship between biomedical disease-free survival rates and preoperative PSA was 81% for PSA less than 10, 74% for PSA between 10 and 20, and 16% for PSA greater than 20 ng/mL. The average operation time for the outpatient procedure using epidural anesthesia is 2 hours and 18 minutes. The limitation of this machine is that it is ineffective in prostates greater than 50 mL in volume.

Ablatherm is approved in Europe, Canada, Russia, and South Korea. It uses a built-in 7.5-MHz imaging probe and a treatment transducer with 4-cm focal length, operated at 2.25 to 3.00 MHz. A recent study using Ablatherm[93] showed that 93.4% of patients had negative biopsies and 87% had stable PSA levels (<1.0) at 5 years after treatment. The long-term follow-up studies are continuing in Europe.

A technology review was undertaken to guide patients and physicians as to its suitability,[94] which reveals that the mean follow-up for most prostate studies is 2 years. Complications include impotence rates of 44% to 61%, urethral strictures (rectal fistulae 0.7% to 3.2%), and grade 2 to 3 incontinence 0% to 14%. There are no randomized studies. The quality of evidence is poor. Efficacy outcomes cannot be concluded. A number of other reviews were given.[95–97] New investigations include phased-array transrectal probe design for improvement of the performance of prostate treatment[98] and an extracorporeal treatment system that has now been built up for clinical trials.[99]

Breast

Hynynen and colleagues[100] developed a clinical HIFU technique guided and monitored by MRI. Recently, they reported the results of HIFU treatment of 11 breast fibroadenomas in nine patients.[101] MRI showed that eight lesions were ablated successfully. Huber and colleagues[102] published the first focused ultrasound study on breast cancer treatment. They concluded that this MRI-guided therapy may become a new strategy for treatment in selected patients with breast cancer. Recently, Gianfelice and colleagues[103] published their promising findings on the MRI-guided HIFU treatment of 12 patients with small breast cancer tumors (<3.5 cm). Three patients were treated with the InSightec-TxSonics Mark 1 system (Insightec-TxSonics, Dallas, TX) and nine with the InSightec-TxSonics Mark 2 system. A mean of 46.7% tumor was within the targeted zone and a mean of 43.3% of the cancerous tissue was ablated in the first group; these values were 95.6% and 88.3% in the second group, respectively. Results from a phase I study using ExAblate 2000 (InSightec Ltd, Haifa, Israel) in Israel was just published, and more studies are still on going.[104] Considering the largest number of patients studied to date, 106 patients with breast cancer and 28 patients with benign breast tumors underwent extracorporeal HIFU ablation using the Chongqing HIFU system in China.[57] At a 1- to 2-year follow-up, it was observed that half of the patients had the total resorption of their ablated tumor, but longer follow-up is needed before drawing a conclusion. They recently reported comparable treatment results on 22 breast cancer patients, in which the survival rates of 5-year disease-free and recurrence-free patients were 95% and 89%, respectively.[105] Although they concluded that HIFU therapy for breast cancer was safe and feasible, they also pointed out that more clinical trials are necessary to validate this noninvasive method.

Kidney

A number of animal studies have been under way to investigate the efficiency of HIFU treatment for renal tumors.[106–113] Susani and colleagues[114] studied the effect of HIFU ablation on the morphologic change of renal tissue in a phase I trial. Their histologic evidence indicated that thermal lesions were precisely induced in the target regions and HIFU is feasible for renal tumor therapy. Kohrmann[115] studied renal tumors (sized 2.3 cm, 1.4 cm, and 2.8 cm), applying HIFU. Ultrasound pulses were applied at minimum intervals of 15 seconds with pulse duration of 4 seconds. A follow-up MRI showed necrosis in the two lower-pole tumors within 17 and 48 days, respectively. One upper-pole renal tumor was not affected by treatment because of absorption of ultrasound energy by the interposed ribs. At a 6-month follow-up MRI, the two lower-pole tumors had shrunk in size to 8 mm and 11 mm, respectively. In a recent report, 27 patients with advanced renal cell cancer received HIFU therapy, and 9 patients were successfully treated.[57] Clinical trials in Oxford, United Kingdom, were also performed and results supported the conclusion that HIFU treatment of renal tumors in a western population is safe and feasible.[60] Detailed reviews on HIFU therapy of renal cancer and a comprehensive comparison between HIFU and other minimally invasive approaches were given.[116,117]

Bladder

HIFU has also been considered as a potential noninvasive therapy for superficial bladder tumors. Preclinical studies on cultured bladder carcinoma cells and in rats showed the feasibility of HIFU for the treatment of bladder cancers, especially using ultrasound imaging as a guidance.[118–123] Another feasibility study successfully ablated the bladder wall tissue of 25 large white pigs by using HIFU.[124] In the same year, a clinical phase II study was reported,[125] which enrolled 25 patients with a single, low-grade bladder tumor. Seventy-five percent of the patients had a normal bladder ultrasonography and cytoscopy after 1 month. In a 1-year follow-up, 67% did not have recurrence and no tumor invasion or metastasis was found during the next 3 to 21 months. In Japan, researchers also demonstrated in rabbits that the bladder cancer can be destroyed by successive focused high-energy shock waves (HESW).[126–128] Although HIFU was established to treat bladder cancers, it is still a case-based selective technique, and long-term studies are required to confirm its efficacy.[129]

Hemostasis

Preliminary results of HIFU applications for hemostasis have shown that HIFU can occlude blood vessels, stop internal bleeding, and control hemorrhage in arteries. Hynynen and colleagues[130] examined arterial occlusion by HIFU within deep tissues such as kidney. They concluded that complete occlusion of blood flow was achieved, and HIFU has a significant potential for clinical therapies.

Vaezy and colleagues[131] have been systematically investigating the capability of HIFU to control bleeding from parenchymal and vascular injuries. In their animal studies, moderate to profuse bleeding induced by incision or needle puncture in liver, spleen, and blood vessels was stopped completely after about a 1-minute HIFU application, during which real-time B-mode or Doppler ultrasound imaging was integrated with HIFU for targeting and monitoring the therapy.[45,132–137] Their recent studies indicate that HIFU may provide long-term (up to 60 days) safety in liver and splenic hemostasis.[138,139] A current animal study on hemorrhage control in arteries showed that hemostasis was achieved in all 15 HIFU-treated arteries, and that successful long-term (up to 60 days) hemostasis was found without destroying normal blood flow and vessel wall structure in most vessels.[140] In addition, Cornejo and colleagues[141] reported that HIFU was valuable for the treatment of injured solid organs in blunt trauma.

Liver and other organ biopsies are very commonly performed and bleeding is the main complication of the procedure. HIFU can be used to induce coagulation at the biopsy needle entry site on the liver capsule. Ultrasound imaging was used to confirm hemostasis.[142] They found that the HIFU-treated samples (n = 44) showed virtually no blood loss; for the 14-gauge needle (n = 18), the mean blood loss in controls was 1.79 g (range 0.32–4.97 g) and for the 18-gauge needle biopsies (n = 10), the blood loss was 1.22 g (range 0.2–2.8 g). Their preliminary results demonstrated that HIFU-induced thermal coagulation can be used to control post-biopsy hemorrhage. Results are demonstrated in **Figs. 4–7**. More work is needed to demonstrate that this technique is clinically effective.

Other Current Clinical Uses of High-Intensity Focused Ultrasound

Before the clinical implementation many studies demonstrated of HIFU for the treatment of uterine fibroids,[143–145] demonstrated that HIFU effectively reduced the volume of uterine fibroids and had a potential to treat the recurrent uterine leiomyosarcoma in animal models. In parallel,[43,44] developed an ultrasound-guided HIFU device which was evaluated by in vitro phantom, in vivo ergonomic, and animal model testing. Although further safety issues need to be considered, this device shows promise for clinical use. In the past few years, ExAblate 2000 (**Fig. 8**) has been investigated in the clinical phase I/II/III trials in several institutions. It uses MRI for real-time targeting and imaging of uterine fibroids. More than 100 MR-guided focused ultrasound surgeries (MRgFUS) have taken place worldwide. The results confirmed the feasibility and safety of the MRgFUS system.[42,146–148] More importantly, this

A

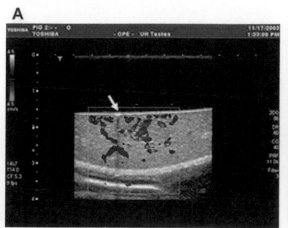

B

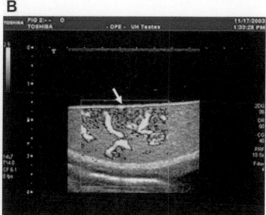

Fig. 4. 14 MHz linear array transducer of a control biopsy site using an 18-gauge needle show the biopsy needle entry site (*arrow*) with blood flow present in and around the biopsy site seen on color flow Doppler (*A*) and power Doppler (*B*). (*Data from* Deng CX, Dogra V, Exner AA, et al. A feasibility study of high intensity focused ultrasound for liver biopsy hemostasis. Ultrasound Med Biol 2004;30:1531–7.)

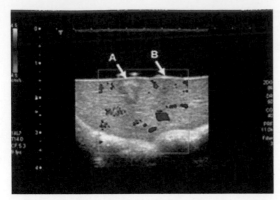

Fig. 5. Color flow Doppler image of HIFU treated biopsy sites (*arrows*, A, 14-gauge needle site; B, 18-gauge needle site). Both sites after HIFU treatment demonstrate absence of color flow and altered echogenicity. (*Data from* Deng CX, Dogra V, Exner AA, et al. A feasibility study of high intensity focused ultrasound for liver biopsy hemostasis. Ultrasound Med Biol 2004;30:1531–7.)

through an intact skull by using large surface area phased arrays.[150–152] These multielement arrays can avoid severe skull heating by distributing energy over a large skull area and then finally being focused on the target tissue. In particular, with the physical skull characteristics derived from modern imaging modalities such as MRI and CT,[151] proposed the phase correction method to overcome the field distortion caused by the bone. Later, Clement and Hynynen[153,154] refined the technique by using a 320-element hemisphere-shaped array on 10 human skulls with the use of CT-image-based phase correction. They also successfully produced HIFU lesions by using a 500-element phase array transducer through a human skull into an in vivo rabbit brain with MRI thermometry. A trans-skull adaptive focusing technique, based on time reversal technology, has been used successfully to achieve necrosis in a sheep brain.[155] Moreover, in a recent study,[156] developed a resonance ultrasound method for noninvasively determining the ultrasound phase shift and restoring the transcranial ultrasound focus. These techniques allow HIFU to be used in many brain applications. At present, the primary practice of HIFU is for cerebral metastasis. The researchers at Brigham and Women's Hospital (BWH) are now collaborating with InSightec to develop an integrated MRgFUS system for brain tumor treatment. Recently, InSightec received FDA approval for a phase I clinical trial at BWH, to evaluate the feasibility of MRgFUS in the noninvasive treatment of the brain tumors. However, the problem in this technique is that it cannot treat superficial tumors close to the skull, and alternative techniques are being sought to solve this problem.

system had a 6-month success rate of 71%, going beyond the trial's goal of 50%, which ultimately led to FDA approval in October 2004. Further trials are warranted for minimizing its side effects. In recent times, Jacobs and colleagues[149] proposed a diffusion-weighted (DW) MRI technique for monitoring the HIFU therapy of uterine fibroids, which also identified the necrotic lesions successfully.

In the brain, because of the strong ultrasound attenuation and distortion caused by the bony skull, noninvasive HIFU treatment is considered difficult to achieve in early studies. Recent research has demonstrated the capability of inducing HIFU into deep-seated brain targets

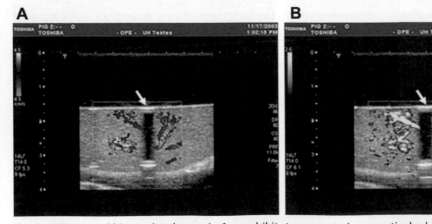

Fig. 6. HIFU-treated biopsy sites (*arrows*) often exhibit strong posterior acoustic shadowing as shown in (*A*) color flow Doppler and (*B*) power Doppler ultrasound images. (*Data from* Deng CX, Dogra V, Exner AA, et al. A feasibility study of high intensity focused ultrasound for liver biopsy hemostasis. Ultrasound Med Biol 2004;30:1531–7.)

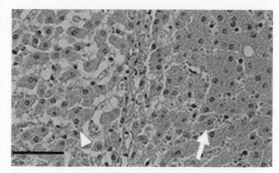

Fig. 7. Liver section stained with hematoxylin and eosin. Light microscopy (×40) demonstrates an area of coagulation necrosis (*arrowhead*) and normal liver parenchyma (*arrow*). There is loss of cellular and nuclear detail in the HIFU-treated liver typical of coagulation necrosis. Disrupted hepatocyte structure (erythrocyte infiltration, disruption of cytoplasmic borders) is also evident. The scale bar in the image is 200 μm in length. (*Data from* Deng CX, Dogra V, Exner AA, et al. A feasibility study of high intensity focused ultrasound for liver biopsy hemostasis. Ultrasound Med Biol 2004;30:1531–7.)

HIFU is also being used for selective ablation in functional disorders. It has been demonstrated that HIFU is capable of selectively opening the blood-brain barrier (BBB) within a targeted region of the brain. An early animal study[157] investigated the threshold of HIFU exposure for increasing the permeability of the BBB. Two mechanisms underlying HIFU-induced cell destruction in brain were also proposed in this study: direct effect by ultrasound and indirect effect by drugs delivered through ultrasound-modified BBB. Mesiwala and colleagues[158] later showed experimental evidence that the HIFU-induced BBB opening was reversible with little tissue damage. Their electron microscopy findings suggested that the possible

mechanism behind this effect was the HIFU-induced disruption of tight junctions between capillary endothelial cells of the BBB. Another method developed by Hynynen and colleagues[159] introduced a contrast agent to this study. MRI was used to monitor the temperature elevation and tissue changes followed by a whole brain histologic evaluation. Their results indicated that at the frequency of 1.63 MHz, the reversible BBB disruption was generated with minimal damage to the surrounding brain tissue. In the subsequent publication, Hynynen and colleagues refined their techniques and demonstrated the ability of focused ultrasound to disrupt the BBB in a frequency range suitable for noninvasive transskull sonications.[160] However, in several cases endothelial damage was observed, which suggests additional investigations are necessary to verify the long-term effects after HIFU exposure in the brain. This noninvasive technique potentially can be used for drug or gene delivery. Currently, a phase I trial is taking place for selective opening of the BBB for local drug delivery. Therefore, the use of HIFU on increasing cell permeability is now gaining more attention.

As early as the 1980s, several preliminary studies claimed that focused ultrasound was able to change the bioelectrical activity of the brain by changing the permeability of neuronal membranes.[161,162] This effect was further verified by studies on cultured cell lines and animals.[163–165] It indicated that HIFU could help cell uptake of cytotoxic drugs and somewhat overcome multidrug resistance (MDR) of tumor cells.[165] HIFU seemed to be a valuable technique facilitating drug delivery to tumor tissue.[164] The current trend is to use focused ultrasound to produce acoustic cavitation. By now the combination has shown outcomes comparable to

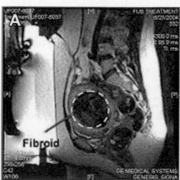
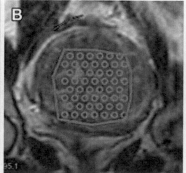
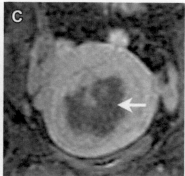

Fig. 8. MRI-guided focused ultrasound (MRgFUS) using the ExAblate 2000 (*A*) demonstrates pretherapy imaging of the uterine fibroid, (*B*) shows the area covered by the HIFU beam, and (*C*) demonstrates gadolinium-enhanced T1-weighted magnetic resonance image with lesion with no enhancement (*arrow*) corresponding to HIFU-treated uterine fibroid.

the abovementioned results.[166–170] Sheikov and colleagues[170] reported four possible mechanisms as (1) transcytosis; (2) endothelial cell cytoplasmic openings; (3) tight junction openings; and (4) free pathway through injured endothelium.

Ultrasound-guided HIFU has been investigated in the eye to treat refractory glaucoma (Sonocare, FDA approved, 1988), ocular tumors, incipient cataracts, retinal detachment or reattachment, vitreous hemorrhage, and to reshape the cornea. Moreover, after a successful study on the treatment of ocular tumors in an animal model[171] used HIFU clinically to treat choroidal melanoma, and such studies are still ongoing.

HIFU is also FDA approved for bone fracture healing, including Collie's and tibial fractures. The use of HIFU has already been broadened to the modification of cardiac tissue structure and function, pain relief, and even cosmetic surgery.

SUMMARY

The research examined in this review has yielded many important noninvasive HIFU therapies for the treatment of biologic tissue. The potential for clinical use of HIFU has expanded because of advances in medical imaging technology. For example, Lizzi and colleagues[35,36] started HIFU eye applications in the late 1970s, which led to research and development of more advanced applications for the treatment of glaucoma, ocular tumors, incipient cataracts, retinal detachment or reattachment, vitreous hemorrhage, and cornea reshaping. Building upon Lizzi's early studies of the eye, researchers have continued to refine and improve HIFU therapy techniques to the point that they can even be used for brain applications. Additional work needs to be done as HIFU research broadens into other important areas such as wound healing and cardiac tissue modification.

REFERENCES

1. Lele PP. Application of ultrasound in medicine. N Engl J Med 1972;286(24):1317–8.
2. Kremkau FW. Cancer therapy with ultrasound: a historical review. J Clin Ultrasound 1979;7(4): 287–300.
3. Lynn JG, Zwemer RL, Chick AJ. The biological application of focused ultrasonic waves. Science 1942;96(2483):119–20.
4. Ballantine HT Jr, Bell E, Manlapaz J. Progress and problems in the neurological applications of focused ultrasound. J Neurosurg 1960;17:858–76.
5. Ballantine HT Jr, Hueter TF, Nauta WJ, et al. Focal destruction of nervous tissue by focused ultrasound: biophysical factors influencing its application. J Exp Med 1956;104(3):337–60.
6. Barnard JW, Fry WJ, Fry FJ, et al. Effects of high intensity ultrasound on the central nervous system of the cat. J Comp Neurol 1955;103(3): 459–84.
7. Fry FJ, Ades HW, Fry WJ. Production of reversible changes in the central nervous system by ultrasound. Science 1958;127(3289):83–4.
8. Fry WJ. Intense ultrasound: a new tool for neurological research. J Ment Sci 1954;100(418):85–96.
9. Fry WJ. Use of intense ultrasound in neurological research. Am J Phys Med 1958;37(3):143–7.
10. Fry WJ. Intense ultrasound in investigations of the central nervous system. Adv Biol Med Phys 1958; 6:281–348.
11. Fry WJ, Barnard JW, Fry EJ, et al. Ultrasonic lesions in the mammalian central nervous system. Science 1955;122(3168):517–8.
12. Fry WJ, Barnard JW, Fry FJ, et al. Ultrasonically produced localized selective lesions in the central nervous system. Am J Phys Med 1955;34(3): 413–23.
13. Fry WJ, Mosberg WH Jr, Barnard JW, et al. Production of focal destructive lesions in the central nervous system with ultrasound. J Neurosurg 1954;11(5):471–8.
14. Lele PP. A simple method for production of trackless focal lesions with focused ultrasound: physical factors. J Physiol 1962;160:494–512.
15. Lele PP. Concurrent detection of the production of ultrasonic lesions. Med Biol Eng 1966;4(5):451–6.
16. Lele PP. Production of deep focal lesions by focused ultrasound—current status. Ultrasonics 1967;5:105–12.
17. Wall PD, Fry FJ, Stephens R, et al. Changes produced in the central nervous system by ultrasound. Science 1951;114(2974):686–7.
18. Warwick R, Pond J. Trackless lesions in nervous tissues produced by high intensity focused ultrasound (high-frequency mechanical waves). J Anat 1968;102(Pt 3):387–405.
19. Fry FJ. Precision high intensity focusing ultrasonic machines for surgery. Am J Phys Med 1958; 37(3):152–6.
20. Burov AK. High-intensity ultrasonic vibrations for action on animal and human malignant tumours. Dokl Akad Nauk SSSR 1956;106:239–41.
21. Bamber JC, Hill CR. Ultrasonic attenuation and propagation speed in mammalian tissues as a function of temperature. Ultrasound Med Biol 1979; 5(2):149–57.
22. Chivers RC, Hill CR. Ultrasonic attenuation in human tissue. Ultrasound Med Biol 1975;2(1): 25–9.
23. Frizzell LA. Threshold dosages for damage to mammalian liver by high intensity focused

ultrasound. IEEE Trans Ultrason Ferroelectr Freq Control 1988;35(5):578–81.

24. Goss SA, Frizzell LA, Dunn F. Ultrasonic absorption and attenuation in mammalian tissues. Ultrasound Med Biol 1979;5(2):181–6.

25. Parker KJ. Ultrasonic attenuation and absorption in liver tissue. Ultrasound Med Biol 1983;9(4): 363–9.

26. Fry FJ, Johnson LK. Tumor irradiation with intense ultrasound. Ultrasound Med Biol 1978;4(4): 337–41.

27. ter Haar G, Sinnett D, Rivens I. High intensity focused ultrasound—a surgical technique for the treatment of discrete liver tumours. Phys Med Biol 1989;34(11):1743–50.

28. Zeiss E. Uber Linsenueranderungen An Heraus Genommenen Rinderlinsen durch Ultra-schallein Wirkung. Arch F Ophth 1938;139:301–22.

29. Lavine O, Langenstrass KH, Bowyer CM, et al. Effects of ultrasonic waves on the refractive media of the eye. AMA Arch Ophthalmol 1952;47(2): 204–19.

30. Baum J, Singer S, Jolesz FA. MR imaging-guided focused ultrasound surgery of fibroadenomas in the breast: a feasibility study. Radiology 2001; 219(1):176–85.

31. Purnell EW. Ultrasonic biometry of the posterior ocular coats. Trans Am Ophthalmol Soc 1980;78: 1027–78.

32. Purnell EW, Sokollu A, Holasek E. The production of focal chorioretinitis by ultrasound. A preliminary report. Am J Ophthalmol 1964;58:953–7.

33. Purnell EW, Sokollu A, Torchia R, et al. Focal chorioretinitis produced by ultrasound. Invest Ophthalmol 1964;3:657–64.

34. Coleman DJ, Lizzi FL, Jakobiec FA. Therapeutic ultrasound in the production of ocular lesions. Am J Ophthalmol 1978;86(2):185–92.

35. Lizzi FL, Coleman DJ, Driller J, et al. Experimental, ultrasonically induced lesions in the retina, choroid, and sclera. Invest Ophthalmol Vis Sci 1978;17(4): 350–60.

36. Lizzi FL, Packer AJ, Coleman DJ. Experimental cataract production by high frequency ultrasound. Ann Ophthalmol 1978;10(7):934–42.

37. Coleman DJ, Lizzi FL, Driller J, et al. Therapeutic ultrasound in the treatment of glaucoma. II. Clinical applications. Ophthalmology 1985;92(3):347–53.

38. Coleman DJ, Lizzi FL, Driller J, et al. Therapeutic ultrasound in the treatment of glaucoma. I. Experimental model. Ophthalmology 1985;92(3):339–46.

39. Coleman DJ, Lizzi FL, Silverman RH, et al. Therapeutic ultrasound. Ultrasound Med Biol 1986; 12(8):633–8.

40. Lizzi FL, Driller J, Ostromogilsky M. Thermal model for ultrasonic treatment of glaucoma. Ultrasound Med Biol 1984;10(3):289–98.

41. Clement GT. Perspectives in clinical uses of high-intensity focused ultrasound. Ultrasonics 2004; 42(10):1087–93.

42. Hindley J, Gedroyc WM, Regan L, et al. MRI guidance of focused ultrasound therapy of uterine fibroids: early results. AJR Am J Roentgenol 2004;183(6):1713–9.

43. Chan AH, Fujimoto VY, Moore DE, et al. In vivo feasibility of image-guided transvaginal focused ultrasound therapy for the treatment of intracavitary fibroids. Fertil Steril 2004;82(3):723–30.

44. Chan AH, Fujimoto VY, Moore DE, et al. An image-guided high intensity focused ultrasound device for uterine fibroids treatment. Med Phys 2002; 29(11):2611–20.

45. Vaezy S, Shi X, Martin RW, et al. Real-time visualization of high-intensity focused ultrasound treatment using ultrasound imaging. Ultrasound Med Biol 2001;27(1):33–42.

46. Parker KJ, Fu D, Graceswki SM, et al. Vibration sonoelastography and the detectability of lesions. Ultrasound Med Biol 1998;24(9):1437–47.

47. Kallel F, Stafford RJ, Price RE, et al. The feasibility of elastographic visualization of HIFU-induced thermal lesions in soft tissues. Image-guided high-intensity focused ultrasound. Ultrasound Med Biol 1999;25(4):641–7.

48. Righetti R, Kallel F, Stafford RJ, et al. Elastographic characterization of HIFU-induced lesions in canine livers. Ultrasound Med Biol 1999;25(7): 1099–113.

49. Souchon R, Rouvière O, Gelet A, et al. Visualisation of HIFU lesions using elastography of the human prostate in vivo: preliminary results. Ultrasound Med Biol 2003;29(7):1007–15.

50. Lizzi FL, Muratore R, Deng CX, et al. Radiation-force technique to monitor lesions during ultrasonic therapy. Ultrasound Med Biol 2003;29(11): 1593–605.

51. Bercoff J, Pernot M, Tanter M, et al. Monitoring thermally-induced lesions with supersonic shear imaging. Ultrason Imaging 2004;26(2):71–84.

52. Cheng SQ, Zhou XD, Tang ZY, et al. High-intensity focused ultrasound in the treatment of experimental liver tumour. J Cancer Res Clin Oncol 1997;123(4):219–23.

53. Prat F, Centarti M, Sibille A, et al. Extracorporeal high-intensity focused ultrasound for VX2 liver tumors in the rabbit. Hepatology 1995;21(3): 832–6.

54. Sibille A, Prat F, Chapelon JY, et al. Extracorporeal ablation of liver tissue by high-intensity focused ultrasound. Oncology 1993;50(5):375–9.

55. Yang R, Reilly CR, Rescorla FJ, et al. High-intensity focused ultrasound in the treatment of experimental liver cancer. Arch Surg 1991;126(8): 1002–9 [discussion: 1009–10].

56. Yang R, Sanghvi NT, Rescorla FJ, et al. Liver cancer ablation with extracorporeal high-intensity focused ultrasound. Eur Urol 1993;23(Suppl 1): 17–22.

57. Wu F, Wang ZB, Chen WZ, et al. Extracorporeal high intensity focused ultrasound ablation in the treatment of 1038 patients with solid carcinomas in China: an overview. Ultrason Sonochem 2004; 11(3–4):149–54.

58. Wu F, Wang ZB, Chen WZ, et al. Advanced hepatocellular carcinoma: treatment with high-intensity focused ultrasound ablation combined with transcatheter arterial embolization. Radiology 2005; 235(2):659–67.

59. Wu F, Chen WZ, Bai J, et al. Pathological changes in human malignant carcinoma treated with high-intensity focused ultrasound. Ultrasound Med Biol 2001;27(8):1099–106.

60. Illing RO, Kennedy JE, Wu F, et al. The safety and feasibility of extracorporeal high-intensity focused ultrasound (HIFU) for the treatment of liver and kidney tumours in a Western population. Br J Cancer 2005;93(8):890–5.

61. Kennedy JE, ter Haar GR, Wu F, et al. Contrast-enhanced ultrasound assessment of tissue response to high-intensity focused ultrasound. Ultrasound Med Biol 2004;30(6):851–4.

62. Kennedy JE, Wu F, ter Haar GR, et al. High-intensity focused ultrasound for the treatment of liver tumours. Ultrasonics 2004;42(1–9):931–5.

63. Bihrle R, Foster RS, Sanghvi NT, et al. High-intensity focused ultrasound in the treatment of prostatic tissue. Urology 1994;43(2 Suppl):21–6.

64. Foster RS, Bihrle R, Sanghvi NT, et al. High-intensity focused ultrasound in the treatment of prostatic disease. Eur Urol 1993;23(Suppl 1): 29–33.

65. Gelet A, Chapelon JY, Margonari J, et al. High-intensity focused ultrasound experimentation on human benign prostatic hypertrophy. Eur Urol 1993;23(Suppl 1):44–7.

66. Ebert T, Graefen M, Miller S, et al. High-intensity focused ultrasound (HIFU) in the treatment of benign prostatic hyperplasia (BPH). Keio J Med 1995;44(4):146–9.

67. Nakamura K, Baba S, Fukazawa R, et al. Treatment of benign prostatic hyperplasia with high intensity focused ultrasound: an initial clinical trial in Japan with magnetic resonance imaging of the treated area. Int J Urol 1995;2(3):176–80.

68. Nakamura K, Baba S, Saito S, et al. High-intensity focused ultrasound energy for benign prostatic hyperplasia: clinical response at 6 months to treatment using Sonablate 200. J Endourol 1997;11(3): 197–201.

69. Sanghvi NT, Foster RS, Bihrle R, et al. Noninvasive surgery of prostate tissue by high intensity focused ultrasound: an updated report. Eur J Ultrasound 1999;9(1):19–29.

70. Sullivan L, Casey RW, Pommerville PJ, et al. Canadian experience with high intensity focused ultrasound for the treatment of BPH. Can J Urol 1999; 6(3):799–805.

71. Uchida T, Muramoto M, Kyunou H, et al. Clinical outcome of high-intensity focused ultrasound for treating benign prostatic hyperplasia: preliminary report. Urology 1998;52(1):66–71.

72. Uchida T, Yokoyama E, Iwamura M, et al. High intensity focused ultrasound for benign prostatic hyperplasia. Int J Urol 1995;2(3):181–5.

73. Madersbacher S, Schatzl G, Djavan B, et al. Long-term outcome of transrectal high-intensity focused ultrasound therapy for benign prostatic hyperplasia. Eur Urol 2000;37(6):687–94.

74. Kour NW. Minimally invasive surgery for benign prostatic hyperplasia—a review. Ann Acad Med Singap 1995;24(4):619–26.

75. Mulligan ED, Lynch TH, Mulvin D, et al. High-intensity focused ultrasound in the treatment of benign prostatic hyperplasia. Br J Urol 1997;79(2):177–80.

76. Hegarty NJ, Fitzpatrick JM. High intensity focused ultrasound in benign prostatic hyperplasia. Eur J Ultrasound 1999;9(1):55–60.

77. Chapelon JY, Margonari J, Vernier F, et al. In vivo effects of high-intensity ultrasound on prostatic adenocarcinoma Dunning R3327. Cancer Res 1992;52(22):6353–7.

78. Madersbacher S, Pedevilla M, Vingers L, et al. Effect of high-intensity focused ultrasound on human prostate cancer in vivo. Cancer Res 1995; 55(15):3346–51.

79. Beerlage HP, Pedevilla M, Vingers L, et al. Transrectal high-intensity focused ultrasound using the Ablatherm device in the treatment of localized prostate carcinoma. Urology 1999;54(2):273–7.

80. Chapelon JY, Ribault M, Vernier F, et al. Treatment of localised prostate cancer with transrectal high intensity focused ultrasound. Eur J Ultrasound 1999;9(1):31–8.

81. Chaussy C, Thuroff S. High-intensity focused ultrasound in prostate cancer: results after 3 years. Mol Urol 2000;4(3):179–82.

82. Chaussy C, Thuroff S. Results and side effects of high-intensity focused ultrasound in localized prostate cancer. J Endourol 2001;15(4):437–40 [discussion: 447–8].

83. Chaussy C, Thuroff S. The status of high-intensity focused ultrasound in the treatment of localized prostate cancer and the impact of a combined resection. Curr Urol Rep 2003;4(3):248–52.

84. Gelet A, Chapelon JY, Bouvier R, et al. Transrectal high-intensity focused ultrasound: minimally invasive therapy of localized prostate cancer. J Endourol 2000;14(6):519–28.

85. Gelet A, Chapelon JY, Bouvier R, et al. Transrectal high intensity focused ultrasound for the treatment of localized prostate cancer: factors influencing the outcome. Eur Urol 2001;40(2):124–9.

86. Gelet A, Chapelon JY, Bouvier R, et al. Treatment of prostate cancer with transrectal focused ultrasound: early clinical experience. Eur Urol 1996; 29(2):174–83.

87. Madersbacher S, Kratzik C, Marberger M. Prostatic tissue ablation by transrectal high intensity focused ultrasound: histological impact and clinical application. Ultrason Sonochem 1997;4(2): 175–9.

88. Rebillard X, Gelet A, Davin JL, et al. Transrectal high-intensity focused ultrasound in the treatment of localized prostate cancer. J Endourol 2005; 19(6):693–701.

89. Thuroff S, Chaussy C, Vallancien G, et al. High-intensity focused ultrasound and localized prostate cancer: efficacy results from the European multicentric study. J Endourol 2003;17(8):673–7.

90. Uchida T. High-intensity focused ultrasound for localized prostate cancer. Nippon Rinsho 2005; 63(2):345–9.

91. Uchida T, Sanghvi NT, Gardner TA, et al. Transrectal high-intensity focused ultrasound for treatment of patients with stage T1b-2n0m0 localized prostate cancer: a preliminary report. Urology 2002; 59(3):394–8 [discussion: 398–9].

92. Vallancien G, Prapotnich D, Cathelineau X, et al. Transrectal focused ultrasound combined with transurethral resection of the prostate for the treatment of localized prostate cancer: feasibility study. J Urol 2004;171(6 Pt 1):2265–7.

93. Blana A, Walter B, Rogenhofer S, et al. High-intensity focused ultrasound for the treatment of localized prostate cancer: 5-year experience. Urology 2004;63(2):297–300.

94. Pickles T, Goldenberg L, Steinhoff G. Technology review: high-intensity focused ultrasound for prostate cancer. Can J Urol 2005;12(2):2593–7.

95. Beerlage HP, Thüroff S, Madersbacher S, et al. Current status of minimally invasive treatment options for localized prostate carcinoma. Eur Urol 2000;37(1):2–13.

96. Colombel M, Gelet A. Principles and results of high-intensity focused ultrasound for localized prostate cancer. Prostate Cancer Prostatic Dis 2004;7(4):289–94.

97. Madersbacher S, Marberger M. High-energy shockwaves and extracorporeal high-intensity focused ultrasound. J Endourol 2003;17(8): 667–72.

98. Saleh KY, Smith NB. A 63 element 1.75 dimensional ultrasound phased array for the treatment of benign prostatic hyperplasia. Biomed Eng Online 2005;4(1):39.

99. Hacker A, Köhrmann KU, Back W, et al. Extracorporeal application of high-intensity focused ultrasound for prostatic tissue ablation. BJU Int 2005; 96(1):71–6.

100. Hynynen K, Freund WR, Cline HS, et al. A clinical, noninvasive, MR imaging-monitored ultrasound surgery method. Radiographics 1996;16(1): 185–95.

101. Hynynen K, Pomeroy O, Smith DN, et al. MR imaging-guided focused ultrasound surgery of fibroadenomas in the breast: a feasibility study. Radiology 2001;219(1):176–85.

102. Huber PE, Jenne JW, Rastert R, et al. A new noninvasive approach in breast cancer therapy using magnetic resonance imaging-guided focused ultrasound surgery. Cancer Res 2001;61(23): 8441–7.

103. Gianfelice D, Khiat A, Amara M, et al. MR imaging-guided focused ultrasound surgery of breast cancer: correlation of dynamic contrast-enhanced MRI with histopathologic findings. Breast Cancer Res Treat 2003;82(2):93–101.

104. Zippel DB, Papa MZ. The use of MR imaging guided focused ultrasound in breast cancer patients: a preliminary phase one study and review. Breast Cancer 2005;12(1):32–8.

105. Wu F, Wang ZB, Zhu H, et al. Extracorporeal high intensity focused ultrasound treatment for patients with breast cancer. Breast Cancer Res Treat 2005;92(1):51–60.

106. Adams JB, Moore RG, Anderson JH, et al. High-intensity focused ultrasound ablation of rabbit kidney tumors. J Endourol 1996;10(1):71–5.

107. Chapelon JY, Margonari J, Theillère Y, et al. Effects of high-energy focused ultrasound on kidney tissue in the rat and the dog. Eur Urol 1992; 22(2):147–52.

108. Damianou C. In vitro and in vivo ablation of porcine renal tissues using high-intensity focused ultrasound. Ultrasound Med Biol 2003;29(9):1321–30.

109. Damianou C. MRI monitoring of the effect of tissue interfaces in the penetration of high intensity focused ultra sound in kidney in vivo. Ultrasound Med Biol 2004;30(9):1209–15.

110. Damianou C, Pavlou M, Velev O, et al. High intensity focused ultrasound ablation of kidney guided by MRI. Ultrasound Med Biol 2004;30(3):397–404.

111. Daum DR, Smith NB, King R, et al. In vivo demonstration of noninvasive thermal surgery of the liver and kidney using an ultrasonic phased array. Ultrasound Med Biol 1999;25(7):1087–98.

112. Frizzell LA, Linke CA, Carstensen EL, et al. Thresholds for focal ultrasonic lesions in rabbit kidney, liver, and testicle. IEEE Trans Biomed Eng 1977; 24(4):393–6.

113. Watkin NA, Morris SB, Rivens IH, et al. High-intensity focused ultrasound ablation of the kidney in

a large animal model. J Endourol 1997;11(3): 191–6.

114. Susani M, Madersbacher S, Kratzik C, et al. Morphology of tissue destruction induced by focused ultrasound. Eur Urol 1993;23(Suppl 1): 34–8.

115. Kohrmann KU, Michel MS, Gaa J, et al. High intensity focused ultrasound as noninvasive therapy for multilocal renal cell carcinoma: case study and review of the literature. J Urol 2002;167(6): 2397–403.

116. Roberts WW. Focused ultrasound ablation of renal and prostate cancer: current technology and future directions. Urol Oncol 2005;23(5):367–71.

117. Trabulsi EJ, Kalra P, Gomella LG. New approaches to the minimally invasive treatment of kidney tumors. Cancer J 2005;11(1):57–63.

118. Chartier-Kastler E, Chopin D, Vallancien G. The effects of focused extracorporeal pyrotherapy on a human bladder tumor cell line (647 V). J Urol 1993;149(3):643–7.

119. Vallancien G, Chartier-Kastler E, Bataille N, et al. Focused extracorporeal pyrotherapy. Eur Urol 1993;23(Suppl 1):48–52.

120. Vallancien G, Chartier-Kastler E, Chopin D, et al. Focussed extracorporeal pyrotherapy: experimental results. Eur Urol 1991;20(3):211–9.

121. Vallancien G, Chopin D, Davila C, et al. Focused extracorporeal pyrotherapy. Initial experimental results. Prog Urol 1991;1(1):149–53.

122. Vallancien G, Veillon B, Charton M, et al. Can transabdominal ultrasonography of the bladder replace cystoscopy in the followup of superficial bladder tumors? J Urol 1986;136(1):32–4.

123. Wang GM, Yang YF, Sun LA, et al. [An experimental study on high intensity focused ultrasound combined with mitomycin treatment of bladder tumor]. Zhonghua Wai Ke Za Zhi 2003;41(12): 897–900 [in Chinese].

124. Watkin NA, Morris SB, Rivens IH, et al. A feasibility study for the non-invasive treatment of superficial bladder tumours with focused ultrasound. Br J Urol 1996;78(5):715–21.

125. Vallancien G, Harouni M, Guillonneau B, et al. Ablation of superficial bladder tumors with focused extracorporeal pyrotherapy. Urology 1996;47(2): 204–7.

126. Hoshi S, Orikasa S, Kuwahara M, et al. Shock wave and THP-adriamycin for treatment of rabbit's bladder cancer. Jpn J Cancer Res 1992;83(3): 248–50.

127. Hoshi S, Orikasa S, Kuwahara M, et al. High energy underwater shock wave treatment on implanted urinary bladder cancer in rabbits. J Urol 1991; 146(2):439–43.

128. Hosi S, Orikasa S, Kuwahara M, et al. The effect of high-energy underwater shock waves on implanted

urinary bladder cancer in rabbits. Jpn J Cancer Res 1990;81(4):317–9.

129. Uchida T, Ohori M, Egawa S. [Minimally invasive therapy for bladder and prostate cancer]. Gan To Kagaku Ryoho 2001;28(8):1094–8 [in Japanese].

130. Hynynen K, Colucci V, Chung A, et al. Noninvasive arterial occlusion using MRI-guided focused ultrasound. Ultrasound Med Biol 1996;22(8):1071–7.

131. Vaezy S, Martin R, Crum L. High intensity focused ultrasound: a method of hemostasis. Echocardiography 2001;18(4):309–15.

132. Martin RW, Vaezy S, Kaczkowski P, et al. Hemostasis of punctured vessels using Doppler-guided high-intensity ultrasound. Ultrasound Med Biol 1999;25(6):985–90.

133. Vaezy S, Marti R, Mourad P, et al. Hemostasis using high intensity focused ultrasound. Eur J Ultrasound 1999;9(1):79–87.

134. Vaezy S, Martin R, Kaczkowski P, et al. Use of high-intensity focused ultrasound to control bleeding. J Vasc Surg 1999;29(3):533–42.

135. Vaezy S, Martin R, Keilman G, et al. Control of splenic bleeding by using high intensity ultrasound. J Trauma 1999;47(3):521–5.

136. Vaezy S, Martin R, Schmiedl U, et al. Liver hemostasis using high-intensity focused ultrasound. Ultrasound Med Biol 1997;23(9):1413–20.

137. Vaezy S, Martin R, Yaziji H, et al. Hemostasis of punctured blood vessels using high-intensity focused ultrasound. Ultrasound Med Biol 1998; 24(6):903–10.

138. Noble ML, Vaezy S, Keshavarzi A, et al. Spleen hemostasis using high-intensity ultrasound: survival and healing. J Trauma 2002;53(6): 1115–20.

139. Vaezy S, Noble ML, Keshavarzi A, et al. Liver hemostasis with high-intensity ultrasound: repair and healing. J Ultrasound Med 2004;23(2):217–25.

140. Zderic V, Keshavarzi A, Noble ML, et al. Hemorrhage control in arteries using high-intensity focused ultrasound: a survival study. Ultrasonics 2006;44(1):46–53.

141. Cornejo CJ, Vaezy S, Jurkovich GJ, et al. High-intensity ultrasound treatment of blunt abdominal solid organ injury: an animal model. J Trauma 2004;57(1):152–6.

142. Deng CX, Dogra V, Exner AA, et al. A feasibility study of high intensity focused ultrasound for liver biopsy hemostasis. Ultrasound Med Biol 2004; 30(11):1531–7.

143. Keshavarzi A, Vaezy S, Noble ML, et al. Treatment of uterine leiomyosarcoma in a xenograft nude mouse model using high-intensity focused ultrasound: a potential treatment modality for recurrent pelvic disease. Gynecol Oncol 2002;86(3):344–50.

144. Keshavarzi A, Vaezy S, Noble ML, et al. Treatment of uterine fibroid tumors in an in situ rat model

using high-intensity focused ultrasound. Fertil Steril 2003;80(Suppl 2):61–7.

145. Vaezy S, Fujimoto VY, Walker C, et al. Treatment of uterine fibroid tumors in a nude mouse model using high-intensity focused ultrasound. Am J Obstet Gynecol 2000;183(1):6–11.

146. Jolesz FA, Hynynen K, McDannold N, et al. MR imaging-controlled focused ultrasound ablation: a noninvasive image-guided surgery. Magn Reson Imaging Clin N Am 2005;13(3):545–60.

147. Stewart EA, Gedroyc WM, Tempany CM, et al. Focused ultrasound treatment of uterine fibroid tumors: safety and feasibility of a noninvasive thermoablative technique. Am J Obstet Gynecol 2003; 189(1):48–54.

148. Tempany CM, Stewart EA, McDannold N, et al. MR imaging-guided focused ultrasound surgery of uterine leiomyomas: a feasibility study. Radiology 2003;226(3):897–905.

149. Jacobs MA, Herskovits EH, Kim HS. Uterine fibroids: diffusion-weighted MR imaging for monitoring therapy with focused ultrasound surgery–preliminary study. Radiology 2005;236(1):196–203.

150. Hynynen K, Jolesz FA. Demonstration of potential noninvasive ultrasound brain therapy through an intact skull. Ultrasound Med Biol 1998;24(2): 275–83.

151. Sun J, Hynynen K. The potential of transskull ultrasound therapy and surgery using the maximum available skull surface area. J Acoust Soc Am 1999;105(4):2519–27.

152. Tanter M, Thomas JL, Fink M. Focusing and steering through absorbing and aberrating layers: application to ultrasonic propagation through the skull. J Acoust Soc Am 1998;103(5 Pt 1):2403–10.

153. Clement GT, Hynynen K. Correlation of ultrasound phase with physical skull properties. Ultrasound Med Biol 2002;28(5):617–24.

154. Clement GT, Hynynen K. A non-invasive method for focusing ultrasound through the human skull. Phys Med Biol 2002;47(8):1219–36.

155. Aubry JF, Tanter M, Pernot M, et al. Experimental demonstration of noninvasive transskull adaptive focusing based on prior computed tomography scans. J Acoust Soc Am 2003;113(1):84–93.

156. Aarnio J, Clement GT, Hynynen K. A new ultrasound method for determining the acoustic phase shifts caused by the skull bone. Ultrasound Med Biol 2005;31(6):771–80.

157. Patrick JT, Nolting MN, Goss SA, et al. Ultrasound and the blood-brain barrier. Adv Exp Med Biol 1990;267:369–81.

158. Mesiwala AH, Farrell L, Wenzel HJ, et al. High-intensity focused ultrasound selectively disrupts the blood-brain barrier in vivo. Ultrasound Med Biol 2002;28(3):389–400.

159. Hynynen K, McDannold N, Vykhodtseva N, et al. Noninvasive MR imaging-guided focal opening of the blood-brain barrier in rabbits. Radiology 2001; 220(3):640–6.

160. Hynynen K, McDannold N, Sheikov NA, et al. Local and reversible blood-brain barrier disruption by noninvasive focused ultrasound at frequencies suitable for trans-skull sonications. Neuroimage 2005;24(1):12–20.

161. Velling VA, Shkliaruk SP. [Modulation of the functional state of the brain using focused ultrasound]. Fiziols Zh SSSR Im I M Sechenova 1987;73(6): 708–14 [in Russian].

162. Velling VA, Shklyaruk SP. Modulation of the functional state of the brain with the aid of focused ultrasonic action. Neurosci Behav Physiol 1988;18(5): 369–75.

163. Bednarski MD, Lee JW, Callstrom MR, et al. In vivo target-specific delivery of macromolecular agents with MR-guided focused ultrasound. Radiology 1997;204(1):263–8.

164. Yuh EL, Shulman SG, Mehta SA, et al. Delivery of systemic chemotherapeutic agent to tumors by using focused ultrasound: study in a murine model. Radiology 2005;234(2):431–7.

165. Zhai BJ, Shao ZY, Wu F, et al. [Reversal of multidrug resistance of human hepatocarcinoma HepG2/Adm cells by high intensity focused ultrasound]. Ai Zheng 2003;22(12):1284–8 [in Chinese].

166. Kinoshita M, Hynynen K. A novel method for the intracellular delivery of siRNA using microbubble-enhanced focused ultrasound. Biochem Biophys Res Commun 2005;335(2):393–9.

167. Miller DL, Pislaru SV, Greenleaf JE. Sonoporation: mechanical DNA delivery by ultrasonic cavitation. Somat Cell Mol Genet 2002;27(1–6):115–34.

168. Rapoport N. Combined cancer therapy by micellar-encapsulated drug and ultrasound. Int J Pharm 2004;277(1–2):155–62.

169. Rapoport NY, Christensen DA, Fain HD, et al. Ultrasound-triggered drug targeting of tumors in vitro and in vivo. Ultrasonics 2004;42(1–9): 943–50.

170. Sheikov N, McDannold N, Vykhodtseva N, et al. Cellular mechanisms of the blood-brain barrier opening induced by ultrasound in presence of microbubbles. Ultrasound Med Biol 2004; 30(7):979–89.

171. Lizzi FL, Deng CX, Lee P, et al. A comparison of ultrasonic beams for thermal treatment of ocular tumors. Eur J Ultrasound 1999;9(1):71–8.

Quasi-Static Ultrasound Elastography

Tomy Varghese, PhD

KEYWORDS

- Elastography • Elasticity • Strain • Young's modulus
- Viscoelastic • Ultrasound • Imaging

Imaging the viscoelastic properties of tissue for diagnosis and treatment has gained popularity over the last decade because of its ability to provide noninvasive and new diagnostic information.[1–29] Elastography has been likened to manual palpation of tissue, used by clinicians for centuries to aid in clinical diagnosis. The clinical popularity of manual palpation is due to the fact that pathologic and stiffness changes in the body are generally well correlated,[30] and irregular and stiffer masses commonly present as warning signs of diseases in organs such as the breast, liver, and prostate. For example, breast scirrhous carcinomas on palpation are felt to be extremely hard nodules,[31,32] while liver tissue with cirrhosis is also known to be significantly stiffer than normal healthy liver tissue.[31] However, manual palpation is generally limited to superficial structures and depends largely on the ability of the physician performing the examination. Stiffer masses located deep in the body almost certainly cannot be detected by surface manual palpation. The biggest advancement in tissue elasticity imaging has come with the advent and advances in "elastography" over the last 2 decades. The motivation for the use of elastographic techniques stems from the existence of large differences in stiffness or modulus contrast between surrounding normal and pathologic tissues that may otherwise possess similar image contrasts with conventional clinical imaging modalities.

The term "Elastography" was coined by Ophir and colleagues,[6] to refer to an ultrasound-based imaging technique whereby local axial strains were estimated by computing the gradient of axial shifts in echo arrival times along the ultrasound beam direction following a quasi-static tissue deformation. Elastography, however, has now become used as a more general term to identify methods that image tissue stiffness using different imaging modalities, for example, ultrasound, magnetic resonance imaging, optical coherence tomography, x-ray computed tomography,[6,26–29] different perturbation techniques to deform tissue,[5,6,15,24,33–36] and based on the elasticity parameter being measured or imaged.[6,37–39] In this review, the author focuses on quasi-static ultrasound-based elastography, since this group of methods form the more commonly used approaches for clinical elasticity imaging.

The practice of quasi-static ultrasound elastography was initially based on the estimation of the axial tissue displacement and strain (corresponding to displacements estimated along both the direction of insonification and tissue deformation) by analyzing ultrasonic radiofrequency echo signals obtained from standard clinical ultrasound diagnostic equipment. Frames of radiofrequency echo-signals acquired before and after a small amount (about 1%) of quasi-static deformation were correlated to estimate differential displacements along small data segments or regions of interest using classic time-delay estimation techniques.[40,41] Finally, the axial strain distribution was computed from the gradient of the time delays or tissue displacements.[6]

This work was funded in part by NIH grants R01 CA112192-02, R21 CA140939-01, and Komen Foundation grant BCTR0601153.

Department of Medical Physics, The University of Wisconsin-Madison, 1159 WIMR, 1111 Highland Avenue, Madison, WI 53706, USA

E-mail address: tvarghese@wisc.edu

Ultrasound Clin 4 (2009) 323–338
doi:10.1016/j.cult.2009.10.009

Algorithms for displacement and strain estimation have progressed from 1-dimensional (1D) tracking of the displacement along the insonification and deformation direction,[6,9,42–46] to 2-dimensional (2D) tracking of the displacement vector within the scan plane,[47–51] to 3-dimensional (3D)[52–54] methods for tracking the complete displacement vector. These methods can also be classified based on whether they use phase information present in the radiofrequency data, namely time-domain cross-correlation,[6,55] phase-tracking techniques,[7] and phase root tracking methods.[24] Estimators that do not use phase information include optical flow-based speckle tracking,[12] analysis of envelope or B-mode signals,[56] power spectral methods,[44,57,58] and methods like sum amplitude or sum-squared difference that mimic cross-correlation.[59,60] Algorithms to reduce signal decorrelation such as temporal stretching[4–7] of the postdeformation signal to align the radiofrequency peaks with the predeformation signal, and multi-compression averaging,[6–9] which reduces signal decorrelation by using small deformations, have been used. Displacement estimates from the multiple small deformations have been accumulated,[8,9] averaged, or compounded[6–9] to improve strain and modulus images. Displacement estimates obtained from multiple angular insonifications have also been averaged to improve the noise properties of the strain images.[61,62] 2D signal processing methods to estimate the displacement vector for data acquired using curvilinear arrays have also been developed,[63] because most of the previous algorithms catered to data acquired using linear arrays.[47–51] Displacement estimation in areas where the tissue continuity assumption does not hold, namely for vascular tissue, have also been developed,[64,65] by processing data using a coarse to a fine approach in multiple estimation stages.[47,49,50] Real-time implementations of strain imaging on both custom[24] and clinical ultrasound scanners,[48] for direct visualization of the strain distribution while scanning the patient, has been reported.

Only the axial-strain distribution (ie, strains along the insonification and deformation) were imaged until recently,[6] while lateral (perpendicular to the beam propagation direction and within the same scan plane) and elevational (perpendicular to the beam propagation direction and scan plane) displacements were usually not estimated. Algorithms have been developed for the estimation of the complete displacement vector and consequently the strain tensor components.[66–68] Because the components of the strain tensor are coupled, accurate estimations of all components are necessary for a complete visualization of the 3D strain distribution incurred in tissue. Lubinski and colleagues[69] computed local lateral displacements from axial displacements assuming tissue incompressibility (Poisson ratio of 0.495). Konofagou and Ophir[66] describe a method that used weighted interpolation between neighboring radiofrequency A-lines in the lateral direction, along with iterative corrections of lateral and axial displacements to estimate displacement vectors. Another method using radiofrequency data acquired along multiple angular insonification directions (using data from a phased array transducer) was described by Techavipoo and colleagues[68] to estimate components of the displacement vector, which was later adapted to linear array transducers with electronic beam steering.[67]

The normal strain tensor components are also essential in the estimation of other important parameters such as the shear strains[67,70,71] and lateral to axial strain ratios (equivalent to the Poisson ratio under specific conditions).[38] Imaging of the shear strain distribution has been used to evaluate lesion mobility, to differentiate between benign masses such as fibroadenomas that are surrounded by a capsule and loosely attached to background normal tissue and malignant masses that are firmly attached to the normal background tissue through infiltration and the accompanying desmoplastic reaction.[72,73] The lateral to axial strain ratio has been used as a marker to characterize poroelastic tissue enabling differentiation, for example, between normal and edematous tissues.[74]

However, the strain tensor distribution does not indicate the absolute elastic properties of tissue, because it is significantly dependent on the applied deformation or stress distribution.[75,76] The additional information with the complete strain tensor distribution can be used to obtain unique solutions for the inverse problem.[37,77] Many investigators have focused on the estimation of the Young modulus in tissue, which if estimated accurately would provides an absolute or quantitative distribution of the underlying tissue elastic properties. However, there are many challenges that have to be addressed for accurate estimation of the Young modulus, including accurate estimation of the stress distribution and the associated boundary conditions.

Techniques to obtain the local stress distribution patterns using force sensor arrays during tissue deformation have been reported.[78] Temporal and spatial maps of the stress distribution have been obtained to evaluate breast masses. The major limitation is the absence of depth-dependent information that is being addressed using analytical and finite element methods to model the stress distribution.

The improvements in the quality of the strain and modulus images have dramatically improved over the last 2 decades. This improvement has led to the commercialization of quasi-static elastography, with 4 manufacturers currently offering strain imaging modes on commercial clinical systems. The following sections lead the reader through a classification of quasi-static elastographic techniques and provide a brief description of the fundamental principles underpinning quasi-static elastography. The review then concludes with a description of the current clinical applications of quasi-static strain and modulus imaging.

CLASSIFICATION OF QUASI-STATIC ELASTOGRAPHY

Elastographic techniques can be broadly classified based on the mechanical stimuli applied to quasi-static and dynamic techniques. Under quasi-static techniques, which are the focus of this article, the approaches can be further classified into 3 categories, namely: (1) steady-state quasi-static excitation,[6–14] (2) steady-state quasi-static low-frequency excitation on the order of 5 to 10 Hz, and (3) imaging of steady-state quasi-static deformations due to physiologic excitation,[34–36] as illustrated in **Fig. 1**. Dynamic methods can also be further classified into approaches that use (1) harmonic excitations on the order of 10 to 1000 Hz,[3–5,23,79] and (2) transient dynamic excitation and subsequent estimation of the transient response.[20–22,80]

Steady-State Quasi-Static Excitation

Techniques that use a steady-state quasi-static excitation of tissue using the ultrasound transducer represent some of the most commonly used perturbation approaches to elastographic imaging. Radiofrequency data are collected before and after a known applied deformation, applied as a single deformation step or as multiple deformation steps.[6,7,9,81] The pre- and postdeformation data are then compared using different algorithms to estimate differential local displacements between the 2 tissue states.[40,41,82,83] Local strains are then estimated from the gradient of the displacement using forward differences or least-square based methods.

Steady-state quasi-static deformations have been applied using either stepper motor control (with the transducer held in a fixture) or freehand compression using the transducer. Approaches in which the deformations are applied using intracavitary probes and ablation electrodes have also been described.[84] Reports on the significant improvement in the strain contrast with electrode displacement when compared with external deformation methods for quasi-static elastography have been presented.[85] In addition, 3D strain imaging[86] and modulus reconstruction (solution of the inverse problem)[87] have also been demonstrated using this approach.

Steady-State Quasi-Static Low-Frequency Excitation

The methods described in this category use low-frequency deformations on the order of 1 to 10 Hz to perturb tissue. Because the deformation frequencies are low, these are considered to be quasi-static in nature, and do not generate appreciable shear waves in tissue. Both well-controlled[24,33] and freehand-based[15] approaches have been described. Hall and colleagues[15] described an approach that coupled real-strain strain imaging (7 frames per second) and visualization with freehand deformations termed "palpation imaging". This approach was implemented initially on the Siemens Elegra, and later on the Antares and the S2000 (Siemens Ultrasound, Seattle, WA, USA), and constitutes one of the earliest commercially available clinical elastography systems on the market.

Steady-State Quasi-Static Physiologic Excitation

Physiologic stimuli due to respiratory,[34] cardiac muscle deformation,[35,36] and cardiovascular sources[9,18,44,88–92] have been used for elastographic imaging. Investigators have used physiologic stimuli to obtain both forward[34–36] and inverse problem[93] solutions for elastography. Physiologic deformation sources, however, introduce challenges due to the nonuniform deformations introduced and the need for gating of the data to obtain reproducible results.

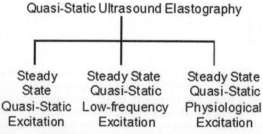

Quasi-Static Ultrasound Elastography

| Steady State Quasi-Static Excitation | Steady State Quasi-Static Low-frequency Excitation | Steady State Quasi-Static Physiological Excitation |

Fig. 1. Classification of quasi-static ultrasound elastography based on the tissue deformation used.

FUNDAMENTAL PRINCIPLES UNDERLYING QUASI-STATIC ELASTOGRAPHY

The success of elastographic imaging is predicated primarily on the several orders of the Young modulus contrast that exist between normal and abnormal tissue types.[1,2,6] This concept is shown as the initial modulus distribution in **Fig. 2**, whose depiction on an image is sought by all the elasticity imaging methods. A singular advantage of techniques based on exploiting these modulus variations is that pathologic changes in tissue generally alter the underlying elasticity of tissue. However, these same pathologic changes may not alter the contrast mechanisms used by conventional imaging modalities.

The practice of elastography can be framed either as the solution of the forward problem, which relies on the estimation of the displacement vector, strain tensor, or other related parameters, or the inverse problem that attempts to reconstruct the initial modulus distribution as shown in **Fig. 2**. In general, both the forward and inverse problem solutions require accurate and precise estimation of the local displacements, with high spatial resolution and signal-to-noise ratio.[11] This procedure contrasts with dynamic methods for tissue elasticity measurement, which use variations in the velocity of the shear waves generated in tissue to obtain modulus distributions.[22,94,95] Dynamic methods for elasticity imaging and reconstruction are not discussed in this article, which focuses primarily on quasi-static elastography.

TISSUE-BASED MODULUS CONTRAST

Several groups have reported results on the Young modulus of soft tissues such as the lung, tendon, breast, prostate, liver, uterus, and brain tissue. However, the measurement methods used vary as widely as the values reported.[96–101] Fewer published results exist on human tissues such as breast, prostate, liver, and uterus, which are of interest for quasi-static elastography.[32,102–106] Measurements on human tissue stiffness by Sarvazyan and colleagues,[107] Parker and colleagues,[5] Walz and colleagues,[108] Wellman and colleagues,[75] Krouskop and colleagues,[32] and Kiss and colleagues[109] demonstrate the existence of stiffness contrast among normal tissues, and between normal and pathologic tissues in the breast, prostate, thyroid, liver, and uterus.

Krouskop and colleagues[32] presented initial reproducible results on the modulus variations on breast and prostate tissue, and also reported on their nonlinear stress strain behavior. These results were corroborated by Wellman and colleagues,[75] indicating that fibrous breast tissue was stiffer than glandular tissues, which were stiffer than adipose or fatty infiltrated tissues. Krouskop and colleagues[32] also reported on the Young modulus values of tumors in the breast with infiltrating ductal carcinomas being significantly stiffer than

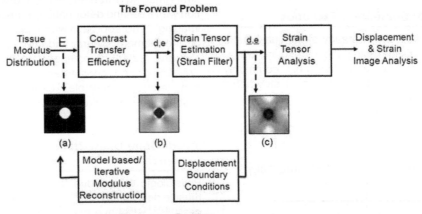

Fig. 2. Block diagram illustrating the forward and inverse problem solutions to obtain strain or modulus distributions for quasi-static elastography. The quasi-static deformation coupled with the underlying tissue elastic modulus distribution (a) and the boundary conditions, cause a strain distribution to be set up in the tissue (b) based on the contrast transfer efficiency. The statistical properties of the ultrasound-based tissue motion estimation process give rise to the strain filter. The ideal strain distribution filtered by the strain filter is the estimated displacement and strain distributions, respectively. (c) The estimated displacement coupled with the boundary conditions can be used to solve the inverse problem to obtain an estimated modulus distribution.

in situ ductal tumors, which were in turn softer than the glandular, fibrous, and fatty tissue in most instances. He also reported on prostate tissue, with normal prostate tissue being stiffer than benign prostate hyperplasia and cancers of the prostate being significantly stiffer than the normal prostate.

Young modulus measurements on liver tissue by Yeh and colleagues[103] show that liver tissue stiffness increases with cirrhosis. Hepatic tumors such as cholangiocarcinomas, focal nodular hyperplasia, and hemangiomas also exhibit increased stiffness. However, hepatocellular carcinomas were found to be softer than healthy liver.[103] Elastic modulus variations of liver tissue with different fibrosis grades were reported by Wen-Chun and colleagues.[103]

This section and associated references provides a glimpse into the several orders of magnitude in the Young modulus of normal and pathologic tissue types that has been used to provide new information on either the modulus or strain distribution in tissue.

CONTRAST TRANSFER EFFICIENCY

The solution of the forward problem in elastography is based on the use of displacement vector and strain tensor images for clinical diagnosis. However, to obtain the strain distribution, the underlying tissue has to be deformed or stressed for the modulus distribution to be converted to a strain distribution. The contrast transfer efficiency concept describes the manner by which the modulus distribution is converted to an ideal strain distribution based on purely mechanical considerations, as illustrated in **Fig. 2**. The contrast transfer efficiency concept was used by Ponnekanti and colleagues[110] to illustrate that the axial strain distribution was more efficient in depicting the modulus distribution of stiffer inclusions embedded in a softer background when compared with softer inclusions in a stiffer background. This study was corroborated by Kallel and colleagues,[111] who also developed an analytical model to verify the finite element results presented by Ponnekanti and colleagues.[110]

STATISTICAL ANALYSIS OF STRAIN ESTIMATION

Tradeoffs in the displacement vector and strain tensor estimation process from the noisy pre- and postdeformed ultrasound radiofrequency signals has been described statistically using the "Strain Filter" concept.[11,46,112] The strain filter has been defined as the statistical upper bound

of the variation in the elastographic signal-to-noise ratio (SNR_e) (ratio of the mean strain estimate to the theoretical lower bound of the standard deviation[40,41,82,83]) as a function of the applied deformation. The strain filter provides a transfer characteristic that describes the filtering process in the strain domain that enables visualization of only a limited range of the local strains generated in tissue as a function of the applied deformation. The strain filter concept allows prediction of this limited range of strains, based on the ultrasound system parameters and the signal processing algorithms and parameters used for strain estimation.[11]

The forward problem in quasi-static elastography, as illustrated in **Fig. 2**, is based on the 3 concepts or principles discussed in the preceding paragraphs.[11] Conversion of the underlying modulus distribution to the strain distribution is clearly elucidated using the contrast transfer efficiency concept to obtain the ideal strain distribution. The statistical analysis of strain estimation described using the strain filter concept demonstrates the tradeoffs between the system parameters and signal processing approaches in depicting the strain visualized in the estimated strain image. Finally, the combination of the contrast transfer efficiency and the strain filter principles leads to the prediction of the upper bound on the contrast-to-noise ratios (CNR_e) obtainable in strain images, which quantifies the forward problem.[113,114]

SPATIAL RESOLUTION FOR QUASI-STATIC STRAIN IMAGING

The cross-correlation window length and the overlap between adjacent processing windows are 2 of the primary signal-processing parameters that impact the axial resolution obtained with quasi-static strain imaging.[10,115–117] The length of the cross-correlation window at a fixed overlap was initially used as a measure of the axial resolution.[10] Alam and colleagues[115] demonstrated that axial resolution can be expressed as a bilinear function of the window length and overlap, with the overlap being the more important factor. Longer duration windows also provide improved sensitivity to strain estimation, and the ability to estimate a larger range of local strains and improved SNR_e and CNR_e (as long as the increased signal decorrelation within the gated window was negated by the increased information content) at the expense of spatial resolution.[46] In general, reductions in the spatial resolution can be traded off to make significant improvements in the SNR_e and CNR_e, and vice versa.[11,118] In a recent article,

Righetti and colleagues[116] illustrated that the ultimate limit on the axial resolution was directly proportional to the wavelength or inversely proportional to the fractional bandwidth of the ultrasound system. On the other hand, the ultrasound lateral beam width limits the achievable lateral resolution for quasi-static strain imaging.[119] In a similar manner, the elevational beam-width would impact the elevational resolution. The axial, lateral, and elevational resolution become important with the use of 2D transducers for 3D strain imaging.[54]

THE INVERSE PROBLEM IN QUASI-STATIC ELASTOGRAPHY

The solution to the inverse problem in quasi-static elastography involves the use of the estimated displacement vector and strain tensor information to reconstruct the underlying modulus distribution illustrated in **Fig. 2**. Accurate and reproducible determination of the modulus distribution would be the preferred image for clinical diagnosis because it would provide a direct image of the underlying modulus distribution. In addition, it would provide quantitative information as opposed to the qualitative information provided with displacement vector and strain tensor images, which depend to a large extent on the applied deformation.

However, the solution to the inverse problem is not straightforward, and requires additional information on both the boundary conditions in effect during the applied deformation and the local stress distribution in tissue. Unfortunately, the local stress distribution is generally unknown other than at the tissue surface where the deformation is applied. The difficulty in the computation of the local stress distribution within the tissue is a major stumbling block for modulus reconstruction. This problem has led to 2 different approaches for modulus reconstruction described in the literature, namely (1) iterative modulus reconstruction[37,87,120] based on assumption on the uniformity of the stress distribution,[37] and (2) model (finite element or analytical) based reconstruction[93,121] approaches.

Iterative methods[37,87,120] attempt to converge to a final modulus distribution, based on the estimated displacement field using assumptions on the boundary conditions and uniformity of the stress distribution. Kallel and colleagues[37] used a Newton-Raphson algorithm to find the modulus distribution that provides the best reproduction of the estimated axial displacement field using Tikhonov regularization to achieve convergence in 8 to 10 steps. Model-based methods,[93,121] on the other hand, use prior information on the

geometry of the imaged object to obtain analytical or finite element solutions that are used to aid in the convergence.

The ill-posed nature of the inverse solutions also introduce large noise artifacts, and may result in nonunique solutions of the underlying modulus distribution.[77] Barbone and Bamber[77] demonstrate that knowledge of only the displacement and boundary conditions remains insufficient to obtain unique solutions for the modulus distribution. Additional information, such as the modulus itself or its derivatives on the boundary and stress distributions, or additional strain tensor information, are essential for unique modulus reconstruction.[37,77]

CLINICAL APPLICATIONS OF QUASI-STATIC ELASTOGRAPHY

Although quasi-static elastography has been under development over the last 2 decades, it is only recently that commercial clinical ultrasound system manufacturers have introduced clinical products based on elastography. The availability of elastography modes on clinical systems will rapidly increase clinical applications and organs systems for which elastography will be used in the future.

In general, 2 criteria have to be satisfied for successful clinical elastographic imaging, namely, the ability to apply a quasi-static deformation and the ability to ultrasonically image the tissue being deformed. Superficial organs such as skin, breast, neck, thyroid, lymph nodes, and deep vein thrombi are some of the best candidates for strain or modulus imaging.[13,15,16,72,73,122–124] Approaches to deform organs located deeper in the body have been reported, which use intracavitary ultrasound transducers, intracavitary balloons for imaging the prostate gland,[125,126] saline infusion for imaging the uterus,[127] and so forth. As described previously, physiologic stimuli have been used to image the heart, vasculature, liver, and the coronary and carotid arteries.[35,36,50,128–133] In the following paragraphs some of the clinical applications of quasi-static strain and modulus imaging are discussed.

Breast

Strain[13,15,16,72,73,122,123] and modulus[39] imaging of masses in the breast have been widely reported in the literature. Strain imaging in the breast was one of the first reported clinical applications of quasi-static elastography,[13] because many breast lesions are superficial and are known to be significantly stiffer than surrounding normal breast tissue.[32] Strain imaging of the breast has been reported using well-controlled stepper motor based deformations (both single and multiple deformation steps),[13] real-time freehand palpation,[15] and also the use of physiologic deformation of the left breast due to cardiac activity.

Some of the early parameters used to differentiate benign from malignant masses were also reported for breast masses to differentiate malignant breast tumors from benign fibroadenomas. Because breast tumors are significantly stiffer (depicted in a darker gray scale as opposed to the lighter gray scale used for softer tissue) than surrounding normal tissue, the stiffness or strain contrast was initially used to differentiate breast masses,[13] as shown in **Fig. 3** for a patient with an invasive ductal carcinoma. Note that although the margins of the mass are not clearly visualized in the B-mode image in **Fig. 3**A, it is clearly seen in the axial strain image in **Fig. 3**B as a darker (stiffer) region. In addition, invasive cancers in the breast were depicted as larger areas of stiffness in the strain images when compared with the corresponding B-mode images,[13] observed from comparing **Fig. 3**A and B. The increased stiffer regions observed in the strain images were hypothesized to be due to the desmoplastic reaction from the infiltration of the tumor into surrounding breast tissue. A second parameter referred to as the "size ratio," derived from the ratio of the lesion dimensions derived from the strain and B-mode images, was then proposed to differentiate benign fibroadenomas from malignant tumors.[13,15] Another parameter used in the differentiation is related to lesion mobility; because cancers are firmly attached to surrounding tissue, compared with fibroadenomas that are more mobile and hence slip during the applied deformation.[72,73] Parameters related to the normalized shear strain around the breast masses haven

been used to quantify the attachment of the mass or lesion to the surrounding tissue, as shown in **Fig. 3**C. The large shear strain areas (blue and red regions) that are clearly seen toward the top of the mass margins indicate firmly attached masses.[72,73] Elastography also provides clear classification of cystic masses, which are depicted with a central decorrelation spot appearing as a bright spot or region on the strain image. Finally, methods to assess the viscoelastic response by evaluating tissue creep have also been described.[134]

Thyroid

The thyroid gland is another superficial gland that is a viable target for quasi-static elastography. Due to the accessibility of the thyroid gland, external deformation of the thyroid using the ultrasound transducer has been used by several groups.[124,135,136] Deformations introduced from pulsations due to blood flow through the carotid artery have also been used as a deformation source.[91]

Lymph Nodes

Assessments of the stiffness of lymph nodes represent another clinical application area for quasi-static elastography, due to the superficial nature of these nodes enabling application of external deformations for strain imaging.[137]

Deep Vein Thrombosis

Deep vein thrombi or blood clots are known to progressively increase in stiffness with age, and a means to stage thrombi age is essential in their treatment. Quasi-static modulus imaging has been used to determine the thrombi age, because

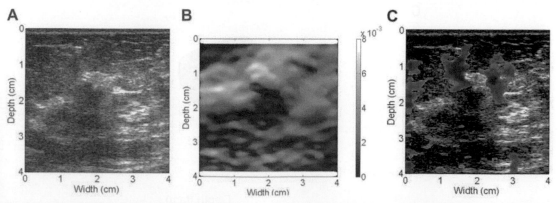

Fig. 3. In vivo ultrasound B-mode (A), axial strain (B), and shear strain (C) images for a patient diagnosed with an invasive ductal carcinoma. The composite image in (C) is formed by superimposing the axial-shear strains on top of the B-mode image. Radiofrequency data were acquired using a Siemens Antares scanner during real-time palpation imaging at the breast center, University of Wisconsin-Madison Hospitals and Clinics.

newer clots can be treated more effectively than older clots.[138]

Prostate

Another area where in vivo strain imaging has made inroads is in the imaging of the prostate gland. The prostate gland presents a more challenging environment for the application of strain imaging, due to its location, primarily for the application of the deformation required for strain imaging. Deformation states of the prostate have been varied using different levels of saline within the balloon,[139] and deformations applied using the transrectal ultrasound transducer (TRUS).[140] The TRUS transducer also provides data in a curvilinear format compared with linear array transducers used for the breast, small parts, and the carotid.

Uterine Strain Imaging

Evaluation of focal uterine masses has also been explored using the transvaginal ultrasound transducer (TVUS) and using saline infusion to provide the deformation.[127] Ex vivo quasi-static strain imaging of different uterine pathology has been

reported in the literature.[141] Another application area for strain and modulus imaging is the evaluation of cervical stiffness,[142,143] which may have implications for the evaluation of patients at risk for preterm labor.

Treatment Monitoring of Ablative Therapies

Treatment monitoring of ablative therapies is probably one of the more natural applications for strain and modulus elastography, because heating tissue induces denaturation of proteins which, in turn, elevates the Young modulus of ablated tissue. Strain imaging has been used to monitor ablative therapies such as high-intensity focused ultrasound,[139] radiofrequency, and microwave ablation procedures.[84] An interesting offshoot is the use of the radiofrequency or microwave electrode itself to introduce the quasi-static deformation for both strain[84] and modulus[87] imaging. This method has been used for in vivo imaging of thermal lesions in the kidney and liver.[125,126] 3D strain imaging has also been reported with electrode displacement elastography.[86] An example of in vivo electrode displacement based strain imaging is illustrated in **Fig. 4**, for a thermal lesion

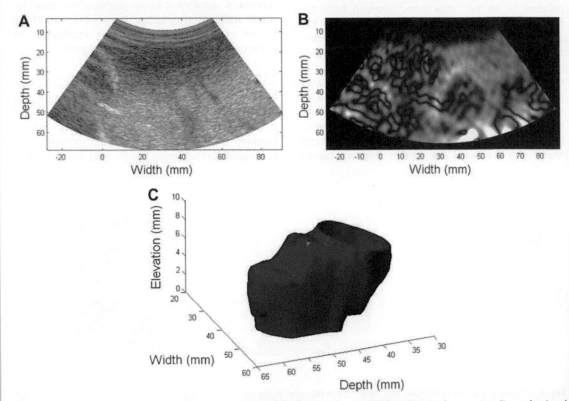

Fig. 4. B-mode (*A*), 2D axial strain (*B*), and 3D image (*C*) of an in vivo ablated region in the porcine liver obtained using quasi-static electrode displacement elastography. Radiofrequency data were collected using a Siemens Antares scanner equipped with a C7F2 fourSight 4-dimensional ultrasound transducer.

created in the liver of a porcine animal model using a Cool-tip radiofrequency ablation system (Valleylab, Boulder, CO).

Monitoring of Edema

Quasi-static elastography has also been used for imaging the poroelastic properties of tissue that accumulates fluid, for example, for evaluating lymphedema, which involves an abnormal interstitial accumulation of lymphatic fluid causing tissue swelling.[38,74,144] Variations in the ratio of the lateral to axial strain values with deformation provide estimates of the fluid content and the ability to differentiate between normal and edematous tissues.[74]

Intravascular Strain Imaging

Intravascular ultrasound (IVUS) based strain imaging of coronary arteries using pulsations introduced due to cardiac activity has been widely described in the literature, and is probably the most common clinical application involving physiologic stimuli.[9,18,44,88,89] The most common implementation uses radiofrequency data acquired at 2 different intraluminal pressure levels near diastole. IVUS elastography involves the acquisition of high-frequency (20 MHz or higher) radiofrequency data from single-element or array transducers located at the tip of a catheter that is inserted into the coronary artery to be evaluated. In addition to the strain distribution modulus, maps have also been generated.[145] One of the challenges in intravascular elastography and carotid strain imaging described in the next subsection is the identification and differentiation of "vulnerable plaque" or plaque prone to rupture.[132]

Carotid Strain Imaging

Most of the reported strain and modulus imaging studies for plaque characterization use IVUS on coronary arteries[132,133] as described earlier. However, the carotid artery is another superficial location that provides easy access to clinical ultrasound equipment with linear array transducers,[50,128–131] and is also amenable to strain imaging. **Fig. 5** presents a B-mode and axial strain image for a patient with a strip of softer plaque observed at a depth of 2 cm and extending from 1.5 to 4 cm. The strain image also classifies the remainder of the plaque in the vessel as relatively stiffer plaque, visualized as the mid-gray scale in **Fig. 5**B.[50,128,131] Investigators have reported on estimation of the Young modulus by solving the inverse problem using the estimated strains and mechanical models of the carotid artery.[130] However, both the carotid and coronary artery models have to account for hemodynamic parameters that vary significantly with stenosis for inverse problem solutions.

Cardiac Elastography

Cardiac-elastography or myocardial strain imaging, whereby the strain distribution is imaged over the entire contraction and relaxation of the heart (cardiac cycle),[35,36] is another clinical application that uses physiologic stimuli. B-mode

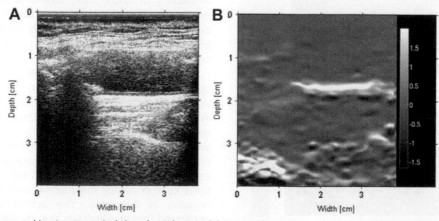

Fig. 5. Ultrasound in vivo B-mode (*A*) and axial strain (*B*) images from the carotid of a patient with atherosclerotic plaque. Brighter or darker regions around the vessel wall indicate softer plaque, while the mid-gray regions denote stiffer plaque. Note the softer plaque region attached to the bottom wall of the artery from 1.5 to 4 cm at a depth of 2 cm. Hyperechogenic regions around the vessel wall along with the areas of shadowing appear mid-gray, denoting stiffer plaque regions. Radiofrequency data were acquired using a Siemens Antares scanner, University of Wisconsin-Madison Hospitals and Clinics.

speckle tracking for strain imaging is currently used, primarily due to limitations associated with tissue Doppler-derived velocity and strain estimates.[146–148] Both General Electric Medical Systems (GE Healthcare, Milwaukee, WI) and Siemens (Siemens Ultrasound, Mountain View, CA) have rolled out clinical cardiac ultrasound systems equipped with 2D speckle tracking methods for strain imaging. Strain imaging that uses radiofrequency signals would provide significantly improved strain sensitivity compared with the B-mode based approaches.[35,36] A short-axes B-mode and strain image obtained using radiofrequency data, estimated using a hybrid 2D algorithm developed for curvilinear transducers,[63] is shown in **Fig. 6**. The strains depicted in the image for the cardiac muscle are mostly compressive (blue color), because this image was obtained during systole. However, the frame rates at which radiofrequency data are acquired is an important factor in obtaining unbiased and robust estimation of tissue displacements and strain.[149] Frame rates for B-mode data are significantly higher than those for radiofrequency data. Approaches to obtain high-precision radial, circumferential, and longitudinal strains are also necessary for the widespread clinical application of this modality. Estimation of principal strain components, which are angle-independent, is one such approach that may provide reproducible diagnostic measures for evaluating cardiac disease.[150]

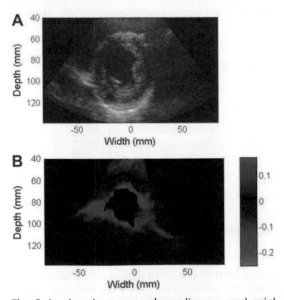

Fig. 6. In vivo short-axes echocardiogram and axial strain image for a patient in systole. Data were acquired using a GE Vivid 7 scanner, University of Wisconsin-Madison Hospitals and Clinics.

Respiratory and Cardiac Stimuli for Abdominal Strain Imaging

Deformations of the liver and other abdominal organs introduced due to respiration, for example, diaphragmatic deformations, have been used for imaging thermal lesions created in the liver.[34] Cardiovascular motion[90] has also been used for in vivo elastographic imaging of the liver. However, all of these approaches require gating of the data acquisition to the respiratory or cardiac waveform to ensure similar deformation increments and for reproducible imaging.

SUMMARY

The last 2 decades have seen tremendous advances in the development and clinical practice of quasi-static ultrasound elastography in the depiction of quality displacement vector, strain tensor, and modulus distributions. At present, 4 different commercial ultrasound system manufacturers offer quasi-static based strain imaging modes on their clinical systems. Palpation-based strain imaging is currently available on both the Siemens Antares and the S2000 systems (Siemens Ultrasound, Seattle, WA). Hitachi Medical systems (Hitachi Ltd, Tokyo, Japan) provide elastography modes on their scanners. Ultrasonix Medical Corporation (Vancouver, BC, Canada) recently introduced the SonixTOUCH system with an elastography mode. General Electric Medical Systems (GE Healthcare, Milwaukee, WI) and Siemens have also introduced 2D speckle tracking on their cardiac ultrasound systems. The availability of quasi-static based strain imaging modes on clinical systems will further spur the development of this new imaging modality, as it provides additional information not present with current clinical imaging modalities.

Although quantitative (ie, modulus) imaging with quasi-static elastography would provide the best visualization of the underlying modulus distribution in tissue, this mode requires additional development to reduce noise artifacts and to obtain unique solutions. This advance would require the development of techniques for accurate and precise estimation of the local strain and stress distributions at high spatial resolutions, and research is ongoing in this area. The author anticipates continued improvements in the spatial resolution and signal-to-noise ratios in the estimated strain tensor distribution, with improved algorithms and processing techniques. Development of methods for accurate estimation of the local stress distribution need to be developed, with techniques that use force sensors on ultrasound transducers under evaluation.

This article does not review dynamic elastography based methods, which have also made significant strides over the last decade. Commercialization of these approaches include the FibroScan system developed by Echosens (Echosens SA, Paris, France), a device that tracks shear wave speed for monitoring and staging hepatic fibrosis,[151] and the S2000 (Siemens Ultrasound, Seattle, WA) equipped with the Virtual Touch software acoustic radiation force based imaging mode. Recently SuperSonic Imagine announced FDA approval for their shear wave elastography system called Aixplorer based on the supersonic shear wave imaging concept. Some of these recent developments to obtain modulus estimates of small regions in tissue may enable more accurate staging of diffuse diseases. Several excellent review articles exist in the literature that would provide the interested reader with additional insights into this novel imaging modality.[152–156]

ACKNOWLEDGMENTS

I would like to thank Dr Min Rao, PhD, Dr Hao Chen PhD, Mr Matthew McCormick, Mr Nick Rubert, and Ms Haiyan Xu for providing the results used in this article.

REFERENCES

1. Dickinson RJ, Hill CR. Measurement of soft tissue motion using correlation between A-scans. Ultrasound Med Biol 1982;8:263–71.

2. Wilson LS, Robinson DE. Ultrasonic measurement of small displacements and deformations of tissue. Ultrason Imaging 1982;4:71–82.

3. Krouskop TA, Dougherty DR, Vinson FS. A pulsed Doppler ultrasonic system for making noninvasive measurements of the mechanical properties of soft tissue. J Rehabil Res Dev 1987;24:1–8.

4. Yamakoshi Y, Sato J, Sato T. Ultrasonic Imaging of internal vibration of soft tissue under forced vibration. IEEE Trans Ultrason Ferroelectr Freq Control 1990;37:45–53.

5. Parker KJ, Huang SR, Musulin RA, et al. Tissue response to mechanical vibrations for 'sonoelasticity imaging'. Ultrasound Med Biol 1990;16:241–6.

6. Ophir J, Cespedes I, Ponnekanti H, et al. Elastography: a quantitative method for imaging the elasticity of biological tissues. Ultrason Imaging 1991; 13:111–34.

7. O'Donnell M, Skovoroda AR, Shapo BM. Measurement of arterial wall motion using Fourier based speckle tracking algorithms. Proc IEEE Ultrason Sympos 1991;2:1101–4.

8. Ophir J, Cespedes EI, Garra BS, et al. Elastography: ultrasonic imaging of tissue strain and elastic modulus in vivo. Invited paper & review. Eur J Ultrasound 1996;3:49–70.

9. O'Donnell M, Skovoroda AR, Shapo BM, et al. Internal displacement and strain imaging using ultrasonic speckle tracking. IEEE Trans Ultrason Ferroelectr Freq Control 1994;41:314–25.

10. Cespedes EI. Elastography: imaging of biological tissue elasticity. Ann Arbor (MI): University of Houston; 1993.

11. Varghese T, Ophir J, Konofagou E, et al. Tradeoffs in elastographic imaging. Ultrason Imaging 2001; 23:216–48.

12. Bertrand M, Meunier M, Doucet M, et al. Ultrasonic biomechanical strain gauge based on speckle tracking. IEEE Ultrasonics Symposium 1989;2: 859–64.

13. Garra BS, Cespedes EI, Ophir J, et al. Elastography of breast lesions: initial clinical results. Radiology 1997;202:79–86.

14. Ophir J, Garra B, Kallel F, et al. Elastographic imaging. Ultrasound Med Biol 2000;26(Suppl):S23–9.

15. Hall TJ, Zhu Y, Spalding CS. In vivo real-time free-hand palpation imaging. Ultrasound Med Biol 2003;29:427–35.

16. Hiltawsky KM, Kruger M, Starke C, et al. Freehand ultrasound elastography of breast lesions: clinical results. Ultrasound Med Biol 2001;27:1461–9.

17. Insana MF, Hall TJ, Chaturvedi P, et al. Ultrasonic properties of random media under uniaxial loading. J Acoust Soc Am 2001;110:3243–51.

18. de Korte CL, Ignacio Cespedes EI, van der Steen AF, et al. Intravascular elasticity imaging using ultrasound: feasibility studies in phantoms. Ultrasound Med Biol 1997;23:735–46.

19. Bamber JC, Bush NL. Freehand elasticity imaging using speckle decorrelation rate. Acoust Imag 1996;22:285–92.

20. Walker WF. Internal deformation of a uniform elastic solid by acoustic radiation force. J Acoust Soc Am 1999;105:2508–18.

21. Nightingale KR, Nightingale RW, Palmeri ML, et al. A finite element model of remote palpation of breast lesions using radiation force: factors affecting tissue displacement. Ultrason Imaging 2000;22:35–54.

22. Sarvazyan AP, Rudenko OV, Swanson SD, et al. Shear wave elasticity imaging: a new ultrasonic technology of medical diagnostics. Ultrasound Med Biol 1998;24:1419–35.

23. Fatemi M, Greenleaf JF. Probing the dynamics of tissue at low frequencies with the radiation force of ultrasound. Phys Med Biol 2000;45:1449–64.

24. Pesavento A, Lorenz A, Siebers S, et al. New real-time strain imaging concepts using diagnostic ultrasound. Phys Med Biol 2000;45:1423–35.

25. Lizzi FL, Muratore R, Deng CX, et al. Radiation-force technique to monitor lesions during ultrasonic therapy. Ultrasound Med Biol 2003;29:1593–605.

26. Plewes DB, Betty I, Urchuk SN, et al. Visualizing tissue compliance with MR imaging. J Magn Reson Imaging 1995;5:733–8.

27. Muthupillai R, Lomas DJ, Rossman PJ, et al. Magnetic resonance elastography by direct visualization of propagating acoustic strain waves. Science 1995;269:1854–7.

28. Fowlkes JB, Emelianov SY, Pipe JG, et al. Magnetic-resonance imaging techniques for detection of elasticity variation. Med Phys 1995;22:1771–8.

29. Schmitt JM. OCT elastography: imaging microscopic deformation and strain of tissue. Opt Express 1998;3:199–211.

30. Fung YG. Biomechanical properties of living tissues. New York: Springer Verlag; 1981. chapter 7.

31. Anderson WAD. Pathology. St. Louis (MO): C.V. Mosby Co; 1953.

32. Krouskop TA, Wheeler TM, Kallel F, et al. Elastic moduli of breast and prostate tissues under compression. Ultrason Imaging 1998;20:260–74.

33. Turgay E, Salcudean S, Rohling R. Identifying the mechanical properties of tissue by ultrasound strain imaging. Ultrasound Med Biol 2006;32:221–35.

34. Varghese T, Shi H. Elastographic imaging of thermal lesions in liver in-vivo using diaphragmatic stimuli. Ultrason Imaging 2004;26:18–28.

35. Varghese T, Zagzebski JA, Rahko P, et al. Ultrasonic imaging of myocardial strain using cardiac elastography. Ultrason Imaging 2003;25:1–16.

36. Konofagou EE, D'Hooge J, Ophir J. Myocardial elastography-a feasibility study in vivo. Ultrasound Med Biol 2002;28:475–82.

37. Kallel F, Bertrand M. Tissue elasticity reconstruction using linear perturbation method. IEEE Trans Med Imaging 1996;15:299–313.

38. Konofagou EE, Harrigan TP, Ophir J, et al. Poroelastography: imaging the poroelastic properties of tissues. Ultrasound Med Biol 2001;27:1387–97.

39. Oberai AA, Gokhale NH, Goenezen S, et al. Linear and nonlinear elasticity imaging of soft tissue in vivo: demonstration of feasibility. Phys Med Biol 2009;54:1191–207.

40. Quazi AH. An overview of the time delay estimate in active and passive systems for target localization. IEEE Trans Acoust Speech Sig Proc 1981;29:527–33.

41. Weinstein E, Weiss A. Fundamental limitations in passive time delay estimation Part II: Wideband systems. IEEE Trans Acoust Speech Sig Proc 1984;32:1064–78.

42. Bilgen M, Insana MF. Deformation models and correlation analysis in elastography. J Acoust Soc Am 1996;99:3212–24.

43. Chen EJ, Adler RS, Carson PL, et al. Ultrasound tissue displacement imaging with application to breast cancer. Ultrasound Med Biol 1995;21:1153–62.

44. Talhami HE, Wilson LS, Neale ML. Spectral tissue strain: a new technique for imaging tissue strain using intravascular ultrasound. Ultrasound Med Biol 1994;20:759–72.

45. Pesavento A, Perrey C, Krueger M, et al. A time-efficient and accurate strain estimation concept for ultrasonic elastography using iterative phase zero estimation. IEEE Trans Ultrason Ferroelectr Freq Control 1999;46:1057–67.

46. Varghese T, Bilgen M, Ophir J. Multiresolution imaging in elastography. IEEE Trans Ultrason Ferroelectr Freq Control 1998;45:65–75.

47. Chaturvedi P, Insana MF, Hall TJ. 2-D companding for noise reduction in strain imaging. IEEE Trans Ultrason Ferroelectr Freq Control 1998;45:179–91.

48. Zhu Y, Hall T. A modified block matching method for real-time freehand strain imaging. Ultrason Imaging 2002;24:161–76.

49. Pellot-Barakat C, Frouin F, Insana MF, et al. Ultrasound elastography based on multiscale estimations of regularized displacement fields. IEEE Trans Med Imaging 2004;23:153–63.

50. Shi H, Varghese T. Two-dimensional multi-level strain estimation for discontinuous tissue. Phys Med Biol 2007;52:389–401.

51. Jiang J, Hall TJ. A parallelizable real-time motion tracking algorithm with applications to ultrasonic strain imaging. Phys Med Biol 2007;52:3773–90.

52. Patil AV, Garson CD, Hossack JA. 3D prostate elastography: algorithm, simulations and experiments. Phys Med Biol 2007;52:3643–63.

53. Chen X, Xie H, Erkamp R, et al. 3-D correlation-based speckle tracking. Ultrason Imaging 2005;21:21–36.

54. Rao M, Varghese T. Correlation analysis of three-dimensional strain imaging using ultrasound two-dimensional array transducers. J Acoust Soc Am 2008;124:1858–65.

55. Cespedes I, Ophir J, Ponnekanti H, et al. Elastography: elasticity imaging using ultrasound with application to muscle and breast in vivo. Ultrason Imaging 1993;15:73–88.

56. Varghese T, Ophir J. Characterization of elastographic noise using the envelope of echo signals. Ultrasound Med Biol 1998;24:543–55.

57. Varghese T, Konofagou EE, Ophir J, et al. Direct strain estimation in elastography using spectral cross-correlation. Ultrasound Med Biol 2000;26:1525–37.

58. Konofagou EE, Varghese T, Ophir J, et al. Power spectral strain estimators in elastography. Ultrasound Med Biol 1999;25:1115–29.

59. Hoyt K, Forsberg F, Ophir J. Comparison of shift estimation strategies in spectral elastography. Ultrasonics 2006;44:99–108.

60. Bohs LN, Friemel BH, McDermott BA, et al. A real time system for quantifying and displaying two-dimensional velocities using ultrasound. Ultrasound Med Biol 1993;19:751–61.

61. Rao M, Chen Q, Shi H, et al. Spatial-angular compounding for elastography using beam steering on linear array transducers. Med Phys 2006;33:618–26.

62. Techavipoo U, Chen Q, Varghese T, et al. Noise reduction using spatial-angular compounding for elastography. IEEE Trans Ultrason Ferroelectr Freq Control 2004;51:510–20.

63. Chen H, Varghese T. Multi-level hybrid 2-D strain imaging algorithm for ultrasound sector/phased arrays. Med Phys 2009;36:2098–106.

64. Zhu Y, Chaturvedi P, Insana MF. Strain imaging with a deformable mesh. Ultrason Imaging 1999;21:127–41.

65. Maurice RL, Bertrand M. Lagrangian speckle model and tissue-motion estimation-theory. [ultrasonography]. IEEE Trans Med Imaging 1999;18:593–603.

66. Konofagou E, Ophir J. A new elastographic method for estimation and imaging of lateral displacements, lateral strains, corrected axial strains and Poisson's ratios in tissues. Ultrasound Med Biol 1998;24:1183–99.

67. Rao M, Chen Q, Shi H, et al. Normal and shear strain estimation using beam steering on linear-array transducers. Ultrasound Med Biol 2007;33:57–66.

68. Techavipoo U, Chen Q, Varghese T, et al. Estimation of displacement vectors and strain tensors in elastography using angular insonifications. IEEE Trans Med Imaging 2004;23:1479–89.

69. Lubinski MA, Emelianov SY, Raghavan KR, et al. Lateral displacement estimation using tissue incompressibility. IEEE Trans Ultrason Ferroelectr Freq Control 1996;43:247–56.

70. Konofagou EE, Harrigan T, Ophir J. Shear strain estimation and lesion mobility assessment in elastography. Ultrasonics 2000;38:400–4.

71. Rao M, Varghese T, Madsen EL. Shear strain imaging using shear deformations. Med Phys 2008;35:412–23.

72. Thitaikumar A, Mobbs LM, Kraemer-Chant CM, et al. Breast tumor classification using axial shear strain elastography: a feasibility study. Phys Med Biol 2008;53:4809–23.

73. Rao M, Baker S, Sommer AM, et al. Shear strain elastography for breast mass differentiation [abstract]. In: 7th International Conference on the ultrasonic measurement and imaging of tissue elasticity. Austin (TX), October 27–30, 2008.

74. Righetti R, Garra BS, Mobbs LM, et al. The feasibility of using poroelastographic techniques for distinguishing between normal and lymphedematous tissues in vivo. Phys Med Biol 2007;52:6525–41.

75. Wellman PS, Dalton EP, Krag D, et al. Tactile imaging of breast masses: first clinical report. Arch Surg 2001;136:204–8.

76. Sarvazyan A. Mechanical imaging: a new technology for medical diagnostics. Int J Med Inform 1998;49:195–216.

77. Barbone PE, Bamber JC. Quantitative elasticity imaging: what can and cannot be inferred from strain images. Phys Med Biol 2002;47:2147–64.

78. Egorov V, Sarvazyan AP. Mechanical imaging of the breast. IEEE Trans Med Imaging 2008;27:1275–87.

79. Dutt V, Kinnick RR, Muthupillai R, et al. Acoustic shear-wave imaging using echo ultrasound compared to magnetic resonance elastography. Ultrasound Med Biol 2000;26:397–403.

80. Sandrin L, Catheline S, Tanter M, et al. Time-resolved pulsed elastography with ultrafast ultrasonic imaging. Ultrason Imaging 1999;21:259–72.

81. Ophir J, Kallel F, Varghese T, et al. Elastography: a systems approach. Int J Imag Syst Technol 1997;8:89–103.

82. Knapp CH, Carter GC. The generalized correlation method for estimation of time delay. IEEE Trans Acoust Speech Sig Proc 1976;24:320–7.

83. Walker FW, Trahey GE. A fundamental limit on delay estimation using partially correlated speckle signals. IEEE Trans Ultrason Ferroelectr Freq Control 1995;42:301–8.

84. Varghese T, Zagzebski JA, Lee FT Jr. Elastographic imaging of thermal lesions in the liver in vivo following radiofrequency ablation: preliminary results. Ultrasound Med Biol 2002;28:1467–73.

85. Bharat S, Varghese T. Contrast-transfer improvement for electrode displacement elastography. Phys Med Biol 2006;51:6403–18.

86. Bharat S, Fisher TG, Varghese T, et al. Three-dimensional electrode displacement elastography using the Siemens C7F2 fourSight four-dimensional ultrasound transducer. Ultrasound Med Biol 2008;34:1307–16.

87. Jiang J, Varghese T, Brace C, et al. Young's modulus reconstruction for radio-frequency ablation electrode-induced displacement fields: a feasibility study. IEEE Trans Med Imaging 2009;28:1325–34.

88. de Korte CL, van der Steen AF, Cespedes EI, et al. Intravascular ultrasound elastography in human arteries: initial experience in vitro. Ultrasound Med Biol 1998;24:401–8.

89. Ryan LK, Foster FS. Ultrasonic measurement of differential displacement and strain in a vascular model. Ultrason Imaging 1997;19:19–38.

90. Kolen AF, Miller NR, Ahmed EE, et al. Characterization of cardiovascular liver motion for the eventual application of elasticity imaging to the liver in vivo. Phys Med Biol 2004;49:4187–206.

91. Bae U, Dighe M, Dubinsky T, et al. Ultrasound thyroid elastography using carotid artery pulsation: preliminary study. J Ultrasound Med 2007; 26:797–805.

92. Kolen AF, Bamber JC, Ahmed EE. Analysis of cardiovascular induced liver motion for application to elasticity imaging of the liver in-vivo [abstract]. J Ultrasound Med 2003;21:S53.

93. Baldewsing RA, Danilouchkine MG, Mastik F, et al. An inverse method for imaging the local elasticity of atherosclerotic coronary plaques. IEEE Trans Inf Technol Biomed 2008;13:277–89.

94. Landau LD, Lifshitz EM. Theory of elasticity. New York: Elsevier; 1986.

95. Palmeri ML, Wang MH, Dahl JJ, et al. Quantifying hepatic shear modulus in vivo using acoustic radiation force. Ultrasound Med Biol 2008;34:546–58.

96. Suki B, Barabasi AL, Lutchen KR. Lung tissue viscoelasticity: a mathematical framework and its molecular basis. J Appl Physiol 1994;76:2749–59.

97. Arbogast KB, Margulies SS. Material characterization of the brainstem from oscillatory shear tests. J Biomech 1998;31:801–7.

98. Kim SM, McCulloch TM, Rim K. Comparison of viscoelastic properties of the pharyngeal tissue: human and canine. Dysphagia 1999;14:8–16.

99. Lakes RS, Vanderby R. Interrelation of creep and relaxation: a modeling approach for ligaments. J Biomech Eng 1999;121:612–5.

100. Yuan H, Kononov S, Cavalcante FS, et al. Effects of collagenase and elastase on the mechanical properties of lung tissue strips. J Appl Physiol 2000;89:3–14.

101. Darvish KK, Crandall JR. Nonlinear viscoelastic effects in oscillatory shear deformation of brain tissue. Med Eng Phys 2001;23:633–45.

102. Chen EJ, Novakofski J, Jenkins WK, et al. Young's modulus measurements of soft tissues with application to elasticity imaging. IEEE Trans Ultrason Ferroelectr Freq Control 1996;43:191–4.

103. Yeh WC, Li PC, Jeng YM, et al. Elastic modulus measurements of human liver and correlation with pathology. Ultrasound Med Biol 2002;28:467–74.

104. Han L, Noble JA, Burcher M. A novel ultrasound indentation system for measuring biomechanical properties of in vivo soft tissue. Ultrasound Med Biol 2003;29:813–23.

105. Sammani A, Bishop J, Luginbuhl C, et al. Measuring the elastic modulus of ex vivo small tissue samples. Phys Med Biol 2003;48:2183–98.

106. Ishihara M, Sato M, Sato S, et al. Viscoelastic characterization of biological tissue by photoacoustic measurement. Jpn J Appl Phys 2003;42:L556–8.

107. Sarvazyan AP, Skovorada AR, Vucelic D. Utilization of surface acoustic waves and shear acoustic properties for imaging and tissue characterization. Proc Acoust Imag 1991;19:463–7.

108. Walz, M, Teubner J, Georgi M. Elasticity of benign and malignant breast lesions, imaging, application and results in clinical and general practice. In: Eight International Congress on the Ultrasonic Examination of the Breast. 56, 1993, p. 56.

109. Kiss MZ, Hobson MA, Varghese T, et al. Frequency-dependent complex modulus of the uterus: preliminary results. Phys Med Biol 2006; 51:3683–95.

110. Ponnekanti H, Ophir J, Huang Y, et al. Fundamental mechanical limitations on the visualization of elasticity contrast in elastography. Ultrasound Med Biol 1995;21:533–43.

111. Kallel F, Bertrand M, Ophir J. Fundamental limitations on the contrast-transfer efficiency in elastography: an analytic study. Ultrasound Med Biol 1996;22:463–70.

112. Varghese T, Ophir J. A theoretical framework for performance characterization of elastography: the strain filter. IEEE Trans Ultrason Ferroelectr Freq Control 1997;44:164–72.

113. Varghese T, Ophir J. An analysis of elastographic contrast-to-noise ratio performance. Ultrasound Med Biol 1998;24:915–24.

114. Bilgen M. Target detectability in acoustic elastography. IEEE Trans Ultrason Ferroelectr Freq Control 1999;46:1128–33.

115. Alam SK, Ophir J, Varghese T. Elastographic axial resolution criteria: an experimental study. IEEE Trans Ultrason Ferroelectr Freq Control 2000;47:304–9.

116. Righetti R, Ophir J, Ktonas P. Axial resolution in elastography. Ultrasound Med Biol 2002;28: 101–13.

117. Bilgen M, Insana MF. Error analysis in acoustic elastography. II. Strain estimation and SNR analysis. J Acoust Soc Am 1997;101:1147–54.

118. Srinivasan S, Righetti R, Ophir J. Trade-offs between the axial resolution and the signal-to-noise ratio in elastography. Ultrasound Med Biol 2003;29: 847–66.

119. Righetti R, Srinivasan S, Ophir J. Lateral resolution in elastography. Ultrasound Med Biol 2003;29: 695–704.

120. Doyley MM, Meaney PM, Bamber JC. Evaluation of an iterative reconstruction method for quantitative elastography. Phys Med Biol 2000;45:1521–40.

121. Aglyamov S, Skovoroda AR, Rubin JM, et al. Model-based reconstructive elasticity imaging of deep venous thrombosis. IEEE Trans Ultrason Ferroelectr Freq Control 2004;51:521–31.

122. Burnside ES, Hall TJ, Sommer AM, et al. Differentiating benign from malignant solid breast masses

with US strain imaging. Radiology 2007;245: 401–10.

123. Regner DM, Hesley GK, Hangiandreou NJ, et al. Breast lesions: evaluation with US strain imaging—clinical experience of multiple observers. Radiology 2006;238:425–37.

124. Lyshchik A, Higashi T, Asato R, et al. Thyroid gland tumor diagnosis at US elastography. Radiology 2005;237:202–11.

125. Bharat S. Electrode displacement strain imaging for thermally ablative therapies [PhD dissertation]. Ann Arbor (MI): University Microfilms International (UMI); 2009.

126. Kolokythas O, Gauthier T, Fernandez AT, et al. Ultrasound-based elastography: a novel approach to assess radio frequency ablation of liver masses performed with expandable ablation probes: a feasibility study. J Ultrasound Med 2008;27: 935–46.

127. Hobson MA, Madsen EL, Frank GR, et al. Anthropomorphic phantoms for assessment of strain imaging methods involving saline-infused sonohysterography. Ultrasound Med Biol 2008;34: 1622–37.

128. Shi H, Mitchell CC, McCormick M, et al. Preliminary in vivo atherosclerotic carotid plaque characterization using the accumulated axial strain and relative lateral shift strain indices. Phys Med Biol 2008;53: 6377–94.

129. Ribbers H, Lopata RG, Holewijn S, et al. Noninvasive two-dimensional strain imaging of arteries: validation in phantoms and preliminary experience in carotid arteries in vivo. Ultrasound Med Biol 2007;33:530–40.

130. Schmitt C, Soulez G, Maurice RL, et al. Noninvasive vascular elastography: toward a complementary characterization tool of atherosclerosis in carotid arteries. Ultrasound Med Biol 2007;33:1841–58.

131. Maurice RL, Soulez G, Giroux MF, et al. Noninvasive vascular elastography for carotid artery characterization on subjects without previous history of atherosclerosis. Med Phys 2008;35:3436–43.

132. de Korte CL, Schaar JA, Mastik F, et al. Intravascular elastography: from bench to bedside. J Interv Cardiol 2003;16:253–9.

133. de Korte CL, van der Steen AF, Cepedes EI, et al. Characterization of plaque components and vulnerability with intravascular ultrasound elastography. Phys Med Biol 2000;45:1465–75.

134. Sridhar M, Insana MF. Ultrasonic measurements of breast viscoelasticity. Med Phys 2007;34:4757–67.

135. Wilson T, Chen Q, Zagzebski JA, et al. Initial clinical experience imaging scatterer size and strain in thyroid nodules. J Ultrasound Med 2006;25:1021–9.

136. Meixner D, Hangiandreou NJ, Charboneau JW, et al. Initial clinical experience with real-time ultrasound strain imaging of the thyroid [abstract]. RSNA 2002;225:713.

137. Alam F, Naito K, Horiguchi J, et al. Accuracy of sonographic elastography in the differential diagnosis of enlarged cervical lymph nodes: comparison with conventional B-mode sonography. AJR Am J Roentgenol 2008;191:604–10.

138. Rubin JM, Xie H, Kim K, et al. Sonographic elasticity imaging of acute and chronic deep venous thrombosis in humans. J Ultrasound Med 2006; 25:1179–86.

139. Souchon R, Rouviere O, Gelet A, et al. Visualisation of HIFU lesions using elastography of the human prostate in vivo: preliminary results. Ultrasound Med Biol 2003;29:1007–15.

140. Lorenz A, Ermert H, Sommerfeld HJ, et al. Ultrasound elastography of the prostate. A new technique for tumor detection. Ultraschall Med 2000; 21:8–15 [in German].

141. Hobson MA, Kiss MZ, Varghese T, et al. In vitro uterine strain imaging: preliminary results. J Ultrasound Med 2007;26:899–908.

142. Thomas A, Kümmel S, Gemeinhardt O, et al. Real-time sonoelastography of the cervix: tissue elasticity of the normal and abnormal cervix. Acad Radiol 2007;14:193–200.

143. Mazza E, Nava A, Bauer M, et al. Mechanical properties of the human uterine cervix: an in vivo study. Med Image Anal 2006;10:125–36.

144. Berry GP, Bamber JC, Armstrong CG, et al. Towards an acoustic model-based poroelastic imaging method: I. Theoretical foundation. Ultrasound Med Biol 2006;32:547–67.

145. Baldewsing RA, Schaar JA, Mastik F, et al. Local elasticity imaging of vulnerable atherosclerotic coronary plaques. Adv Cardiol 2007; 44:35–61.

146. Becker M, Bilke E, Kuhl H, et al. Analysis of myocardial deformation based on pixel tracking in two dimensional echocardiographic images enables quantitative assessment of regional left ventricular function. Heart 2005;92:1102–8.

147. Reisner S, Lysyansky P, Agmon Y, et al. Global longitudinal strain: a novel index of left ventricular systolic function. J Am Soc Echocardiogr 2004; 17:630–3.

148. Suffoletto MS, Dohi K, Cannesson M, et al. Novel speckle-tracking radial strain from routine black-and-white echocardiographic images to quantify dyssynchrony and predict response to cardiac resynchronization therapy. Circulation 2006;113: 960–8.

149. Chen H, Varghese T, Rahko PS, et al. Ultrasound frame rate requirements for cardiac elastography: experimental and in vivo results. Ultrasonics 2009;49:98–111.

150. Lee WN, Qian Z, Tosti CL, et al. Preliminary validation of angle-independent myocardial elastography using MR tagging in a clinical setting. Ultrasound Med Biol 2008;34:1980–97.

151. Sandrin L, Fourquet B, Hasquenoph JM, et al. Transient elastography: a new noninvasive method for assessment of hepatic fibrosis. Ultrasound Med Biol 2003;29:1705–13.

152. Ophir J, Alam SK, Garra B, et al. Elastography: ultrasonic estimation and imaging of the elastic properties of tissues. Proc Inst Mech Eng H 1999; 213:203–33.

153. Parker KJ, Taylor LS, Gracewski SM, et al. A unified view of imaging the elastic properties of tissue. J Acoust Soc Am 2005;117:2705–12.

154. Garra BS. Imaging and estimation of tissue elasticity by ultrasound. Ultrasound Q 2007;23:255–68.

155. Greenleaf JF, Fatemi M, Insana MF. Selected methods for imaging elastic properties of biological tissues. Annu Rev Biomed Eng 2003;5: 57–78.

156. Hall TJ. AAPM/RSNA physics tutorial for residents: topics in US: beyond the basics: elasticity imaging with US. Radiographics 2003;23:1657–71.

Contrast-enhanced Ultrasound: Past, Present, and Future

Michele Bertolotto, MD[a],*, Orlando Catalano, MD[b]

KEYWORDS

• Contrast media • Microbubbles • Ultrasound • Liver

The introduction of ultrasound contrast agents (UCAs) is the major advance in sonographic imaging since the development of Doppler techniques. Various clinical applications have been introduced or at least suggested for contrast-enhanced ultrasound (CEUS), in radiological and cardiologic imaging. Nevertheless, the commercialization of various UCAs in different countries and the development of several scanning technologies have created confusion, with a consistent need for standardization of methodology and terminology.[1]

This article reviews the historical and physical basis of CEUS, then illustrates the hepatic and extrahepatic applications, and finally discusses the major forthcoming developments.

HISTORICAL PERSPECTIVE

Attempts to use pharmacologic agents have come together with the application of sonographic beams to diagnostic imaging. In the 1960s cardiologists were still trying to detect right-to-left heart shunts by administering a substance intravenously (which was unable to pass the pulmonary filter) and recognizing its presence within the left cardiac chambers. Transpulmonary agents (3–5 μm diameter), capable of passing into the main circulation to reach all body parenchymas, were developed only in the 1990s.[2] These UCAs, the so-called first generation, consisted of air encapsulated within a tiny supporting shell (proteic, lipidic, or polymeric) (ie, microbubbles). First-generation UCAs

were mostly used to improve the Doppler signal from vessels of large to intermediate diameter, allowing increased detection of arteries and veins, greater depiction of their course and relationships, and improved demonstration of their luminal abnormalities.[3] As an example, a difficult Doppler differentiation between obstruction and near-obstructive stenosis could be obtained with greater confidence by injecting a UCA. Also for nodules and masses, contrast-enhanced power and color Doppler techniques allowed depiction of more slow-flow, small-caliber vessels with an improved display of the angioarchitecture and with more data available for tumor characterization. A benefit was the lack of alteration of the flow velocity at spectral analysis performed after UCA injection.[4]

Nevertheless, especially if injected as a bolus, UCAs caused signal artifacts, particularly the over-amplification artifact called blooming, which could cause signal noise interference with lesion assessment. In addition, first-generation UCAs were substantially unable to demonstrate signal from small vessels located within tumors. To depict intratumoral microcirculation, the blood should have an adequate intensity and speed. By using a UCA it is possible to increase the signal intensity but it is not possible to improve the flow velocity.

In the subsequent decade the sensitivity of Doppler scanners for slow flows improved and the need for signal enhancement decreased. Consequently, researchers' interest returned to gray-scale applications.[5–7] Various technologies

[a] Department of Radiology, University of Trieste, Ospedale di Cattinara, Strada di Fiume 449, I-34149, Trieste, Italy
[b] Department of Radiology, National Cancer Institute "Fondazione G.Pascale," via M.Semmola, I-80131, Naples, Italy
* Corresponding author.
E-mail address: bertolot@units.it (M. Bertolotto).

Ultrasound Clin 4 (2009) 339–367
doi:10.1016/j.cult.2009.10.011

were introduced by manufacturers, allowing determination of a beam-induced rupture of the microbubbles and recording of the subsequent high intensity, broad-band signal. These high mechanical index (MI >0.2), gray-scale techniques provided intermittent images during the various phases of UCA circulation, similar to multiphase computed tomography (CT) and magnetic resonance imaging (MRI). High MI CEUS allowed a fine depiction of tumor perfusion, detecting signals from small vessels.

The use of high-intensity flashes necessary for microbubble rupture caused consumption of microbubbles ("destructive" CEUS) and was substantially incompatible with real-time scanning, a fundamental aspect of modern US imaging. This incompatibility was overcome by the development of the so-called second generation of UCAs.[8,9] The new microbubbles were filled with injectable gases other than air, which improved stability and elasticity (Table 1). Second-generation UCAs could still be used with high MI technologies but, if stimulated by a low-power beam (MI <0.2), these microbubbles could also produce a detectable perfusion signal (whereas in the same conditions first-generation UCAs fail to determine any relevant change).[10]

Low MI imaging, based on microbubble oscillation without destruction, allows a real-time, gray-scale display of the organ enhancement. This display is because second-generation UCAs oscillate at a frequency of 2 to 3 MHz, which is around the frequency employed in diagnostic US, particularly for the abdomen (this also explains why CEUS exploration of superficial structures has a poorer image quality).[11] When the beam power is set low enough, the microbubble works by resonance, rapidly contracting and expanding in response to the pressure changes of the sound wave. When microbubbles are insonated by a beam of appropriate power and frequency, the oscillation becomes nonlinear (ie, the diameter in the rarefaction phase of the acoustic cycle largely exceeds its compression in the pressure phase). The asymmetric oscillations result in nonlinear echoes containing overtones, or harmonics, of the driving frequency. This phenomenon makes the "nondestructive" contrast-specific imaging in real time possible.[12]

CEUS requires contrast-specific software, suppressing the static signal from background tissues and highlighting the signal from circulating microbubbles. This result is obtained in various modalities. In pulse inversion technique 2 pulses are sent along each scan line, the second being the mirror of the first. Both echoes are summed by the transducer, with no significant signal produced by static, linear reflectors such as the background tissues (sum of the 2 echoes equal to zero) and with intense signals arising from nonlinear reflectors such as the microbubbles (sum of the 2 echoes different from zero).[13–15]

Low MI real-time, gray-scale US is currently the standard procedure based on UCAs and is

Table 1
UCAs available for clinical use in European Union (EU), USA, and other countries. Generic names are given in parentheses

Product Name	Chemical Nature	Availability
Imagent (AF0150)	Perfluorohexane and nitrogen gas in stabilized microbubbles	USA, EU
SonoVue (BR1)	Sulfur hexafluoride gas in polymer with phospholipids	EU, several Asian countries excluding Japan
Definity (ImaRx)	Perflutren lipid microsphere injectable suspension	Canada
Albunex	Air-filled protein shell	USA
Optison (FSO 69)	Perflutren protein-type A microspheres	USA, EU
Echovist (SHU 454)	Galactose-based gas bubbles	EU
Levovist (SHU 508A)	Galactose-based, palmitic acid-stabilized microbubbles	EU, Canada, Japan
Echogen (QW3600)	Dodecafluoropentane in a sucrose solution	EU
Sonazoid (DD723/NC100100)	Perflubutane-based microbubbles	Japan

probably the only one to which the acronym CEUS should be applied.[1,15]

GENERAL ASPECTS

UCAs are now routinely employed in most European and Eastern Asian countries, at least in the main universities and hospitals, although a real capillary spread is still missing. In the United States there is still no approval from the Food and Drug Administration for radiological use, and use is restricted to some cardiological applications.[15]

UCAs are significantly different from CT and MR contrast media. UCAs are intravascular ("blood pool") substances, lacking an interstitial spread; their half-life in blood is typically a few minutes.[11,14] Consequently, CEUS findings overlap CT and MR findings during arterial-phase imaging but diverge when moving to the venous phase.[16] Whereas UCAs recirculate several times until their dissolution, CT and MRI contrast media (being significantly smaller than UCAs) permeate the vessel wall and spread to the interstitium. Because of the lack of an extravascular diffusion, UCAs theoretically fit perfectly as functional traces of organ circulation. Another difference with CT and MR contrast media is that UCAs are modified by the scanning beam, although this does not happen for radiographs or radiofrequencies. The scanning energy itself modifies the microbubbles employed in US but not the contrast media employed for CT and MR imaging (to complicate the problem, each UCA behaves differently when stimulated by ultrasound beams of different MI).[17] A final major difference relates to the imaging phases. Whereas the scanning phases for CT and MRI are intended at the peak of enhancement for each phase, the same does not apply to CEUS. The arterial phase of CEUS starts at the moment of arrival of microbubbles within the arterial pedicle of the scanned organ (10–15 seconds after intravenous [IV] injection) and lasts up to about 40 seconds, when the venous phase becomes prevalent. The venous and late phase lasts from 3 to 6 minutes, depending on the scanned parenchyma (see later discussion). Because of the real-time capabilities of low MI CEUS, the organ of interest is continuously scanned during each contrast phase. Incorrect timing of CT or MR acquisition phases may result in missed detection of focal lesions or in incorrect/impossible characterization, whereas CEUS allows continuous depiction of the lesion through all vascular phases. Some first- and second-generation UCAs show a more or less pronounced postvascular phase, being retained within the liver

and, even more, within the spleen.[18] This is the so-called postvascular or parenchymal phase, which follows the vascular phase.[19,20]

The kidneys show the most rapid, intense, and transient (as a consequence of lacking glomerular filtration) enhancement after IV UCA injection, whereas the spleen has a strong but persistent enhancement (up to 6–8 minutes). The liver and the pancreas behave intermediately, with a progressive and persistent intensity enhancement. Because of the dual vascular supply of the liver, the hepatic phases after the arterial phase include the portal phase (40–120 seconds after contrast injection) and the sinusoidal (or late) phase (120–300 seconds after contrast injection).[21] Whenever there is a need for multiorgan exploration (for example, trauma imaging), the kidney or kidneys should be imaged first, the pancreas or liver next, and the spleen last (also considering that the early-phase inhomogeneous enhancement of the spleen [similar to the "zebra pattern" from CT and MR] may cause an incorrect image interpretation).

UCAs are flexible and well-tolerated tools, and serious reactions are rarely reported. In a retrospective review of European experience on the use of the second-generation UCA SonoVue (Bracco International BV, Amsterdam, The Netherlands) there were only 2 serious adverse events and no deaths among 23,188 patients investigated.[22] Nevertheless, allergy toward contrast medium constituents or other addicted substances should always be considered. There is no special need for starving or for preliminary laboratory testing. Because there is no renal excretion, UCAs can be safely employed in patients with acute or chronic renal insufficiency. Whenever necessary, the small volume of the UCA can be injected again, to clarify an area that was initially unclear or to scan multiple organs. The volume can also be fractioned, to evaluate the arterial-phase behavior of different organs or of multiple lesions in different locations in an organ. Nevertheless, even with these expedients, CEUS lacks the panoramic quality typical of CT and MRI and does not allow a complete abdominal survey. In addition, UCAs do not usually allow the rescue of a nondiagnostic US examination. Difficult patients, such as those who are meteoric, are also difficult to scan with CEUS. It can be difficult to explore fully patients with severe steatosis or fibrosis, because the hepatic penetration of the ultrasound beam is limited.

The need for adequate training of the operator should be considered. In addition, CEUS requires scanners fitted with specific software. Many kinds of probe are available for CEUS, including transcutaneous transducers for abdominal and superficial structures, transvaginal and transrectal transducers, endoscopic transducers, intravascular transducers, and transducers for intraoperative CEUS. Maximum intensity projection images allow tracking of the course of the microbubbles with exquisite depiction of the morphology of the vessels.[15] Valuable contrast-enhanced 3-dimensional and extended field of view images can also be obtained.[20]

At CEUS imaging the baseline background is substantially cleaned, given the absence of significant harmonic signal for tissues at low MI, and only the signal coming from circulating microbubbles is detected. The intrinsic echogenicity of a focal lesion on baseline US does not significantly interfere with the diagnostic performance of CEUS.[23] In addition, different from CT, the echogenicity of the parenchyma surrounding the lesion does not significantly affect the diagnostic accuracy of CEUS.[24] For example, a focal lesion on a bright liver background can be characterized with the same effectiveness as a lesion within a nonsteatosic parenchyma.[21]

CEUS should be intended first as a completion of US examination, which provides additional data not achievable with baseline US. In the authors' practice, when a liver lesion is found indeterminate at US, a CEUS is immediately performed, allowing in most cases a definitive diagnosis and avoiding more sophisticated and expensive imaging modalities. This practice is possible because US is employed in Italy as the initial imaging modality in the work-up of most abdominal clinical issues. In other countries, where CT and MR are performed initially, there is probably less potential for CEUS. In addition to improving an inconclusive US examination, CEUS can act as a problem-solving modality. Frequently, when (or their referring physicians) a discrepancy is found between 2 imaging modalities (eg, CT, MR, or positron emission tomography [PET]) the authors try to solve the problem using CEUS (sometimes immediately, without scheduling the examination). Typical scenarios include discrepancy between a CT study negative for focal liver lesions (FLLs) and a PET study showing some focal uptake; an FLL not adequately characterized with CT because of lack of multiphasic acquisition or because the lesion is smaller than a centimeter; or nonspecific PET uptake within a given organ.

Liver

CEUS is now well established in liver imaging; it has been standardized, it is reproducible, and it relies on defined diagnostic criteria and simple algorithms.[25] CEUS possibilities and limitations are adequately understood, and guidelines for the use of contrast agents in liver ultrasound were published by the European Federation of Societies for Ultrasound in Medicine and Biology in 2004 and in 2008 (also including other organs).[26,27]

Characterization of FLLs

The capability of US in lesion characterization is low. A significant overlap exists between the echo pattern and vascularity of benign and malignant FLLs, and a wide range of accuracy percentages has been reported for gray-scale and color Doppler analysis. Using CEUS, FLLs can be characterized accurately, following diagnostic criteria similar to dynamic CT and MR. By knowing the typical perfusion model of each liver lesion through the various vascular phases it is possible to differentiate it adequately. The characterization ability of CEUS is not significantly affected by the lesion diameter. Benign lesions display a significant contrast enhancement during the portal and sinusoidal phase, appearing as isoechoic or hyperechoic, whereas during the same phases malignant lesions appear as hypoechoic, because of contrast washout.[15,25] However, several exceptions exist: poorly vascularized benign lesions such as macroregenerative nodules, thrombosed or fibrotic hemangiomas, and inflammatory or necrotic lesions may appear hypoechoic in the portal-sinusoidal phase, mimicking malignancy. On the other hand well-differentiated hepatocellular carcinomas (HCCs) can display significant enhancement during the portal and sinusoidal phase. Patient history, clinics, and the appearance of CEUS in the arterial phase may help in the differential diagnosis.

About 80% of liver hemangiomas reveal a globular enhancement (**Fig. 1**) during the arterial phase (peripheral enhancing globes whose size increases progressively) and a centripetal filling-in during the portal-sinusoidal phase.[28] In high-flow hemangiomas the globes merge rapidly into a homogeneously hyperechoic lesion (**Fig. 2**). Some hemangiomas that fill slowly do not show a significant central enhancement in the portal and late phase but their characterization is adequate because of globular enhancement. A small percentage of hemangiomas present with a fair or absent contrast enhancement caused by extensive thrombosis or fibrotic changes and cannot be adequately diagnosed.[28] CEUS was able to characterize 88% of liver hemangiomas with an atypical US appearance.[29]

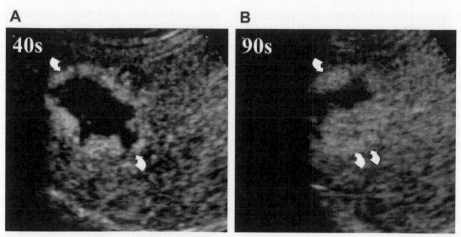

Fig. 1. Typical appearance of liver hemangioma (*arrows*). CEUS shows globular peripheral enhancement 40 seconds after microbubble injection (*A*) and progressive, centripetal fill-in after 90 seconds (*B*). The central portion of the lesions remains unenhanced because of incomplete filling in.

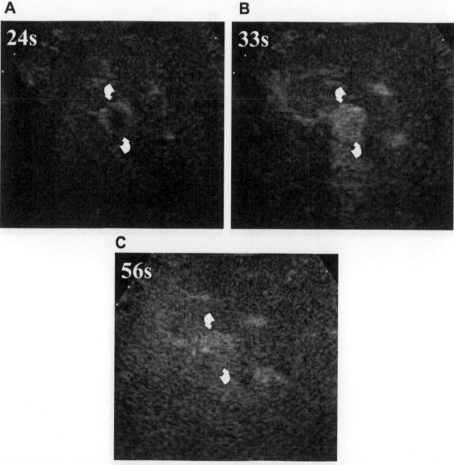

Fig. 2. High flow hemangioma (*arrows*). Images obtained during the arterial phase at 24 seconds (*A*) and 33 seconds (*B*) from microbubble injection show globular peripheral enhancement early after microbubble arrival (*A*) with complete centripetal fill-in within 9 seconds (*B*). The lesion is isoechoic to the liver 56 seconds after the injection (*C*).

The US appearance of focal nodular hyperplasia (FNH) is not specific, although color Doppler US allows effective characterization in up to 80% of cases by demonstrating a central arterial vessel radiating toward the periphery of the lesion.[30] FNH enhances rapidly from the center toward the periphery, and its appearance changes repeatedly within a few seconds.[28] The central feeding artery and the radial branches can be exquisitely appreciated during the early arterial phase, because of the real-time capabilities of CEUS (**Fig. 3**). During the portal-late phase the lesion appears homogeneously hyperechoic or isoechoic to the liver, except for evidence of a hypoechoic central scar (about 25% of cases during the sinusoidal phase).

Hepatic adenoma (**Fig. 4**) enhances markedly and centripetally during the early arterial phase, appearing as hyperechoic compared with the surrounding liver, and then becoming isoechoic, slightly hypoechoic, or slightly hyperechoic during the portal and late phase.[28,31] The enhancement of small adenomas is usually homogeneous, whereas larger lesions show a heterogeneous contrast enhancement caused by nonenhancing hemorrhagic and necrotic areas. The absence of a central feeding artery and the presence of nonenhancing areas can aid in the differential diagnosis between adenoma and FNH, although there is some overlap for small lesions.

Metastases have a blood supply from neoangiogenic arterial vessels, with little or no portal contribution. The arterial enhancement reflects the degree of tumor angiogenesis, with some lesions appearing as hypervascular and others as hypovascular. The metastatic lesion can enhance in a diffuse and homogeneous or heterogeneous manner (**Fig. 5**) or can show some central,

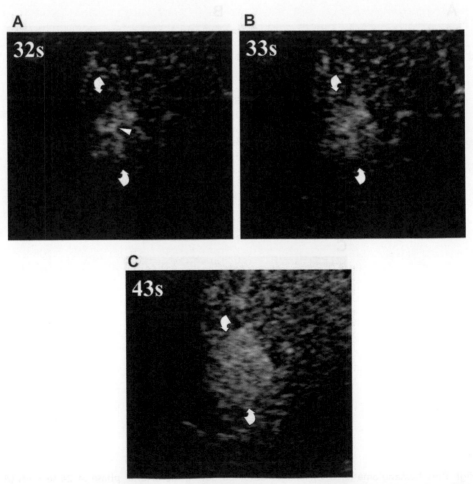

Fig. 3. FNH. (*A*) The central feeding artery (*arrowhead*) of the nodule (*curved arrows*) is seen branching toward the periphery 32 seconds after microbubble injection. Within 1 second, the enhancement progresses from the center to the periphery (*B*). Complete homogeneous enhancement is seen within 10 seconds (*C*).

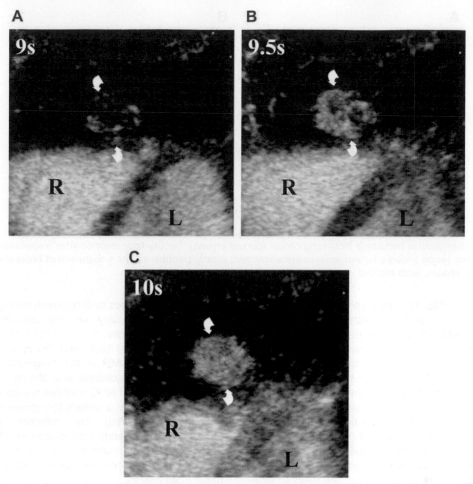

Fig. 4. Hepatic adenoma (*curved arrows*). Peripheral feeding arteries are seen 9 seconds after microbubble injection (A). The enhancement progresses centripetally with complete fill-in of the nodule within 1 second (B, C). R and L, right and left heart ventricles.

nonenhancing necrotic areas; frequently a typical continuous rimlike enhancement of varying size (**Fig. 6**) can be appreciated around the lesion.[5,28] The arterial-dependent enhancement can be transient, and CEUS detects significantly more hypervascularized lesions in comparison with CT and MR, which are not real-time techniques. A perilesional enhancement can be appreciated around the lesion that usually persists for 30 to 60 seconds and disappears during the late phase; this is caused by peritumoral desmoplastic reaction, inflammatory cell infiltration, and vascular proliferation. Typically, liver metastases wash out rapidly, during the arterial phase. At the beginning of the portal phase the lesion enhancement fades and nearly all metastases become increasingly hypoechoic in comparison with the surrounding enhanced parenchyma, with more or less evident

dots (pullulating at real-time assessment), which are considered to express the tumor "microcirculation."[5,28] In the proper clinical setting a hypoperfused lesion in the portal-sinusoidal phase is considered metastasic until proven otherwise, despite its hypervascular or hypovascular appearance during the arterial phase.

The enhancement of intrahepatic cholangiocellular carcinoma is similar to that of hypovascular metastasis; the tumor usually presents with a dotted enhancement of variable intensity during the arterial phase and appears hypoechoic during the portal and late phase. Perilesional enhancement can also be observed, especially in larger nodules.[32]

HCC is typically a hypervascularized tumor. The peripheral feeding vessels are frequently appreciable in the early arterial phase branching toward the center of the lesion with a basketlike

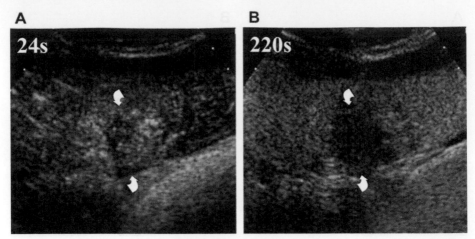

Fig. 5. Hypervascular metastasis from lung cancer (*curved arrows*). Twenty-four seconds after microbubble injection (*A*) the lesion shows a heterogeneous enhancement, mostly peripheral. The enhancement fades during the following phases, with marked washout at 220 seconds (*B*).

distribution (**Fig. 7**). Tumor enhancement immediately follows, which is typically diffuse, intense, and transient. The enhancement of small nodules is usually homogeneous, whereas larger nodules are usually heterogeneous because of necrotic changes. Progressive washout is observed during the portal and late phase, being typically slower, less marked, and less complete than in metastasis (**Fig. 8**). In comparison with the surrounding liver parenchyma, around 60% of HCCs appear as hypoechoic during the portal-sinusoidal phase, whereas 40% of HCCs, particularly those that are small or well differentiated, are seen as isoechoic.[28] This behavior is different from that seen with CT and MR, in which most of the HCC nodules appear as hyperenhancing on the arterial-phase images and hypoenhancing on the portal- and especially on the delayed-phase images; consequently, the accuracy of CEUS in characterizing small HCC nodules is lower than that with CT and MR (if the diagnostic criteria from published guidelines are strictly applied). About 2% to 3% of HCC nodules are poorly vascularized and show a dotted low-grade contrast enhancement during the different vascular phases.[28,33] HCC-related malignant thrombi within the portal vein typically enhance in the arterial phase, whereas cirrhosis-related benign thrombosis does not.[34]

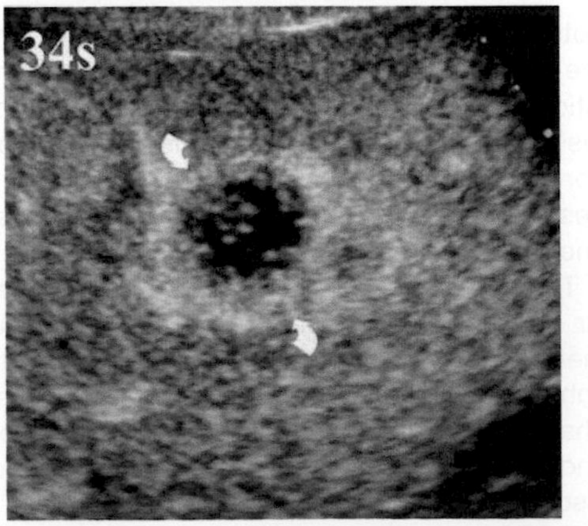

Focal fatty spared areas and focal fatty areas are frequently encountered in hepatic steatosis. Questionable skip areas and focal fatty changes can be easily characterized with CEUS. Unlike liver nodules, these pseudolesions enhance with a speed and intensity equal to the surrounding liver, becoming indistinguishable from it (isoenhanced) through all vascular phases.[28]

Liver abscesses usually appear at US as inhomogeneous and slightly hypoechoic, with ill-defined margins. After microbubble injection the lesion itself and its internal structure are more conspicuous. Typically, the periphery enhances, whereas nonenhancing internal areas correspond to necrotic, liquefied zones. Multiloculated abscesses are characterized by enhancing septa with an overall honeycomb pattern.[35]

CEUS can be helpful in demonstrating the true nature of solid-looking hepatic cysts at conventional US and in differentiating cystic liver metastases from complex benign cysts.[36] Most benign complex cysts show absent enhancement or enhancement through all vascular phases, whereas malignant cysts show a washout during

Fig. 6. Hypovascular metastasis from urinary bladder cancer (*arrows*). Arterial-phase scan showing a rimlike enhancement around the lesion and few spots internally.

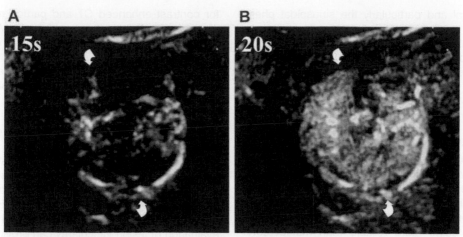

Fig. 7. HCC in a cirrhotic patient (*arrows*). Peripheral feeding arteries are seen during the early arterial phase, 15 seconds after microbubble injection (*A*). This is followed within 5 seconds by an intense and heterogeneous enhancement of the entire lesion (*B*).

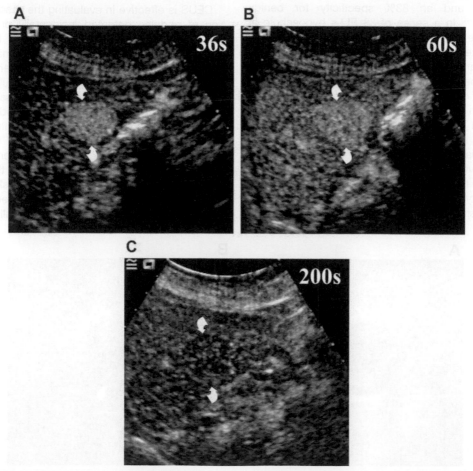

Fig. 8. HCC in a cirrhotic patient (*arrows*). The lesion shows a homogeneous contrast enhancement during the arterial phase (*A*) which persists through the portal phase (*B*). During the late phase (*C*) the lesion is nearly isoechoic to liver.

the portal and particularly the sinusoidal phase (**Fig. 9**).

All studies comparing the diagnostic performance of US and CEUS conclude that the latter improves the characterization of FLLs. The number of correct diagnoses increases from 60%–65% to 86%–95% after contrast injection, and the differentiation between malignant and benign lesions improves from 23%–68% to 92%–95%.[5,37,38] In a French prospective multicenter study of 874 patients with 1034 nodules not fully characterized by conventional US or previous single-phase CT scans, CEUS yielded a sensitivity of 79% and a specificity of 88% in the differentiation between benign and malignant lesions, being more reliable than multidetector CT (MDCT) and MRI in on-site and off-site interobserver agreement.[39] In a German multicenter trial of 1349 patients with a hepatic lesion lacking a definite diagnosis based on conventional US and power Doppler, CEUS showed a 90% overall accuracy, with a 96% sensitivity for malignant lesions and an 83% specificity for benign lesions.[40] In a series of 88 FLLs hypoechoic at baseline US,[41] CEUS was accurate in definitively characterizing 81% of benign lesions and 88% of malignant lesions, and allowed a differential diagnosis between benign and malignant lesions in 95% of cases.

Given the high specificity, use of CEUS can allow a decrease in the number of liver biopsy and of second-level CT and MR examinations, particularly for lesions with a benign pattern. In an activity-based cost analysis study CEUS was shown to be the least expensive second-level modality after baseline US for diagnosis of benign liver lesions.[42] CEUS costs are lower than those for contrast-enhanced CT and particularly lower than those for contrast-enhanced MRI.[39] A CEUS-based algorithm for FLLs indeterminate at unenhanced US is more cost-effective than an algorithm relying on CT or MR. An Italian multicenter study showed CEUS to be cost-saving for the health system and for the hospital.[38]

Detection of nodules in patients with chronic liver disease

The development of an HCC is the most serious complication of liver fibrosis and cirrhosis. US is commonly regarded as the imaging modality of choice for HCC screening because of low cost, availability, and noninvasiveness.[43] Color Doppler evaluation of lesion vascularity can provide useful information, because HCC is usually hypervascularized with a prevalence of peripheral arterial flows. However, using conventional US techniques a high percentage of FLLs detected in a patient with chronic liver disease cannot be reliably characterized.

CEUS is effective in evaluating the vascularization of nodules detected incidentally or during surveillance in the cirrhotic liver.[43,44] Hepatic carcinogenesis is a multistep process characterized by development of large benign regenerating nodules that evolve in dysplastic nodules and eventually in HCC. This process is associated with progressively decreased portal blood supply and increased neoangiogenic arterial flow.[45,46] About 80% of benign regenerative nodules present with persistent dotted contrast enhancement and hypoechoic appearance during the arterial phase, followed by an enhancement similar to the adjacent liver parenchyma. The remaining 20% of benign nodules, which usually have

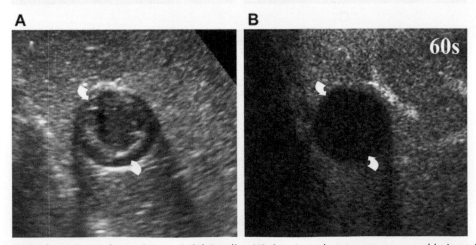

Fig. 9. Complex hepatic cyst (*curved arrows*). (*A*) Baseline US showing a heterogeneous round lesion with well-defined margins but no defined posterior enhancement. (*B*) After microbubble injection the lesion does not enhance in all vascular phases.

a dysplastic pattern on histologic analysis, cannot be differentiated from HCCs.[28] When an FLL is detected by US in a patient with chronic liver disease, CEUS can be performed, distinguishing in most cases between a premalignant and a malignant nodule, although some overlap exists.

CEUS has a limited value in staging patients with a known HCC, and CT or MR should always follow to depict the disease extent adequately and particularly to exclude other nodules.[43] Although most lesions that are visible in US can be characterized effectively by their hypervascular pattern during the arterial phase, as many as 40% of them are barely visible during the portal and late phase. Consequently, because exploring the entire liver parenchyma during the short arterial phase duration is not possible, there is always a need for further staging.

Detection of metastases in patients with extrahepatic malignancies

Gray-scale and color Doppler US have a limited accuracy, because isoechoic metastases and subcentimetral metastases are difficult to detect. In addition, nonmetastatic lesions can occasionally be found in patients who have cancer, and their appropriate characterization is mandatory. CEUS overcomes many limitations of conventional US in detection and characterization of FLLs in the oncologic patient.

When microbubbles are used with the low MI modality, the liver can be continuously explored for up to 4 to 5 minutes from the bolus injection. Virtually all metastases appear as hypoechoic in comparison with the surrounding parenchyma during the portal and delayed phase after microbubble injection, and consequently there is

enough time for a careful search of these lesions (**Fig. 10**). If the liver can be adequately scanned through all its portions CEUS is as effective as CT and MR in detecting metastasis.

Quaia and colleagues[47] evaluated 345 lesions using a first-generation UCA and destructive modes, and 261 lesions using a second-generation UCA and nondestructive modes. Microbubbles markedly enhanced the sensitivity for the number of detected lesions using both CEUS approaches, from 40% and 46% to 83% and 87%, respectively, whereas no statistically significant differences were found between the diagnostic performance of CEUS approaches and CT. Konopke and colleagues[48] evaluated 100 patients with suspected liver lesions before laparotomy and found that UCA injection improved the US sensitivity for the number of detected lesions from 53% to 86%, whereas CT reached a 76% sensitivity. Oldenburg and colleagues[49] evaluated 40 patients with a known malignancy and with at least 1 liver lesion visible on baseline US. Injection of the UCA enhanced the sensitivity of US for lesion detection, compared with reference procedures, from 69% to 90%. Moreover, CEUS showed 13 lesions not seen on the reference imaging.

The cost of generalized use of microbubbles to exclude liver metastases in all patients with a previous or actual extrahepatic cancer is probably excessive. It is necessary to identify subpopulations of patients who may receive a clinical benefit from this approach. For example, patients undergoing surgical or interventional procedures for liver metastasis may benefit from a combined CT and CEUS approach, because assessment of metastatic disease must be as accurate as possible in these patients to avoid inappropriate treatments.

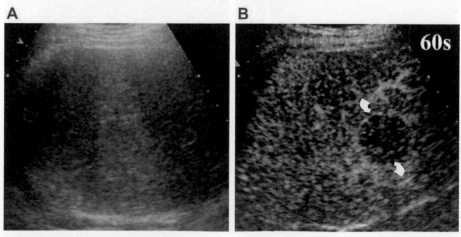

Fig. 10. Metastasis from colon cancer. The lesion is not visible at baseline US (*A*) whereas it is well recognizable 60 seconds after microbubble administration (*B, arrows*).

Assessment of treated liver lesions

CEUS is useful for increasing lesion conspicuity and consequently guiding the diagnostic and therapeutic puncture of FLLs when they are barely appreciable on unenhanced US.[50,51]

Percutaneous ablation has become a widespread technique for the treatment of unresectable liver tumors, particularly HCC and colorectal cancer metastasis. In these cases, posttreatment assessment is important, because detection of residual, viable tumor tissue usually indicates the need for retreatment. CT and MR are commonly used for the assessment of ablation response. A recent study, however, demonstrated that CEUS is as effective as CT in detecting residual or recurrent tumor following ablation therapy.[52] In some institutions CEUS is employed during the ablation procedure itself, to demonstrate immediately the completeness of the treatment. In other institutions CEUS is employed a few days after ablation (**Fig. 11**), to detect a residual tumor early and consequently to plan for retreatment. CEUS is particularly helpful in guiding the targeted ablation of residual or recurrent tumor tissue within necrotic nodules.[53]

CEUS has proven useful in the early assessment of therapeutic effect after intra-arterial transcatheter chemoembolization.[54] CT has been widely used to evaluate these patients but it requires a minimum 15 to 20 days' interval and can be difficult because of oily-agent related artifacts. Together with MR, CEUS is a useful alternative.

Another major indication to CEUS is follow-up of patients undergoing systemic chemotherapy, with conventional agents.[55] CEUS could be particularly useful when using drugs that inhibit tumor angiogenesis. In these patients, the antiangiogenic agents are expected to produce a reduced lesion vascularity that can be recognized with CEUS but not with unenhanced US.[56–59] The lesions treated with antiangiogenic drugs decrease in size slowly, but CEUS can already demonstrate a diminished vascularization a few days after treatment, allowing an early differentiation between responding and nonresponding patients.

Kidney

CEUS of the kidney is an emerging field for UCAs. Microbubbles can be injected without regard for renal function, and the intense enhancement of the renal parenchyma makes it easy to detect hypoperfused lesions such as infarctions or hemorrhages.

Renal ischemia

Doppler US is the first-line imaging modality to detect renal perfusion defects but it has clear limitations because of insensitivity to low-velocity and low-amplitude flows. CEUS has been found effective for depicting focal renal perfusion defects in experimental studies,[60–62] and recent investigations show a diagnostic performance to detect renal ischemia approaching that of contrast-enhanced CT.[63] Moreover, the excellent spatial resolution of CEUS allows an effective differential diagnosis between renal infarction and acute cortical necrosis, which appears as nonenhancing cortical areas with preserved hilar vascularity (**Fig. 12**).

Another important application of CEUS in patients with renal ischemia is differentiation between nonperfused, infarcted areas

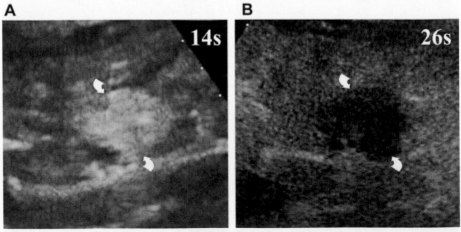

Fig. 11. HCC nodule (*arrows*) treated with radiofrequency ablation. The lesion shows an intense and homogeneous enhancement (*A*, scan obtained 14 seconds from contrast injection) before the treatment whereas it appears completely avascular (*B*, scan obtained 26 seconds after contrast injection) in the CEUS study performed 25 days after percutaneous radiofrequency ablation.

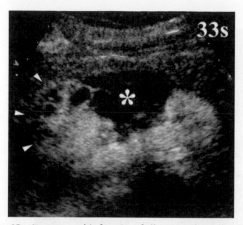

Fig. 12. Acute renal infarction following thromboembolism in a patient with atrial fibrillation. Thirty-three seconds after microbubble injection CEUS reveals a wedge-shaped nonenhancing area (*) in the middle portion of the kidney. Small, nonenhancing cortical areas (*arrowheads*) are also recognizable in the upper pole of the kidney consistent with other regions of cortical infarction.

(irreversible) and hypoperfused parenchymal regions (reversible). Both these conditions appear at color Doppler interrogation as areas lacking color signal, but only infarcted areas lack contrast enhancement after UCA injection.[64]

Solid renal lesions and pseudotumors
After microbubble injection solid renal tumors show diffuse, homogeneous or heterogeneous contrast enhancement during the early corticomedullary phase, often with a hypervascular appearance, and have a variable contrast enhancement in the remaining phases, generally similar to normal renal parenchyma.[65–67] The enhancement is limited to the solid viable regions, sparing intratumoral avascular necrotic, hemorrhagic, or cystic components. Some lesions, usually papillary or chromophobe tumors but also metastases and approximately 13% of clear cell carcinomas, enhance less than the surrounding parenchyma in all vascular phases (**Fig. 13**). Because enhancement of many renal tumors is similar to that of renal parenchyma in most vascular phases, the detection rate of small tumors is unlikely to be much improved by contrast injection.

Ascenti and colleagues[68] suggest that CEUS is effective for visualizing the tumor pseudocapsule, which appears after microbubble injection as a rim of perilesional enhancement increasing in the latter phase of the examination.

Whatever the degree of vascularization, the vascular pattern of renal tumors is different from that of renal parenchyma. This difference could be helpful for differentiating normal variants from real focal lesions (**Fig. 14**).[66,69]

Preliminary investigations suggest that CEUS is more sensitive than contrast-enhanced CT in detecting blood flow in hypovascularized lesions.[66,70] Tamai and colleagues[71] demonstrated enhancement in 5 hypovascular renal tumors with an equivocal enhancement on contrast-enhanced CT.

CEUS has limitations: deep lesion location, bowel gas interposition, and presence of wall

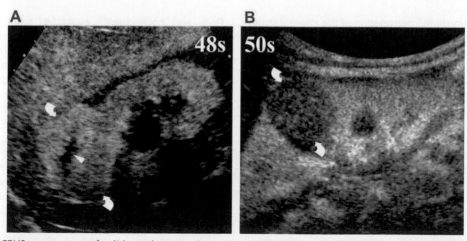

Fig. 13. CEUS appearance of solid renal tumors (*curved arrows*). Images obtained 48 seconds (*A*) and 50 seconds (*B*) after microbubble injection, respectively. (*A*) Clear-cell carcinoma showing intense enhancement and central, necrotic nonenhancing area (*arrowhead*). (*B*) Cromophobe tumor enhancing less than the adjacent renal parenchyma.

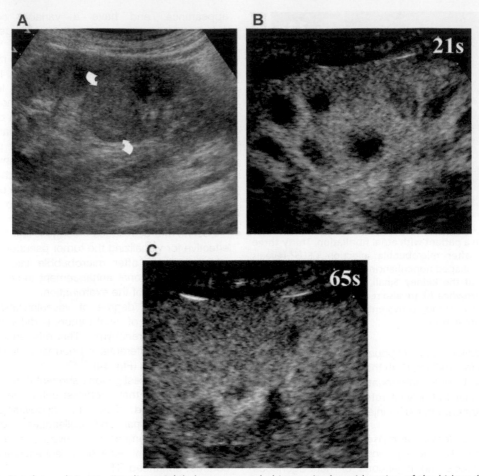

Fig. 14. Renal pseudotumor. Baseline US (*A*) shows a rounded image in the midportion of the kidney (*arrows*), suggesting renal mass. CEUS shows that the image displays enhancement characteristics identical to the other portions of the renal parenchyma 21 seconds (*B*) and 65 seconds (*C*) after microbubble injection, revealing that it is a pseudomass.

calcification limit interrogation of the internal structure, and large size prevents full evaluation of the mass.

Cystic renal lesions

The sensitivity of CEUS in detecting flow in hypovascular renal lesions allows an adequate differential diagnosis between solid tumors and atypical cystic masses. CEUS allows characterization of renal cystic lesions as benign or malignant with at least the same diagnostic accuracy as contrast-enhanced CT (**Fig. 15**).[66,67,72] Quaia and colleagues[73] analyzed a series of 40 consecutive complex cystic renal masses. Three blinded readers found an overall diagnostic accuracy (80%–83%) of CEUS better than CT in the diagnosis of malignancy. In particular, CEUS was more sensitive than CT in detecting enhancement of the cystic wall, septa, and solid components.

Park and colleagues[67] evaluated with CT and CEUS 31 pathologically confirmed cystic renal masses using the Bosniak classification. The diagnostic accuracies of CEUS and CT for malignancy were 74% and 90%, respectively. In 26% of lesions there were differences in the Bosniak score that were upgraded by CEUS. Moreover, for 6 lesions, solid components were detected by CEUS but not by CT. Ascenti and colleagues[74] compared prospectively 40 consecutive cystic renal masses with CEUS and CT using the Bosniak system. For CEUS and CT, the interobserver agreement was high, and a complete concordance was observed between CEUS and CT in the differentiation of surgical and nonsurgical cysts.

CEUS should be used to characterize renal masses with a complex cystic appearance, provided that the lesion can be explored adequately. CT is still necessary for staging

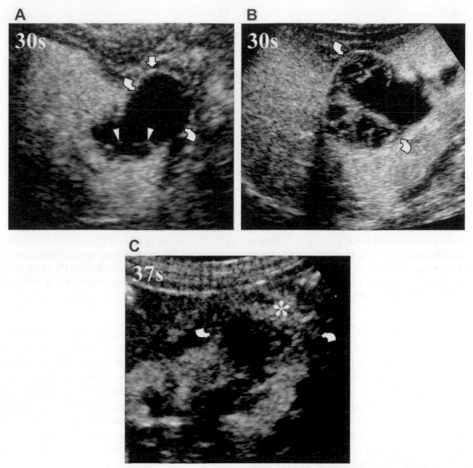

Fig. 15. CEUS characterization of cystic renal lesions (*curved arrows*) in 3 different patients. (*A*) Minimally complicated benign cyst characterized by thin, enhancing wall (*straight arrow*) with no irregularity, and thin septa (*arrowheads*). (*B*) Indeterminate renal lesion, which requires surgical removal because of multiple thick irregular septa and thick enhancing wall. (*C*) Overtly malignant cystic tumor with enhancing irregular wall and vegetations (***).

purposes. Because of its availability and its lack of ionizing radiation CEUS is well suited for follow-up of nonsurgical lesions.

Renal trauma

After microbubble administration renal injuries present as defects of vascularization in a well-perfused parenchyma (**Fig. 16**). Interruption of the renal profile is consistent with a laceration. Renal artery tear or thrombosis presents with absence of parenchymal perfusion. Focal UCA extravasation suggests active hemorrhage.

Although UCA injection improves the sensitivity of US for identification of renal injuries, the role of this technique in the clinical practice is debatable. Injury to the renal collecting system may be overlooked at CEUS because of a lack of microbubbles urinary excretion.[69] In addition, severe trauma patients, even although hemodynamically stable,

usually require a panoramic evaluation with CT of all abdominal organs. CEUS could replace or integrate US in the triage of hemodynamically stable patients with minor abdominal traumas. However, Poletti and colleagues[75] found that even in optimal conditions solid organ injuries may be missed. The authors' experience is in keeping with the results of Valentino and colleagues,[76] who missed no major renal injury in their series. Small and low-grade injuries may be occasionally overlooked, especially in obese patients, and when perirenal hematoma is small or absent. CEUS can be employed in the follow-up of renal injuries that are managed conservatively to reduce the use of CT.

Renal infections

Renal abscesses are depicted effectively after UCA injection, because they do not present with intralesional vessels, which are destroyed or

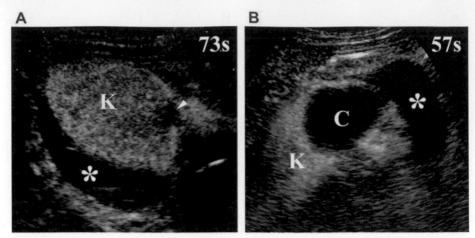

Fig. 16. CEUS appearance of renal injuries in 2 different patients. Images obtained 73 seconds (*A*) and 57 seconds (*B*) after microbubble injection, respectively. (*A*) Small laceration of the renal parenchyma presenting as a perfusion defect interrupting the renal profile (*arrowhead*) with associated perirenal hematoma (*). (*B*) Ruptured renal cyst that appears as an oval, nonenhancing area with well-defined margins communicating with a perirenal hematoma (*). K, kidney; C, cyst.

displaced by the liquefactive process (**Fig. 17**). Focal acute pyelonephritis may improve in conspicuity after microbubble injection if renal vessels are compressed by the adjacent edema, revealing hypoperfused areas.[65]

Mitterberger and colleagues[77] evaluated prospectively 100 consecutive patients with clinical symptoms suggestive of acute pyelonephritis and showed that CEUS and CT are almost equally sensitive and specific for detecting renal changes.

CEUS and renal ablation

Radiofrequency ablation is becoming an alternative therapy in patients with renal cell carcinoma

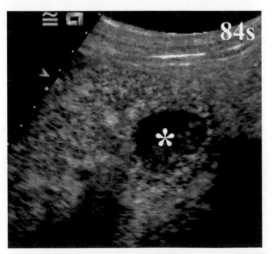

Fig. 17. Renal abscess (*) presenting as a round, hypoechoic lesion with subtle internal debris but lacking enhancement 84 seconds after contrast injection.

who are not candidates for surgery. Preliminary investigation suggests that CEUS can be useful in detecting residual tumor after ablation. Meloni and colleagues[78] evaluated with CEUS and CT or MRI 29 patients with 30 renal tumors before and after radiofrequency ablation. They found that in hypervascular tumor, the accuracy of CEUS in the detection of focal areas of tumor recurrence or progression is similar to that of CT or MRI.

Transplanted kidney

Fischer and colleagues[79] found a delayed enhancement of the renal cortex in patients with graft rejection. This finding, however, was also observed in patients with large perirenal hematomas.[79] Another preliminary investigation showed that in acute tubular necrosis the cortical/medullary ratio of the renal blood volume and mean transit time were significantly lower compared with the control group.[80] The impact of detecting these hemodynamic changes in the management of patients with nonfunctioning transplanted kidney has not been established.

Spleen

Several UCAs exhibit specific hepatosplenic uptake after their disappearance from the blood pool. SonoVue, the most widely used microbubble in Europe, produces a spleen-specific enhancement that lasts longer than the blood pool and liver enhancement phases.[81]

Ectopic splenic tissue

Several studies show that CEUS is useful for characterization of ectopic splenic tissue.[82–86]

Differential diagnosis between benign and malignant lesions is particularly problematic when a peritoneal nodule is identified in tumor patients who have undergone splenectomy. SonoVue is able to characterize the splenic tissue because of the spleen-specific uptake (**Fig. 18**). Splenic hilum lymph nodes, adrenal lesions, pancreatic tail tumors, metastatic deposits, and other lesions have a reduced enhancement in the late phase.[87]

Splenic perfusion defects

In acute splenic infarction CEUS accurately demonstrates the shape and extent of the ischemic area as a region in which contrast enhancement is lacking.[88] CEUS is helpful when the infarction is barely recognizable on baseline US or when it simulates a focal lesion (**Fig. 19**).

According to Valentino and colleagues[76] the sensitivity of CEUS in detection of splenic injuries approaches 100%; according to Poletti and colleagues,[75] however, the sensitivity is lower, and surgical splenic injuries may be missed. Splenic injuries appear as parenchymal portions lacking contrast enhancement. Lacerations are recognizable as hypoechoic bands, linear or branched, perpendicular to the spleen capsule, although lacerocontusive areas and parenchymal hematomas appear as inhomogeneous hypoechoic regions without mass effect or vessel displacement (**Fig. 20**). In patients with splenic trauma CEUS may also display findings that do not appear on conventional US imaging, including perfusion defects and contrast extravasation.[88] In the authors' experience, as a noninvasive, bedside, and repeatable technique, CEUS is ideally suited for the follow-up of splenic traumas

managed conservatively, especially in young patients, because it reduces the number of CT scans.

Focal splenic lesions

Microbubble contrast agents may be helpful in defining the thin wall of splenic cyst and in demonstrating the absence of intralesional enhancement.[86] Hemangioma may present with globular enhancement, as occurs in the liver, or more often with homogeneous, persistent enhancement.[86] Large lesions with cystic/necrotic/thrombotic components, however, may also show heterogeneous enhancement. Splenic hamartomas present with variable enhancement, and are often indistinguishable from hemangiomas or other splenic lesions.[86] Irregular peripheral enhancement is seen in lymphoma, with the lesion appearing as a clear defect in the late phase. In splenic metastases microbubbles may show variable peripheral enhancement, with lesions appearing as defects surrounded by normally enhancing splenic parenchyma. Metastases may be revealed that are not seen on baseline US by increasing their conspicuity.

Prostate

The clear association between increased microvascularity and prostate cancer[89] suggests that the use of CEUS should significantly improve tumor detection (**Fig. 21**). In addition, because increased microvessel density has been correlated with metastatic disease[90] and disease-specific survival,[89,91] the cancers identified with contrast-enhanced imaging techniques are likely to be more aggressive. Several studies have

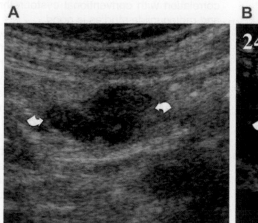
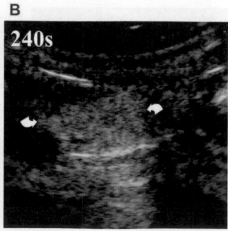

Fig. 18. Islet of peritoneal splenosis (*arrows*) in a patient with multiple endocrine neoplasms syndrome who had undergone splenectomy for trauma. (*A*) Baseline US shows an oval, lobulated nodule with a nonspecific appearance. (*B*) After microbubble administration the nodule typically shows microbubble uptake lasting 240 seconds after the injection.

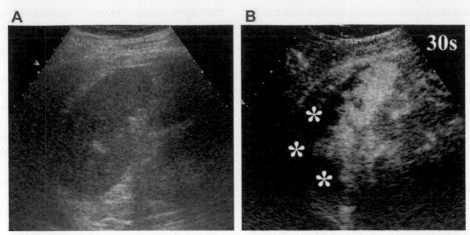

Fig. 19. Acute splenic infarction from septic embolism in a patient with aortic valve prosthesis infection and bacterial endocarditis. (A) No defined abnormalities of the splenic parenchyma are seen on baseline US. (B) CEUS image obtained 30 seconds after microbubble injection shows a large, nonperfused area (*) involving the dome of the spleen.

shown improvements in clinically significant prostate cancer detection using CEUS as a guide for targeted biopsy, and to detect prostate cancer in patients with previous negative biopsies but with persistently increasing prostate-specific antigen (PSA) values.[92,93] The reported sensitivity, however, is variable and therefore CEUS may not be recommended as a routine procedure at present.[93]

Preliminary investigation shows that CEUS can also be useful in evaluating prostate hemodynamics in response to medical treatments.[92] In patients with prostate cancer quantitative analysis of signal intensity after Levovist (Shering, Berlin, Germany) microbubble administration

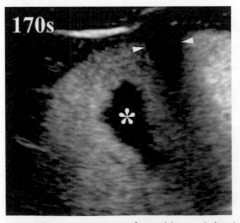

Fig. 20. Splenic hematoma from blunt abdominal trauma presenting as an irregular portion of splenic parenchyma (*) lacking contrast enhancement 170 seconds after microbubble administration. Arrowheads indicate an acoustic shadow produced by a rib.

demonstrated that, following hormonal treatment, signal intensity decrease is correlated with changes in the mean PSA.[94] Administration of tadalafil, a phosphodiesterase type 5 inhibitor, to patients with benign hyperplasia resulted in increased enhancement peak and area under the curve, reflecting changes in prostate vascularity.[95]

Lower Genitourinary Tract

Techniques to evaluate the vesicoureteral reflux have been developed.[96,97] After catheterization, the bladder is filled with saline until the patient has the urge to micturate, and then the UCA is added. Reflux is diagnosed when microbubbles are detected in the ureter or the renal pelvis. The correlation with conventional cystourethrography and radionuclide studies is good.

CEUS allows evaluation of tubal patency without patient exposure to ionizing radiation.[98] After intrauterine injection the passage through the tubes and the spillage into the peritoneal cavity can be assessed. Good correlation with the results of conventional techniques has been shown.

Preliminary investigations show that in patients with scrotal trauma CEUS helps in the evaluation of testicular tissue damage and identification of albugineal tear. Moreover, CEUS improves evaluation of ischemic areas, testicular torsion, and abscess extension. Hypovascular testicular masses, which need surgical removal, can be differentiated from completely avascular lesions such as complex cysts, which may be treated conservatively.

In penile imaging CEUS is useful in the evaluation of congenital abnormalities, trauma, ischemia,

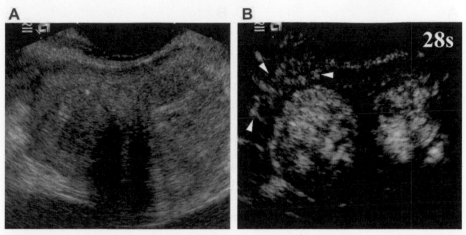

Fig. 21. Appearance of prostate cancer at CEUS. (*A*) Baseline transrectal US of the prostate shows no focal abnormalities in the peripheral portion of the gland. (*B*) Twenty-eight seconds after microbubble injection a hypervascular area is recognized in the right prostate lobe (*arrowheads*). Cancer was found at biopsy.

fibrosis, and detection of isoechoic metastases. It can also be used to assess patency of shunts in patients with ischemic priapism who have undergone surgical shunting.[99–107]

Urinary bladder neoplasms display avid enhancement in the arterial phase persistent in the following phases. CEUS may be useful for detecting tumor in diverticula and for differentiating hypomobile blood clot from tumor tissue. In a preliminary study Caruso and colleagues[102] suggest that CEUS distinguishes the various layers of the bladder wall, and could help to differentiate superficial bladder tumors from those infiltrating the muscle layer.

Pancreas

Inflammatory pancreatic diseases

Koito and colleagues[103] suggest that CEUS improves the diagnosis of pancreatic inflammatory diseases. Identification of regional parenchymal necrosis, which appears as nonvascular areas after UCA injection, is more reliable at CEUS than at baseline US. CEUS is useful for distinguishing inflammatory from neoplastic masses of the pancreas. Enhancement characteristics similar to the adjacent pancreatic parenchyma are consistent with an inflammatory origin. These characteristics are particularly useful in patients with mass-forming pancreatitis, and with autoimmune pancreatitis.[104,105]

Solid pancreatic tumors

Ductal adenocarcinoma is usually hypovascular in all vascular phases.[104,105] Compared with grayscale US a clear depiction of tumor margins is obtained by using CEUS, with better definition of size and of the relationship with the peripancreatic vessels (**Fig. 22A**).

Most endocrine tumors show rapid intense enhancement in the early phases, with exclusion of the necrotic intralesional areas (**Fig. 22B**). Nonfunctioning neuroendocrine tumors may be hypovascularized.[104] The ability of CEUS in demonstrating endocrine tumor vascularization improves identification and characterization of these lesions, compared with US and color Doppler US.

Cystic pancreatic tumors

Differentiation between serous and mucinous cystadenoma of the pancreas is critical, because the former is usually benign, whereas the latter must be removed surgically. CEUS improves characterization of microcystic serous cystadenoma, which presents with multiple small cystic spaces separated by thin septa, well-defined margins, and a central scar.[104] The less common oligocystic and macrocystic types of serous cystadenoma have features indistinguishable from those of the other macrocystic tumors of the pancreas.

In patients with intraductal papillary-mucinous tumors CEUS may allow the identification of intraductal papillary tumor vegetations. However, the definite diagnosis is obtained by demonstrating the communication between the tumor and the pancreatic duct, which is difficult with US.[104]

Pseudocysts lack contrast enhancement and are effectively differentiated from cystic tumors.[104]

Small Bowel

CEUS allows evaluation of bowel wall vascularity in Crohn disease. Different types of enhancement

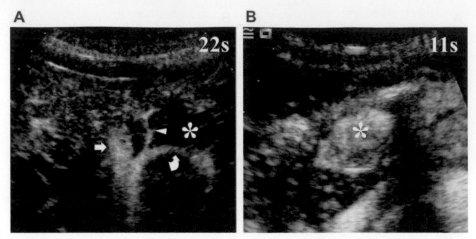

Fig. 22. Solid pancreatic tumor in 2 different patients. Images obtained 22 seconds (*A*) and 11 seconds (*B*) after microbubble injection, respectively. (*A*) Ductal adenocarcinoma presenting as a hypoenhancing lesion (*) infiltrating the splenic artery (*curved arrow*) and the left gastric artery (*arrowhead*), whose lumen is narrowed. The tumor is also in contact with the hepatic artery (*straight arrow*). (*B*) Gastrinoma presenting as an oval nodule (*) with intense and homogeneous enhancement.

of the diseased intestinal wall have been observed, including absent enhancement, prevalent submucosal enhancement, and transparietal enhancement (**Fig. 23**). Serra and colleagues[106] found a significant correlation between the different patterns of enhancement and the Crohn disease activity index (CDAI).

CEUS can help distinguish inflammatory stenoses, which are more responsive to medical treatment and which enhance markedly, from fibrotic stenoses, which are characterized by poor vascularity. In addition, CEUS is helpful in differentiating abscesses and phlegmons, caused by Crohn disease, diverticulitis, or appendicitis.

Preliminary investigation suggests that CEUS can be used in monitoring the clinical course of Crohn disease. In patients with clinical and biochemical remission no enhancement indicates a stable remission, whereas contrast enhancement of the thickened bowel wall suggests a higher risk of relapse and therefore the need for strict follow-up. Quaia and colleagues[107] attempted to correlate quantitatively enhancement of the bowel wall and CDAI during the pharmacologic treatment of Crohn disease and concluded that the quantitative assessment of bowel wall vascularity by CEUS could provide a useful and simple method to assess the effectiveness of medical treatment. In

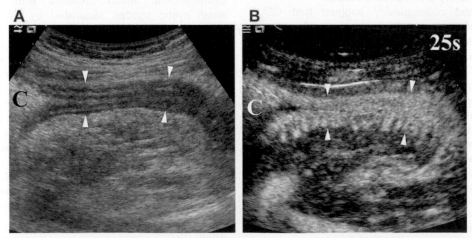

Fig. 23. Crohn disease. (*A*) Baseline US of the terminal ileum shows a thickened bowel wall (*arrowheads*) with layer appearance. (*B*) Twenty-five seconds after microbubble injection the loop shows a diffuse transparietal contrast enhancement. C, cecum.

a preliminary study Guidi and colleagues[108] attempted to compare quantitatively in 8 patients enhancement of the bowel wall after 3 doses of monoclonal antitumor necrosis factor α antibodies (infliximab) with the pretreatment examination, finding a significant reduction of mural vascularization.

Abdominal Aorta

CEUS enables evaluation of several aortic disorders. In patients with abdominal aortic dissection the true lumen can be differentiated from the false lumen because of delayed arrival in the latter of the microbubble bolus.[109] Diagnosis of aortocaval fistula is improved when early synchronous, homogenous enhancement of the aorta and of the inferior vena cava is observed.[110] Endovascular abdominal aortic aneurysm repair is an accepted alternative to open surgery. The most common complication of this procedure is represented by endoleak, which is the persistence of perigraft flow within the aneurysmal sac excluded by the stent graft.[111] Because endoleak is the major cause of enlargement and rupture of the aneurysm after endovascular repair, strict lifelong surveillance is mandatory. CT is the reference imaging procedure for detecting the origin of the perigraft leak, the outflow vessels, and the complications related to endoluminal treatment of aortic aneurysms.[112] Increasing clinical evidence shows that the use of UCAs significantly improves the capability of US to detect endoleaks, overcoming the limitations caused by calcifications, echo reflection by the metallic portion of the stent graft, and slow flow. Iezzi and colleagues[111] showed that CEUS has sensitivity and negative predictive value in endoleak detection similar to CT. Moreover, it seems more specific than CT in the detection of small, low-flow endoleaks.[112] On CEUS images endoleaks appear as enhancing areas beyond the graft but within the aneurysm sac (**Fig. 24**). Delayed scans at 5 to 10 minutes may improve detection of slow-flow endoleaks. Special attention should be paid to the origin and to identification of inflow and outflow collateral vessels that may be identified at the proximal and distal graft attachment site, or outside the lateral tract of the aortic graft through collateral arterial branches, graft disruption, or porosity.

Carotid Artery

UCAs have been used to assess the part of the internal carotid artery immediately outside the cranium, which is difficult to evaluate with conventional Doppler techniques, and to improve quantification of internal carotid artery stenosis.[113] In particular, severe stenoses can be differentiated

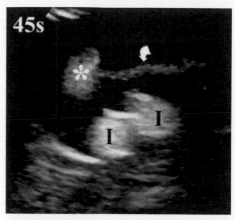

Fig. 24. Endoleak after endovascular aortic aneurysm repair. Image obtained 45 seconds after contrast injection. Partial refilling of the aneurysmal sac (*) beyond the graft (*I*, grafted iliac arteries) through a collateral vessel (*curved arrow*).

from complete occlusion. Moreover, CEUS clearly depicts plaque ulcerations and recanalization not detected on Doppler US images because of the turbulence, flow disturbance, or slow flow. Using state-of-the-art systems, however, carotid arteries are evaluated effectively in virtually all situations using color Doppler US.

An emerging application of CEUS in imaging carotid arteries is to find plaque vascularization.[114–116] Histologic studies have recognized that plaque inflammation, intimal angiogenesis, presence of adventitial vasa vasorum, and plaque neovascularization are strong predictors of instability in atheromatous lesions of cerebrovascular and cardiovascular patients.[117] CEUS is able to visualize adventitial vasa vasorum and plaque neovascularization directly (**Fig. 25**).

Plaque enhancement is found in 80% of symptomatic patients and in 30% of asymptomatic patients. Moreover, intensity of the contrast enhancement is significantly greater in symptomatic patients.[115]

Giannoni and colleagues[118] evaluated with CEUS carotid arteries of 77 consecutive patients before vascular surgery. In all 9 patients undergoing urgent surgery for acute neurologic deficits with hemiparesis CEUS showed enhancement of the plaque, although this pattern was observed in only 1 of 64 asymptomatic patients. On surgical specimens enhancing areas corresponded to regions with an increased number of microvessels staining for vascular endothelial growth factor.

Cerebral Circulation

UCAs have been used to increase the success rate of transcranial Doppler investigation.[119]

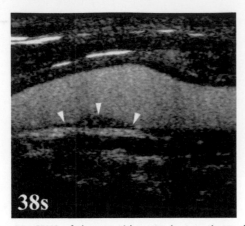

Fig. 25. CEUS of the carotid artery in a patient who had suffered from acute cerebral ischemia 3 days before. A nonstenosing hypoechoic enhancing plaque (*arrowheads*) is recognized at the origin of the internal carotid artery 38 seconds after contrast injection.

Microbubbles offer a new approach to studying the circle of Willis, the venous midline vasculature, and the frontal parenchyma. Recently, low MI perfusion techniques have been introduced that allow detection of UCAs in the cerebral microcirculation.[119] A high frame rate can be applied with excellent time resolution of bolus kinetics. The disadvantage of this technique is the limited investigation depth because of the low MI used.

Joints

Early detection of the pannus and monitoring synovial vascularization are mandatory for appropriate management of patients with rheumatoid arthritis. CEUS has shown promising results in the hands, feet, knees, and, recently, sacroiliac joints. In particular, CEUS allows differentiation between synovial pannus, which is perfused, and fluid.[120] This differentiation is difficult with gray-scale US because both conditions can show hypoechoic to hyperechoic features, and it is clinically important, because the presence of pannus is prognostic for bone damage. CEUS may be of value in the presence of erosive lesions because vascularized erosions are a sign of progressive active disease.[120] Finally, microbubbles can be helpful in detection of hypervascularization in patients with only small or a questionable amount of synovial proliferation, which is not evident with conventional US.[120]

CEUS is substantially better, compared with US and pulsed Doppler US, in differentiating active and inactive synovitis. Measurement of the overall thickness of active synovia is significantly improved.[121]

Objective quantitative analysis of synovial vascularization seems promising for the assessment of response to treatment. Image acquisition procedure, however, has to be standardized and the quality of the examination is dependent on the skill of the operator and use of optimal equipment.

Lymph Nodes

After microbubble administration Rubaltelli and colleagues[122] identified different enhancement patterns in nodal abnormalities. Reactive lymph nodes cause diffuse intense and homogeneous enhancement. Nodal metastases are generally less vascularized than normal nodal tissue and appear as perfusion defects (**Fig. 26**). Lymphomas may be similar to inflammatory lymph nodes or present diffuse heterogeneous contrast enhancement with a dotted appearance during the arterial phase. Although these preliminary results are promising, they necessitate further confirmation from a wider range of cases.

The use of CEUS has been proposed after interstitial injection of UCAs to identify the sentinel lymph node in cancer. According to Goldberg and colleagues,[123,124] using Sonazoid (Amersham, Buckinghamshire, UK) it is possible to trace the lymphatic channels from the injection site up to the draining sentinel lymph nodes, and to identify intranodal metastases, presenting as perfusion defects or heterogeneous enhancement. A preliminary clinical study found similar results.[125] These findings are encouraging, but they are currently experimental and applied mostly to animals. Using SonoVue Wang and colleagues[126] obtained real-time visualization of lymphatic drainage and identified the sentinel lymph nodes in animals, but were not able to detect metastases in the sentinel lymph nodes.

Breast

Breast was 1 of the first organs in which the impact of UCAs was investigated. Initially, CEUS was used to differentiate benign from malignant disease.[127] Contrast-enhanced Doppler US was also tested in the difficult distinction between postoperative scar and tumor recurrence.[128] Although several studies show that microbubble administration improves the ability of US in differentiating benign from malignant breast lesions, sensitivity and specificity are not sufficient to avoid biopsy. Therefore, CEUS has no clinical relevance for this purpose.

Doppler US, even with contrast media, enables visualization of blood vessels at the level of arterioles and venules, but does not reveal flow through

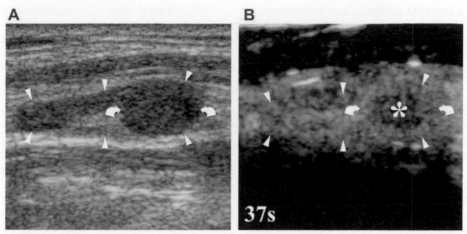

Fig. 26. Metastasis from breast cancer in an axillary lymph node. (*A*) Baseline US showing a lymph node (*arrowheads*) of normal size, but asymmetrical shape caused by an eccentric hypoechoic lump (*curved arrows*). (*B*) Thirty-seven seconds after microbubble injection a hypoenhancing lesion (***) is recognized within the lump (*curved arrows*), consistent with metastatic deposit. Diagnosis was confirmed with targeted biopsy.

the capillary bed, which can be investigated using contrast-specific modes. Using these techniques Liu and colleagues[129] showed that CEUS findings correlated with histologic features of breast masses. In particular, enhancing areas correspond to intraductal carcinoma, invasive carcinoma, intraductal papilloma, fibroadenoma with increased stromal cellularity and epithelial hyperplasia, adenosis rich in acinar and tubular structures or inflammatory cell infiltrate; nonenhancing areas correspond to low cellularity, desmoplastic stroma, dilated ducts, fibrosis, or necrosis. Du and colleagues[130] correlated the enhancement patterns and parameters of the time intensity curve of breast lesions, obtained with real-time CEUS, with microvessel density and vascular endothelial growth factor expression. They found that CEUS has a potential in evaluating microvessel density in breast lesions, but does not allow differential diagnosis between benign and malignant hypervascularized lesions.

FUTURE TRENDS

Targeted microbubbles seem to be the most promising application for the future, with multiple diagnostic and therapeutic clinical applications being investigated.

Agents that bind to specific endothelial molecular markers of angiogenesis such as the integrin $\alpha_v\beta_3$, which is selectively expressed on angiogenic endothelium, could provide a basis for molecular imaging of tumors and drug delivery.[131,132] CEUS may be particularly effective for studying these processes because of its ability to couple selective targeting of vessel phenotype with information on perfusion and microvascular blood volume.

Targeted microbubbles can be detected after circulating microbubbles have disappeared following intravascular injection.

Microbubble targeting to activate leukocytes recruited to the vascular endothelium in regions of injury or inflammation can be accomplished by nonspecific interactions between cells and microbubbles. A more specific method for imaging inflammation has been to target cellular adhesion molecules that are expressed on activated endothelium and that participate in leukocyte recruitment.[132]

Thrombus-targeting microbubbles have been developed to improve the diagnostic accuracy of US for detecting vascular or intracardiac thrombi in animal models. Beyond the detection of thrombi, these microbubbles are being tested as an adjunctive therapy for thrombolysis.[133–135]

Targeted microbubbles can transport to specific sites bioactive materials such as drugs or genes. When microbubbles reach the target site, intracellular delivery can occur with the contribution of endocytosis for compounds of small molecular size, whereas sonoporation (ie, US-induced formation of pores in cell membranes) is the predominant mechanism for larger molecules and plasmids.[134]

A great challenge in sonoporation is to open the blood-brain barrier in a reversible way.[134]

Several researchers are studying US enhanced gene therapy for cardiovascular disorders to control intimal hyperplasia, restore vascular function, or promote angiogenesis.

SUMMARY

With the advent of microbubble contrast agents and contrast-specific techniques, CEUS has become a powerful additional tool for radiological imaging, particularly in the liver. When microbubbles are administered intravenously, the sensitivity and specificity of US in the assessment of FLLs approach those of CT and MR, with the advantages of no radiation and lower cost. The CEUS findings mostly repeat the well-known CT and MR findings, although UCAs behave differently. Functional (perfusional) information can be obtained in addition to morphologic information, often making further imaging unnecessary. Nevertheless, CEUS requires expertise and adequate US equipment. In addition, subjects and organs unsuitable for US are also unsuitable for CEUS, which is not a panoramic imaging modality and consequently not a substitute for comprehensive, whole-body imaging with CT, MR, or PET.

ACKNOWLEDGMENTS

The authors are indebted to Professor Lorenzo Derchi, Genoa, Italy, for his seminal studies on the diagnostic applications of microbubbles and for his encouragement of their work.

REFERENCES

1. Catalano O, Migaleddu V, Quaia E, et al. Terminology for contrast-enhanced sonography: a practical glossary. J Ultrasound Med 2007;26(6):717–30.
2. Goldberg BB, Liu JB, Burns PN, et al. Galactose-based intravenous sonographic contrast agent: experimental studies. J Ultrasound Med 1993;12(8):463–70.
3. Derchi LE, Rizzatto G, Solbiati L. [Contrast media in echography]. Radiol Med 1992;84(3):208–15 [in Italian].
4. Ressner M, Brodin LA, Jansson T, et al. Effects of ultrasound contrast agents on Doppler tissue velocity estimation. J Am Soc Echocardiogr 2006;19(2):154–64.
5. Albrecht T, Hoffmann CW, Schettler S, et al. B-mode enhancement at phase-inversion US with air-based microbubble contrast agent: initial experience in humans. Radiology 2000;216(1):273–8.
6. Harvey CJ, Blomley MJ, Eckersley RJ, et al. Developments in ultrasound contrast media. Eur Radiol 2001;11(4):675–89.
7. Lencioni R, Cioni D, Bartolozzi C. Tissue harmonic and contrast-specific imaging: back to gray scale in ultrasound. Eur Radiol 2002;12(1):151–65.
8. Morel DR, Schwieger I, Hohn L, et al. Human pharmacokinetics and safety evaluation of SonoVue, a new contrast agent for ultrasound imaging. Invest Radiol 2000;35(1):80–5.
9. Schneider M, Arditi M, Barrau MB, et al. BR1: a new ultrasonographic contrast agent based on sulfur hexafluoride-filled microbubbles. Invest Radiol 1995;30(8):451–7.
10. Bauer A, Solbiati L, Weissman N. Ultrasound imaging with SonoVue: low mechanical index real-time imaging. Acad Radiol 2002;9(Suppl 2):S282–4.
11. Martin RP, Lerakis S. Contrast for vascular imaging. Cardiol Clin 2004;22(2):313–20, vii.
12. Burns PN, Wilson SR. Microbubble contrast for radiological imaging: 1. Principles. Ultrasound Q 2006;22(1):5–13.
13. Burns PN, Wilson SR, Simpson DH. Pulse inversion imaging of liver blood flow: improved method for characterizing focal masses with microbubble contrast. Invest Radiol 2000;35(1):58–71.
14. Quaia E. Microbubble ultrasound contrast agents: an update. Eur Radiol 2007;17(8):1995–2008.
15. Wilson SR, Greenbaum LD, Goldberg BB. Contrast-enhanced ultrasound: what is the evidence and what are the obstacles? AJR Am J Roentgenol 2009;193(1):55–60.
16. Burns PN, Wilson SR. Focal liver masses: enhancement patterns on contrast-enhanced images–concordance of US scans with CT scans and MR images. Radiology 2007;242(1):162–74.
17. Sonne C, Xie F, Lof J, et al. Differences in definity and optison microbubble destruction rates at a similar mechanical index with different real-time perfusion systems. J Am Soc Echocardiogr 2003;16(11):1178–85.
18. Mattrey RF, Leopold GR, vanSonnenberg E, et al. Perfluorochemicals as liver- and spleen-seeking ultrasound contrast agents. J Ultrasound Med 1983;2(4):173–6.
19. Bryant TH, Blomley MJ, Albrecht T, et al. Improved characterization of liver lesions with liver-phase uptake of liver-specific microbubbles: prospective multicenter study. Radiology 2004;232(3):799–809.
20. Luo W, Numata K, Morimoto M, et al. Focal liver tumors: characterization with 3D perflubutane microbubble contrast agent-enhanced US versus 3D contrast-enhanced multidetector CT. Radiology 2009;251(1):287–95.
21. Catalano O, Nunziata A, Lobianco R, et al. Real-time harmonic contrast material–specific US of focal liver lesions. Radiographics 2005;25(2):333–49.
22. Piscaglia F, Bolondi L. The safety of Sonovue in abdominal applications: retrospective analysis of 23188 investigations. Ultrasound Med Biol 2006;32(9):1369–75.
23. Liu GJ, Xu HX, Xie XY, et al. Does the echogenicity of focal liver lesions on baseline gray-scale ultrasound interfere with the diagnostic performance

of contrast-enhanced ultrasound? Eur Radiol 2009; 19(5):1214–22.

24. Bartolotta TV, Midiri M, Galia M, et al. Characterization of benign hepatic tumors arising in fatty liver with SonoVue and pulse inversion US. Abdom Imaging 2007;32(1):84–91.

25. Wilson SR, Burns PN. An algorithm for the diagnosis of focal liver masses using microbubble contrast-enhanced pulse-inversion sonography. AJR Am J Roentgenol 2006;186(5):1401–12.

26. Albrecht T, Blomley M, Bolondi L, et al. Guidelines for the use of contrast agents in ultrasound. January 2004. Ultraschall Med 2004;25(4): 249–56.

27. Claudon M, Cosgrove D, Albrecht T, et al. Guidelines and good clinical practice recommendations for contrast enhanced ultrasound (CEUS) – update 2008. Ultraschall Med 2008;29(1):28–44.

28. Quaia E, Calliada F, Bertolotto M, et al. Characterization of focal liver lesions with contrast-specific US modes and a sulfur hexafluoride-filled microbubble contrast agent: diagnostic performance and confidence. Radiology 2004;232(2): 420–30.

29. Bartolotta TV, Midiri M, Quaia E, et al. Liver haemangiomas undetermined at grey-scale ultrasound: contrast-enhancement patterns with SonoVue and pulse-inversion US. Eur Radiol 2005;15(4):685–93.

30. Wang LY, Wang JH, Lin ZY, et al. Hepatic focal nodular hyperplasia: findings on color Doppler ultrasound. Abdom Imaging 1997;22(2):178–81.

31. Ricci P, Cantisani V, D'Onofrio M, et al. Behavior of hepatocellular adenoma on real-time low-mechanical index contrast-enhanced ultrasonography with a second-generation contrast agent. J Ultrasound Med 2008;27(12):1719–26.

32. Xu HX, Lu MD, Liu GJ, et al. Imaging of peripheral cholangiocarcinoma with low-mechanical index contrast-enhanced sonography and SonoVue: initial experience. J Ultrasound Med 2006;25(1): 23–33.

33. Bolondi L, Gaiani S, Celli N, et al. Characterization of small nodules in cirrhosis by assessment of vascularity: the problem of hypovascular hepatocellular carcinoma. Hepatology 2005;42(1): 27–34.

34. Tarantino L, Francica G, Sordelli I, et al. Diagnosis of benign and malignant portal vein thrombosis in cirrhotic patients with hepatocellular carcinoma: color Doppler US, contrast-enhanced US, and fine-needle biopsy. Abdom Imaging 2006;31(5): 537–44.

35. Catalano O, Sandomenico F, Raso MM, et al. Low mechanical index contrast-enhanced sonographic findings of pyogenic hepatic abscesses. AJR Am J Roentgenol 2004;182(2):447–50.

36. Lin MX, Xu HX, Lu MD, et al. Diagnostic performance of contrast-enhanced ultrasound for complex cystic focal liver lesions: blinded reader study. Eur Radiol 2009;19(2):358–69.

37. Lemke AJ, Chopra SS, Hengst SA, et al. [Characterization of hepatic tumors with contrast-enhanced ultrasound and digital grey-scale analysis]. Rofo 2004;176(11):1607–16 [in German].

38. Romanini L, Passamonti M, Aiani L, et al. Economic assessment of contrast-enhanced ultrasonography for evaluation of focal liver lesions: a multicentre Italian experience. Eur Radiol 2007;17(Suppl 6): F99–106.

39. Tranquart F, Le Gouge A, Correas GM, et al. Role of contrast-enhanced ultrasound in the blinded assessment of focal liver lesions in comparison with MDCT and CEMRI: results from a multicentre clinical trial. EJC Supplements 2008;6(11):9–15.

40. Strobel D, Seitz K, Blank W, et al. Contrast-enhanced ultrasound for the characterization of focal liver lesions–diagnostic accuracy in clinical practice (DEGUM multicenter trial). Ultraschall Med 2008;29(5):499–505.

41. D'Onofrio M, Rozzanigo U, Masinielli BM, et al. Hypoechoic focal liver lesions: characterization with contrast enhanced ultrasonography. J Clin Ultrasound 2005;33(4):164–72.

42. Faccioli N, D'Onofrio M, Comai A, et al. Contrast-enhanced ultrasonography in the characterization of benign focal liver lesions: activity-based cost analysis. Radiol Med 2007;112(6):810–20.

43. Nicolau C, Vilana R, Bru C. The use of contrast-enhanced ultrasound in the management of the cirrhotic patient and for detection of HCC. Eur Radiol 2004;14(Suppl 8):P63–71.

44. D'Onofrio M, Rozzanigo U, Caffarri S, et al. Contrast-enhanced US of hepatocellular carcinoma. Radiol Med 2004;107(4):293–303.

45. Ueda K, Terada T, Nakanuma Y, et al. Vascular supply in adenomatous hyperplasia of the liver and hepatocellular carcinoma: a morphometric study. Hum Pathol 1992;23(6):619–26.

46. Efremidis SC, Hytiroglou P. The multistep process of hepatocarcinogenesis in cirrhosis with imaging correlation. Eur Radiol 2002;12(4):753–64.

47. Quaia E, O'Onofrio M, Palumbo A, et al. Comparison of contrast-enhanced ultrasonography versus baseline ultrasound and contrast-enhanced computed tomography in metastatic disease of the liver: diagnostic performance and confidence. Eur Radiol 2006;16(7):1599–609.

48. Konopke R, Kersting S, Saeger HD, et al. [Detection of liver lesions by contrast-enhanced ultrasound – comparison to intraoperative findings]. Ultraschall Med 2005;26(2):107–13 [in German].

49. Oldenburg A, Hohmann J, Foert E, et al. Detection of hepatic metastases with low MI real time

contrast enhanced sonography and SonoVue. Ultraschall Med 2005;26(4):277–84.

50. Meuwly JY, Schnyder P, Gudinchet F, et al. Pulse-inversion harmonic imaging improves lesion conspicuity during US-guided biopsy. J Vasc Interv Radiol 2003;14(3):335–41.

51. Minami Y, Kudo M, Kawasaki T, et al. Treatment of hepatocellular carcinoma with percutaneous radiofrequency ablation: usefulness of contrast harmonic sonography for lesions poorly defined with B-mode sonography. AJR Am J Roentgenol 2004;183(1):153–6.

52. Youk JH, Lee JM, Kim CS. Therapeutic response evaluation of malignant hepatic masses treated by interventional procedures with contrast-enhanced agent detection imaging. J Ultrasound Med 2003;22(9):911–20.

53. Dill-Macky MJ, Asch M, Burns P, et al. Radiofrequency ablation of hepatocellular carcinoma: predicting success using contrast-enhanced sonography. AJR Am J Roentgenol 2006; 186(Suppl 5):S287–95.

54. Kono Y, Lucidarme O, Choi SH, et al. Contrast-enhanced ultrasound as a predictor of treatment efficacy within 2 weeks after transarterial chemoembolization of hepatocellular carcinoma. J Vasc Interv Radiol 2007;18(1 Pt 1):57–65.

55. Krix M. Quantification of enhancement in contrast ultrasound: a tool for monitoring of therapies in liver metastases. Eur Radiol 2005;15(Suppl 5): E104–8.

56. Bertolotto M, Pozzato G, Croce LS, et al. Blood flow changes in hepatocellular carcinoma after the administration of thalidomide assessed by reperfusion kinetics during microbubble infusion: preliminary results. Invest Radiol 2006;41(1):15–21.

57. De Giorgi U, Aliberti C, Benea G, et al. Effect of angiosonography to monitor response during imatinib treatment in patients with metastatic gastrointestinal stromal tumors. Clin Cancer Res 2005; 11(17):6171–6.

58. Lassau N, Lamuraglia M, Chami L, et al. Gastrointestinal stromal tumors treated with imatinib: monitoring response with contrast-enhanced sonography. AJR Am J Roentgenol 2006;187(5): 1267–73.

59. Lassau N, Chami L, Benatsou B, et al. Dynamic contrast-enhanced ultrasonography (DCE-US) with quantification of tumor perfusion: a new diagnostic tool to evaluate the early effects of antiangiogenic treatment. Eur Radiol 2007;17(Suppl 6): F89–98.

60. Girard MS, Mattrey RF, Baker KG, et al. Comparison of standard and second harmonic B-mode sonography in the detection of segmental renal infarction with sonographic contrast in a rabbit model. J Ultrasound Med 2000;19(3):185–92 [quiz 93].

61. Quaia E, Siracusano S, Palumbo A, et al. Detection of focal renal perfusion defects in rabbits after sulphur hexafluoride-filled microbubble injection at low transmission power ultrasound insonation. Eur Radiol 2006;16(1):166–72.

62. Taylor GA, Barnewolt CE, Claudon M, et al. Depiction of renal perfusion defects with contrast-enhanced harmonic sonography in a porcine model. AJR Am J Roentgenol 1999; 173(3):757–60.

63. Bertolotto M, Martegani A, Aiani L, et al. Value of contrast-enhanced ultrasonography for detecting renal infarcts proven by contrast enhanced CT. A feasibility study. Eur Radiol 2008;18(2):376–83.

64. Park BK, Kim SH, Moon MH, et al. Imaging features of gray-scale and contrast-enhanced color Doppler US for the differentiation of transient renal arterial ischemia and arterial infarction. Korean J Radiol 2005;6(3):179–84.

65. Kim JH, Eun HW, Lee HK, et al. Renal perfusion abnormality. Coded harmonic angio US with contrast agent. Acta Radiol 2003;44(2):166–71.

66. Nilsson A. Contrast-enhanced ultrasound of the kidneys. Eur Radiol 2004;14(Suppl 8):P104–9.

67. Park BK, Kim B, Kim SH, et al. Assessment of cystic renal masses based on Bosniak classification: comparison of CT and contrast-enhanced US. Eur J Radiol 2007;61(2):310–4.

68. Ascenti G, Gaeta M, Magno C, et al. Contrast-enhanced second-harmonic sonography in the detection of pseudocapsule in renal cell carcinoma. AJR Am J Roentgenol 2004;182(6):1525–30.

69. Setola SV, Catalano O, Sandomenico F, et al. Contrast-enhanced sonography of the kidney. Abdom Imaging 2007;32(1):21–8.

70. Robbin ML, Lockhart ME, Barr RG. Renal imaging with ultrasound contrast: current status. Radiol Clin North Am 2003;41(5):963–78.

71. Tamai H, Takiguchi Y, Oka M, et al. Contrast-enhanced ultrasonography in the diagnosis of solid renal tumors. J Ultrasound Med 2005;24(12): 1635–40.

72. Clevert DA, Minaifar N, Weckbach S, et al. Multislice computed tomography versus contrast-enhanced ultrasound in evaluation of complex cystic renal masses using the Bosniak classification system. Clin Hemorheol Microcirc 2008; 39(1–4):171–8.

73. Quaia E, Bertolotto M, Cioffi V, et al. Comparison of contrast-enhanced sonography with unenhanced sonography and contrast-enhanced CT in the diagnosis of malignancy in complex cystic renal masses. AJR Am J Roentgenol 2008;191(4): 1239–49.

74. Ascenti G, Mazziotti S, Zimbaro G, et al. Complex cystic renal masses: characterization with contrast-enhanced US. Radiology 2007;243(1):158–65.

75. Poletti PA, Platon A, Becker CD, et al. Blunt abdominal trauma: does the use of a second-generation sonographic contrast agent help to detect solid organ injuries? AJR Am J Roentgenol 2004; 183(5):1293–301.

76. Valentino M, Serra C, Zironi G, et al. Blunt abdominal trauma: emergency contrast-enhanced sonography for detection of solid organ injuries. AJR Am J Roentgenol 2006;186(5):1361–7.

77. Mitterberger M, Pinggera GM, Colleselli D, et al. Acute pyelonephritis: comparison of diagnosis with computed tomography and contrast-enhanced ultrasonography. BJU Int 2008;101(3): 341–4.

78. Meloni MF, Bertolotto M, Alberzoni C, et al. Follow-up after percutaneous radiofrequency ablation of renal cell carcinoma: contrast-enhanced sonography versus contrast-enhanced CT or MRI. AJR Am J Roentgenol 2008;191(4):1233–8.

79. Fischer T, Dieckhofer J, Muhler M, et al. The use of contrast-enhanced US in renal transplant: first results and potential clinical benefit. Eur Radiol 2005;15(Suppl 5):E109–16.

80. Benozzi L, Cappelli G, Granito M, et al. Contrast-enhanced sonography in early kidney graft dysfunction. Transplant Proc 2009;41(4):1214–5.

81. Lim AK, Patel N, Eckersley RJ, et al. Evidence for spleen-specific uptake of a microbubble contrast agent: a quantitative study in healthy volunteers. Radiology 2004;231(3):785–8.

82. Catalano O, Sandomenico F, Matarazzo I, et al. Contrast-enhanced sonography of the spleen. AJR Am J Roentgenol 2005;184(4):1150–6.

83. Gorg C, Bert T. Second-generation sonographic contrast agent for differential diagnosis of peri-splenic lesions. AJR Am J Roentgenol 2006; 186(3):621–6.

84. Kim SH, Lee JM, Lee JY, et al. Contrast-enhanced sonography of intrapancreatic accessory spleen in 6 patients. AJR Am J Roentgenol 2007;188(2): 422–8.

85. Ferraioli G, Di Sarno A, Coppola C, et al. Contrast-enhanced low-mechanical-index ultrasonography in hepatic splenosis. J Ultrasound Med 2006; 25(1):133–6.

86. Gorg C. The forgotten organ: contrast enhanced sonography of the spleen. Eur J Radiol 2007; 64(2):189–201.

87. Bertolotto M, Quaia E, Zappetti R, et al. Differential diagnosis between splenic nodules and peritoneal metastases with contrast-enhanced ultrasound based on signal-intensity characteristics during the late phase. Radiol Med 2009;114(1):42–51.

88. Catalano O, Cusati B, Nunziata A, et al. Real-time, contrast-specific sonography imaging of acute splenic disorders: a pictorial review. Emerg Radiol 2004;11(1):15–21.

89. Bigler SA, Deering RE, Brawer MK. Comparison of microscopic vascularity in benign and malignant prostate tissue. Hum Pathol 1993;24(2): 220–6.

90. Weidner N, Carroll PR, Flax J, et al. Tumor angiogenesis correlates with metastasis in invasive prostate carcinoma. Am J Pathol 1993;143(2): 401–9.

91. Lissbrant IF, Stattin P, Damber JE, et al. Vascular density is a predictor of cancer-specific survival in prostatic carcinoma. Prostate 1997;33(1): 38–45.

92. Wink M, Frauscher F, Cosgrove D, et al. Contrast-enhanced ultrasound and prostate cancer; a multicentre European research coordination project. Eur Urol 2008;54(5):982–92.

93. Seitz M, Gratzke C, Schlenker B, et al. Contrast-enhanced transrectal ultrasound (CE-TRUS) with cadence-contrast pulse sequence (CPS) technology for the identification of prostate cancer. Urol Oncol 2009. [Epub ahead of print].

94. Eckersley RJ, Sedelaar JP, Blomley MJ, et al. Quantitative microbubble enhanced transrectal ultrasound as a tool for monitoring hormonal treatment of prostate carcinoma. Prostate 2002;51(4): 256–67.

95. Bertolotto M, Trincia E, Zappetti R, et al. Effect of Tadalafil on prostate hemodynamics: preliminary evaluation with contrast enhanced US. Radiol Med 2009;114(7):1106–14.

96. Ascenti G, Zimbaro G, Mazziotti S, et al. Harmonic US imaging of vesicoureteric reflux in children: usefulness of a second generation US contrast agent. Pediatr Radiol 2004;34(6):481–7.

97. Valentini AL, De Gaetano AM, Minordi LM, et al. Contrast-enhanced voiding US for grading of reflux in adult patients prior to antireflux ureteral implantation. Radiology 2004;233(1):35–9.

98. Derchi LE, Serafini G, Gandolfo N, et al. Ultrasound in gynecology. Eur Radiol 2001;11(11):2137–55.

99. Bertolotto M, Bucci S, Quaia E, et al. Complete penile corporeal septation: evaluation with contrast enhanced US. Abdom Imaging 2008;33(5):621–5.

100. Bertolotto M, Serafini G, Dogliotti L, et al. Primary and secondary malignancies of the penis: ultrasound features. Abdom Imaging 2005;30(1): 108–12.

101. Bertolotto M, Bucci S, Zappetti R. Contrast-enhanced US of the penis. In: Bertolotto M, editor. Color Doppler US of the Penis. Heidelberg (Berlin): Springer-Verlag; 2008. Chapter 21. p. 183–92.

102. Caruso G, Salvaggio G, Campisi A, et al. Comparison of contrast enhanced ultrasound and gray scale ultrasound in bladder tumor staging. AJR Am J Roentgenol, in press.

103. Koito K, Namieno T, Nagakawa T, et al. Inflammatory pancreatic masses: differentiation from ductal

carcinomas with contrast-enhanced sonography using carbon dioxide microbubbles. AJR Am J Roentgenol 1997;169(5):1263–7.

104. D'Onofrio M, Zamboni G, Faccioli N, et al. Ultrasonography of the pancreas. 4. Contrast-enhanced imaging. Abdom Imaging 2007;32(2):171–81.

105. D'Onofrio M, Zamboni G, Tognolini A, et al. Mass-forming pancreatitis: value of contrast-enhanced ultrasonography. World J Gastroenterol 2006; 12(26):4181–4.

106. Serra C, Menozzi G, Labate AM, et al. Ultrasound assessment of vascularization of the thickened terminal ileum wall in Crohn's disease patients using a low-mechanical index real-time scanning technique with a second generation ultrasound contrast agent. Eur J Radiol 2007;62(1):114–21.

107. Quaia E, Migaleddu V, Baratella E, et al. The diagnostic value of small bowel wall vascularity after sulfur hexafluoride-filled microbubble injection in patients with Crohn's disease. Correlation with the therapeutic effectiveness of specific anti-inflammatory treatment. Eur J Radiol 2009; 69(3):438–44.

108. Guidi L, De Franco A, De Vitis I, et al. Contrast-enhanced ultrasonography with SonoVue after infliximab therapy in Crohn's disease. Eur Rev Med Pharmacol Sci 2006;10(1):23–6.

109. Clevert DA, Weckbach S, Kopp R, et al. Imaging of aortic lesions with color coded duplex sonography and contrast-enhanced ultrasound versus multislice computed tomography (MS-CT) angiography. Clin Hemorheol Microcirc 2008;40(4): 267–79.

110. Bhatia M, Platon A, Khabiri E, et al. Contrast enhanced ultrasonography versus MR angiography in aortocaval fistula: case report. Abdom Imaging 2009. [Epub ahead of print].

111. Iezzi R, Cotroneo AR, Basilico R, et al. Endoleaks after endovascular repair of abdominal aortic aneurysm: value of CEUS. Abdom Imaging 2009. [Epub ahead of print].

112. Carrafiello G, Recaldini C, Lagana D, et al. Endoleak detection and classification after endovascular treatment of abdominal aortic aneurysm: value of CEUS over CTA. Abdom Imaging 2008;33(3): 357–62.

113. Kono Y, Pinnell SP, Sirlin CB, et al. Carotid arteries: contrast-enhanced US angiography–preliminary clinical experience. Radiology 2004;230(2):561–8.

114. Huang PT, Huang FG, Zou CP, et al. Contrast-enhanced sonographic characteristics of neovascularization in carotid atherosclerotic plaques. J Clin Ultrasound 2008;36(6):346–51.

115. Xiong L, Deng YB, Zhu Y, et al. Correlation of carotid plaque neovascularization detected by using contrast-enhanced US with clinical symptoms. Radiology 2009;251(2):583–9.

116. Vicenzini E, Giannoni MF, Benedetti-Valentini F, et al. Imaging of carotid plaque angiogenesis. Cerebrovasc Dis 2009;27(Suppl 2):48–54.

117. Spagnoli LG, Bonanno E, Sangiorgi G, et al. Role of inflammation in atherosclerosis. J Nucl Med 2007; 48(11):1800–15.

118. Giannoni MF, Vicenzini E, Citone M, et al. Contrast carotid ultrasound for the detection of unstable plaques with neoangiogenesis: a pilot study. Eur J Vasc Endovasc Surg 2009;37(6):722–7.

119. Seidel G, Meairs S. Ultrasound contrast agents in ischemic stroke. Cerebrovasc Dis 2009;27(Suppl 2):25–39.

120. De Zordo T, Mlekusch SP, Feuchtner GM, et al. Value of contrast-enhanced ultrasound in rheumatoid arthritis. Eur J Radiol 2007;64(2):222–30.

121. Klauser A, Demharter J, De Marchi A, et al. Contrast enhanced gray-scale sonography in assessment of joint vascularity in rheumatoid arthritis: results from the IACUS study group. Eur Radiol 2005;15(12):2404–10.

122. Rubaltelli L, Khadivi Y, Tregnaghi A, et al. Evaluation of lymph node perfusion using continuous mode harmonic ultrasonography with a second-generation contrast agent. J Ultrasound Med 2004;23(6):829–36.

123. Goldberg BB, Merton DA, Liu JB, et al. Sentinel lymph nodes in a swine model with melanoma: contrast-enhanced lymphatic US. Radiology 2004;230(3):727–34.

124. Goldberg BB, Merton DA, Liu JB, et al. Contrast-enhanced sonographic imaging of lymphatic channels and sentinel lymph nodes. J Ultrasound Med 2005;24(7):953–65.

125. Omoto K, Matsunaga H, Take N, et al. Sentinel node detection method using contrast-enhanced ultrasonography with sonazoid in breast cancer: preliminary clinical study. Ultrasound Med Biol 2009;35(8):1249–56.

126. Wang Y, Wang W, Li J, et al. Gray-scale contrast-enhanced ultrasonography of sentinel lymph nodes in a metastatic breast cancer model. Acad Radiol 2009;16(8):957–62.

127. Moon WK, Im JG, Noh DY, et al. Nonpalpable breast lesions: evaluation with power Doppler US and a microbubble contrast agent-initial experience. Radiology 2000;217(1):240–6.

128. Schroeder RJ, Bostanjoglo M, Rademaker J, et al. Role of power Doppler techniques and ultrasound contrast enhancement in the differential diagnosis of focal breast lesions. Eur Radiol 2003;13(1):68–79.

129. Liu H, Jiang YX, Liu JB, et al. Contrast-enhanced breast ultrasonography: imaging features with histopathologic correlation. J Ultrasound Med 2009;28(7):911–20.

130. Du J, Li FH, Fang H, et al. Correlation of real-time gray scale contrast-enhanced ultrasonography with

microvessel density and vascular endothelial growth factor expression for assessment of angiogenesis in breast lesions. J Ultrasound Med 2008;27(6):821–31.

131. Bohmer MR, Klibanov AL, Tiemann K, et al. Ultrasound triggered image-guided drug delivery. Eur J Radiol 2009;70(2):242–53.

132. Wallez Y, Huber P. Endothelial adherens and tight junctions in vascular homeostasis, inflammation and angiogenesis. Biochim Biophys Acta 2008; 1778(3):794–809.

133. Alonso A, Della Martina A, Stroick M, et al. Molecular imaging of human thrombus with novel abciximab immunobubbles and ultrasound. Stroke 2007;38(5):1508–14.

134. Hernot S, Klibanov AL. Microbubbles in ultrasound-triggered drug and gene delivery. Adv Drug Deliv Rev 2008;60(10):1153–66.

135. Meairs S, Culp W. Microbubbles for thrombolysis of acute ischemic stroke. Cerebrovasc Dis 2009; 27(Suppl 2):55–65.

Advances in Endoscopic Ultrasound

Jason Gutman, MD*, Asad Ullah, MD

KEYWORDS

- Cancer staging • Endoscopic ultrasound
- Fine-needle aspiration • Therapeutic interventions

The use of ultrasonography for medical purposes was first introduced by Karl and Friedrich Dussik of Austria in 1947 to make images of the human brain and ventricles.[1] In 1949, George Ludwig was the first American physician to use ultrasonographic technology, visualizing the gallbladder and foreign bodies.[2] Evaluation of the intestinal wall expanded in the 1950s with research from John J. Wild, when he looked at ultrasound images of gastric cancers and developed a rectal scanner that was able to demonstrate the different layers of the bowel wall.[3–5] In 1968, Hiroka Watanbe of Japan introduced transrectal ultrasonography for prostate examination with the "ultrasonic chair."[6] This device was one of the initial internal probes, and would later become the basis for endoscopic ultrasonography.

At the same time that ultrasonography capabilities and uses were expanding, endoscopy was undergoing a similar development. It was not until 1980, however, that these two technologies finally converged. DiMagno and colleagues[7] described the first use of an endoscope equipped with an ultrasonic probe. The initial prototype had an 8-cm long rigid tip that did not allow use in human subjects. In the canine model, however, they were able to obtain high-resolution images of various anatomic structures. Later that year, Strohm and colleagues[8] described their experiences with "ultrasonic tomography," evaluating 18 patients with various biliary, pancreatic, and hepatic disorders. They were able to demonstrate the capabilities of endoscopic ultrasound (EUS) including the identification of landmarks, such as the aorta and inferior vena cava, and evaluation of the pancreatic bed and distal common bile duct (CBD).

During the 1980s, progress in the field was slow because of several factors. The equipment was still in its infancy, with equipment manufacturers producing a product that was cumbersome and expensive. There was also a lack of training on the part of endoscopists interpreting ultrasonographic images, and even trained radiologists had to learn to interpret these new images from a different point of view. It was not until the 1990s that interest in this field truly began to expand. The development of smaller transducers that could more easily fit the endoscopes and use of the more flexible videoendoscopes allowed for less patient trauma. The use of linear-array technology was the tool needed for a safer method of fine-needle aspiration (FNA). By the mid 1990s there was a large amount of data supporting the use of EUS as an accurate imaging modality for evaluation of abnormalities of the biliary tree and pancreas, and staging and diagnosis of gastrointestinal malignancies by FNA. Indications for EUS include the following:

Staging of esophageal cancer, pancreatic cancer, gastric cancer, bile duct cancer, cancer of papilla of Vater, and cancer of rectum

Evaluation of submucosal lesions

Evaluation of extramural impressions

Evaluation of pancreatic lesions

Evaluation of thickened gastric folds

Evaluation and EUS-guided FNA of lesions adjacent to esophagus, stomach, duodenum, and rectum

Chronic pancreatitis

Detection of CBD stones

Division of Gastroenterology and Hepatology, University of Rochester Medical Center, 601 Elmwood Avenue, Box 646, Rochester, NY 14642, USA
* Corresponding author.
E-mail address: jason_gutman@URMC.Rochester.edu (J. Gutman).

Ultrasound Clin 4 (2009) 369–384
doi:10.1016/j.cult.2009.10.012

EUS-guided drainage of pancreatic pseudocysts
Celiac plexus block
Evaluation of anal sphincters in fecal
incontinence.

EQUIPMENT
Echoendoscopes

Echoendoscopes have an ultrasonic transducer
attached to the tip of the endoscope. These endoscopes are typically side-viewing endoscopes.
There are two types of echoendoscopes: radial
and linear. In the radial echoendoscopes (**Fig. 1**),
the scanning plane is perpendicular to the axis of
the endoscope. The images obtained are similar
to those seen in CT. For many years, the radial
echoendoscopes had a rotating ultrasound transducer driven by a motor. Currently, these scopes
are electronic and do not have rotating parts,
and are less prone to breakdown. There is a small
accessory channel that allows for small mucosal
biopsies to be performed.

In linear echoendoscopes (**Fig. 2**), the scanning
plane is parallel to the long axis of the endoscope.
The advantage of the linear echoendoscope is that
endosonography-guided FNA biopsy can be performed. Linear echoendoscopes show the entire
length of the biopsy needle, whereas radial
echoendoscopes are only capable of showing
a portion of the needle.

EUS Processors

The echoendoscope is connected to an EUS
processor. The processors available are made by
different companies.

Miniprobes

Miniprobes (**Figs. 3** and **4**), also known as "catheter probes," are small-diameter (2–2.6 mm)

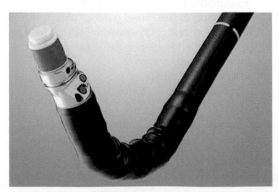

Fig. 1. Radial echoendoscope.

catheters with a mechanical radial ultrasonic
probe at the tip. The mechanical portion is driven
by a small motor. The small size of the probe
allows it to be passed through the accessory
channel of an endoscope. They are especially
useful for examination of small mucosal and
submucosal lesions, because the probes can be
placed on these lesions under direct vision. The
miniprobe has better resolution because of higher
frequency, which ranges from 12 to 30 MHz. Its
clinical use is limited, however, by its shallow
depth of penetration. Wire-guided catheter
probes, which can be passed through the accessory channel, are also available to examine either
the bile duct or the pancreatic duct.

EUS EXAMINATION OF THE GASTROINTESTINAL WALL

The gastrointestinal wall is seen as a five-layered
structure when examined with EUS (**Figs. 5** and **6**).
The mucosa is divided into two layers: superficial
and deep. The superficial mucosa is a hyperechoic
layer, whereas the deep mucosa is hypoechoic.
The third layer is hyperechoic and corresponds
to submucosa. The muscularis propria is the fourth
layer and is hypoechoic. Finally, the fifth layer is
hyperechoic, caused by subserosal or adventitial
fat and connective tissue.

When the gastrointestinal wall is examined with
a miniprobe at higher frequencies (20 MHz), nine
endosonographic layers can be seen. The mucosa
consists of four layers: the first and second layers
represent the epithelium, the third layer identifies
the lamina propria, and the fourth layer is the muscularis mucosa. The fifth layer is the submucosa.
The muscularis propria consists of three layers:
the sixth layer is circular muscle, the seventh layer
is connective tissue between the circular and
longitudinal muscle, and the eighth layer is the
longitudinal muscle. Lastly, the ninth layer is the
adventitia.

LUNG CANCER

Lung cancer is the most common cause of cancer-
related mortality in the world, causing about 1.2
million deaths per year.[9] After lung cancer is diagnosed the next step is staging. In particular, accurate staging is essential to select appropriate
treatment for non–small cell lung cancer. Depending on the stage, non–small cell lung cancer is
treated with surgery alone, downstaging chemotherapy with subsequent surgery, or entirely with
chemoradiation therapy.

Various modalities can be used to stage lung
cancer including CT, positron emission tomography

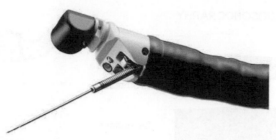

Fig. 2. Linear echoendoscope.

(PET), transesophageal EUS-guided FNA (EUS-FNA), endobronchial ultrasound-guided transbronchial needle aspiration, video-assisted thoracoscopy, or mediastinoscopy. EUS-FNA is increasingly being used for the diagnosis and staging of lung cancer because it provides a minimally invasive alternative to surgical procedures to obtain tissue diagnosis and has a sensitivity and specificity that is better than or at least equal to radiographic imaging alone. EUS-FNA is more sensitive (88% vs 57%) and specific (91% vs 82%) than CT. EUS-FNA and PET have similar sensitivities (88% vs 84%) and specificities (91% vs 89%); however, PET does not provide the potential for a tissue diagnosis. EUS-FNA can also be used as a complimentary study to mediastinoscopy because both techniques provide access to different mediastinal lymph nodes.[10,11] In a study comparing EUS-FNA with mediastinoscopy, both techniques had comparable accuracy, 91% versus 90%, respectively. When EUS-FNA was combined with mediastinoscopy significantly more patients with lymph node metastases were detected.[12]

EUS-FNA has been shown to reduce the need of invasive procedures, such as mediastinoscopy and thoracotomy, in lung cancer patients. In a prospective study of 242 patients with suspected or proved lung cancer, EUS-FNA prevented surgical procedures in 70% of patients because of diagnosis of lymph node metastases, tumor invasion, or benign diagnoses.[13] In another study of 84 patients with mediastinal masses suspected for malignancy, EUS prevented mediastinoscopy in 68% of patients and thorascopy in 48% of patients.[14]

The most common indication for EUS-FNA in lung tumors is evaluation of mediastinal lymph nodes. Non–small cell lung cancer initially spreads by way of the lymphatic system to locoregional lymph nodes (hilar and mediastinal) and then to distant organs by hematogenous route. Mediastinal lymph node enlargement is seen in up to 38% of non–small cell lung cancer at the time of diagnosis. The identification of cancer spread to the mediastinum is critical because this not only determines treatment but also prognosis. Regional lymph nodes in non–small cell lung cancer are classified using the TNM classification according to Mountain and Dresler.[15] Not all mediastinal lymph nodes can be biopsied by EUS. Lymph nodes and their stations that are reliably reachable include low paratracheal on the left (4L), subaortic (5), para-aortic

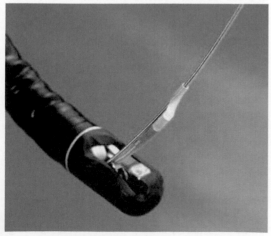

Fig. 3. Wire-guided mini probe.

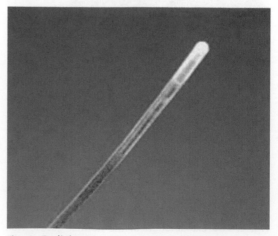

Fig. 4. Radial mini probe.

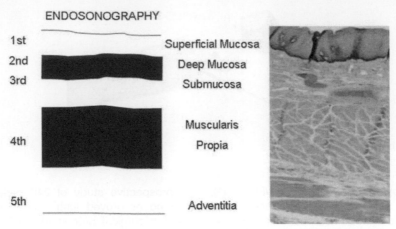

ENDOSONOGRAPHY

1st	Superficial Mucosa
2nd	Deep Mucosa
3rd	Submucosa
4th	Muscularis Propia
5th	Adventitia

Fig. 5. Schematic of gastrointestinal layers seen by endosonography compared with histologic sample (H&E stain at original magnification ×20).

(6), subcarina (7), lower paraesophageal (8), and the pulmonary ligament (9). The more difficult lymph nodes to reach are the right-sided upper and lower paratracheal lymph nodes (2R, 4R).

EUS-FNA can also be used for direct biopsy of lung lesions and determination of mediastinal involvement. Lung masses that are adjacent to the esophagus can be safely biopsied by EUS technique. In a retrospective study of 18 patients with lung masses adjacent to or abutting the esophagus, EUS was able to identify and obtain a tissue diagnosis in all 18 cases.[16] In a prospective study of 32 patients with centrally located lung tumors, EUS-FNA established the diagnosis in 97% of cases.[17] EUS can diagnose direct mediastinal involvement of lung cancer, based on both ultrasonic examination and tissue biopsy. Diagnosis of mediastinal involvement is critical

for treatment options, because if present it is classified as a T4 lesion, which equates to stage IIIb lung cancer, and the patient is not a candidate for surgery. Varadarajulu and colleagues[18] reported that EUS had a sensitivity and specificity of 88% and 98%, respectively, and a positive and negative predictive value of 70% and 99%, respectively, in 308 patients evaluated for T4 staging. In a similar study by Annema,[19] EUS had a sensitivity, specificity, positive predictive value, negative predictive value, and accuracy of 39%, 100%, 100%, 92%, and 92%, respectively, in evaluating T4 tumors.

MEDIASTINAL LESIONS

EUS-FNA can evaluate and biopsy various types of lesions (masses, lymph nodes, cysts, and abscesses) within the mediastinum; however, adequate evaluation is dependent on the location of these lesions. Posterior mediastinal lesions are accessible to EUS-FNA evaluation, whereas lesions in the anterior and middle mediastinum cannot be adequately visualized. The most common indication for EUS of the posterior mediastinum is abnormal lymph nodes. These lymph nodes can be benign or malignant. Benign lymph nodes may be reactive in nature or caused by chronic infections, such as sarcoidosis, histoplasmosis, or tuberculosis. In patients with chronic infections granulomas are often seen. A retrospective study found the sensitivity and specificity of EUS-FNA for diagnosing noncaseating granulomas in suspected sarcoidosis was 89% and 96%, respectively.[20] Another study found that EUS-FNA demonstrated noncaseating granulomas in 41 (82%) of 50 patients with a final diagnosis of sarcoidosis.[21] In addition to granulomas,

1st layer
2nd layer
3rd layer
4th layer
5th layer

Fig. 6. EUS examination of the normal gastric wall showing the five layers of the gastrointestinal wall.

the lymph nodes in histoplasmosis may contain calcifications, which can be seen on EUS. In suspected cases of tuberculosis, EUS-FNA can be used to obtain material from abnormal mediastinal lymph nodes for mycobacterium culture.[22–24] The addition of polymerase chain reaction testing for *Mycobacterium tuberculosis* increases the diagnostic yield compared with cytology and culture in patients suspected of having tuberculosis.[25]

The overall accuracy rate for diagnosing posterior mediastinal malignancy with EUS-FNA is around 93% (**Fig. 7**).[26] EUS-FNA has diagnosed malignant lymph nodes related to lymphoma and metastatic disease from primary lung, breast, colon, renal, testicular, laryngeal, pancreas, and esophageal cancer.[27–29] In suspected cases of lymphoma additional material should be sent for flow cytometry and immunocytochemistry stains. The sensitivity of diagnosing lymphoma increased from 44% to 86% by the addition of flow cytometry and immunocytochemistry.[30] Besides FNA, trucut needles have also been used with EUS equipment for histologic evaluation of lymphomas.[31] Trucut needles have typically been used for percutaneous biopsies, but this role has been expanded to EUS-guided biopsies. These needles are disposable and consist of an outer cannula and inner, notched rod in which the tissue can be cut, trapped, and subsequently withdrawn for evaluation.

Mediastinal cysts account for 10% to 15% of mediastinal masses. They are anechoic when examined by EUS and show acoustic enhancement. Some cysts may appear as more hypoechoic with minimal acoustic shadowing. This appearance may be confused with a mass lesion.[32,33] It should be noted that there is a high risk of mediastinitis if a duplication cyst is aspirated. FNA should only be performed if the suspicion of mass is high, and in these circumstances patients should be given prophylactic antibiotics.

EUS-FNA has also been used in cases of mediastinal abscesses to obtain material for culture and sensitivity. Fritscher-Ravens and colleagues[24] reported a series of 18 patients with clinical mediastinitis who underwent EUS-FNA. There were no apparent complications from performing EUS-FNA into the mediastinal abscesses. There has been a case report of a mediastinal abscess drained by EUS-FNA, followed by placement of a transesophageal pigtail stent.[34]

ESOPHAGEAL CANCER

Treatment and prognosis of patients with esophageal cancer is stage dependant. Accurate staging is necessary for selecting appropriate treatment. CT, PET, and EUS are used for staging of esophageal cancer. CT and PET are best used to exclude the presence of distant metastases. If distant metastases are excluded based on these imaging modalities, patients should undergo EUS for definitive T (depth of invasion and size) and N (nodal involvement) staging, and to determine if endoscopic mucosal resection is possible. Accurate T staging is essential if endoscopic mucosal resection is used for the curative treatment of superficial esophageal cancers. Endoscopic mucosal resection can only be performed if the tumor is confined to the mucosa and has not breached the lamina propria. The accuracy of high-frequency catheter probe in distinguishing between mucosal cancer and cancer invading the submucosa is 81% to 100%.[35] The sensitivity, specificity, and negative predictive values of preoperative EUS for submucosa invasion were 100%, 81%, and 100%, respectively.[36]

The probability of lymph node metastasis depends on the depth of tumor invasion. Lymph node metastases are unlikely to be present if the esophageal tumor does not invade the muscularis mucosa.[37] In contrast, lymph node metastases may be present in up to 10% of patients with involvement of muscularis mucosa.[38] EUS is the best technique and is superior to CT for locoregional staging of esophageal cancer, specifically with tumor size and invasion (T) and lymph node (N) involvement (**Tables 1** and **2**). PET can also be used to evaluate lymph node involvement, but EUS is superior in the detection of peritumoral and celiac involved lymph nodes.[39]

When EUS is combined with CT and PET the number of unnecessary surgeries is decreased. The number of unnecessary surgeries decreased

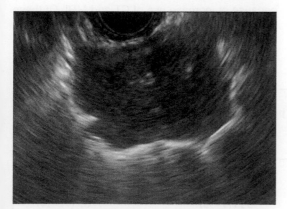

Fig. 7. Hypoechoic mass in the posterior mediastinum. EUS-guided biopsy showed poorly differentiated adenocarcinoma.

Table 1
Preoperative TN staging accuracy of CT and EUS in esophageal carcinoma patients

	Patients (N)	T Stage (%)	N Stage (%)
CT	1154	45 (40–50)	54 (48–71)
EUS	1035	85 (59–92)	77 (50–90)

Data from Rosch T. Endoscopic staging of esophageal cancer: a review of literature results. Gastrointest Endosc 1995;5:537–47.

from 44% to 21% when CT alone was used versus combined CT, PET, and EUS to stage esophageal cancer. There was also decrease in the presence of celiac axis metastasis during surgical exploration in patients who underwent EUS (13%) or PET (7%) compared with CT (32%).[40] EUS can also detect occult liver metastases in patients in whom other imaging studies have been normal.[41]

PANCREATIC CANCER

EUS is the most sensitive method for the detection of benign and malignant pancreatic tumors. The sensitivity of EUS for the detection of pancreatic tumors ranges from 85% to 100% in different studies. EUS is better than conventional CT. Compared with single-detector helical CT, EUS is reported to be either equivalent or superior; however, EUS is shown to be superior to multidetector-row CT.[42–45] Depending on the study, EUS is reported to be both superior[46] and inferior[47] to MRI. Despite the variation of the results in the comparison with CT and MRI, EUS has been found to be especially superior to other imaging modalities in the detection of smaller tumors. EUS detected six of six (100%) tumors less than 15 mm, whereas CT only detected four of six (67%) in one study.[42] The sensitivity of EUS, CT, and MRI for detection of tumors less than 3 cm is 93%, 53%, and 67%, respectively, and for tumors less than 2 cm is 90%, 40%, and 33%, respectively.[46]

Before EUS, definitive diagnosis of pancreatic masses was performed either by surgical or percutaneous CT–ultrasound-guided biopsy (**Figs. 8** and **9**). Currently, pancreatic masses are mostly biopsied by EUS-FNA. The overall sensitivity and specificity of EUS-FNA for the diagnosis of pancreatic tumors is 85% and 98%, respectively. The overall negative predictive value is 55%; a negative biopsy does not necessarily rule out the possibility of pancreatic cancer.[48]

EUS also plays a valuable role in staging of pancreatic tumors. A combination of both multidetector-row CT scan and EUS is probably the most accurate approach for assessing local tumor (T) staging and vascular invasion of pancreatic cancers. Specifically, EUS is best for assessing vascular invasion of the portal vein and splenic vein. The sensitivity of EUS for tumor invasion of the portal vein has been reported to be from 60% to 100% in different studies and is superior to CT scan and angiography.[49–51] The sensitivity of CT scan for staging of superior mesenteric artery and celiac artery seems to be better than EUS, which has a sensitivity of 17% to 83%,[52] 17%,[44] and 50%[49,51] for the superior mesenteric vein, superior mesenteric artery, and celiac artery, respectively.

PANCREATIC CYSTS

Pancreatic cysts are now detected frequently because of increase use of CT and MRI. Of these lesions, 80% to 90% are pseudocysts (**Fig. 10**); 10% are cystic neoplasms (serous cystadenoma, mucinous cystadenoma, mucinous

Table 2
Comparison of accuracy of CT, EUS, and EUS-FNA in preoperative lymph node staging of patients with esophageal cancer

Technique	Sensitivity (%)	Specificity (%)	Accuracy (%)
CT	29 (17–44)	89 (72–98)	51 (40–63)
EUS	71 (56–83)	79 (59–92)	74 (62–83)
EUS-FNA	83 (70–93)	93 (77–99)	87 (77–94)

Data from Vazquez-Sequeiros E, Wiersema MJ, Clain JE, et al. Impact of lymph node staging on the therapy of esophageal cancer. Gastroenterology 2003;125:1626–35.

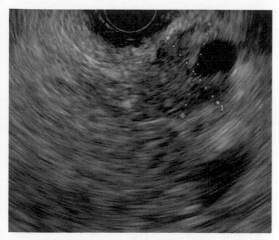

Fig. 8. Hypoechoic mass in the head of pancreas. EUS-guided biopsy showed adenocarcinoma.

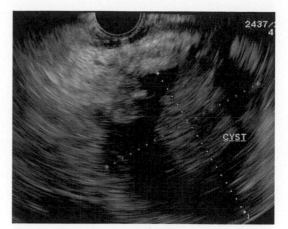

Fig. 10. Pseudocyst with echogenic material in a patient with history of pancreatitis.

cystadenocarcinoma, and intraductal papillary mucinous neoplasia) (**Fig. 11**); and the remaining 10% are congenital or simple cysts.[53] Once a pancreatic cyst is discovered, the next step is to determine if it is a benign, premalignant, or malignant lesion. The ability of CT and MRI to differentiate between benign and malignant pancreatic cysts is limited. EUS has the unique ability of providing high-resolution images of the pancreatic cysts and a means of sampling the cyst and its fluid. During EUS the cyst is carefully examined to determine the wall thickness, mural nodules, papillary projections, or an associated mass. Presence of septations and echogenic material within the cyst is also evaluated. Different features of the cysts have been studied to predict malignancy. Koito and colleagues[54] reported that a thick wall or septa, protruding tumor, or microcystic characteristics were associated with malignancy, whereas thin septa and simple-

looking cysts were benign. They found this system to have an accuracy of 96% and 92% for malignant and benign lesions, respectively. Gress and colleagues[55] reported that mucinous cystadenocarcinoma were more likely to be characterized by a hypoechoic cystic-solid mass or complex cyst, and were frequently associated with a dilated main pancreatic duct. Benign mucinous ductal ectasia (IPMN) is characterized by a dilated main pancreatic duct in conjunction with hyperechoic thickening of the pancreatic duct wall. Intraductal papillary carcinoma has similar features, but additionally reveals a hypoechoic mass.

With EUS-FNA the cystic fluid obtained can be evaluated for malignant cells, mucin stain, amylase, and carcinoembryonic antigen (CEA). The specificity of cytology approaches 100% but the sensitivity varies in reported series. Brugge and colleagues[56] reported sensitivity of 59% for

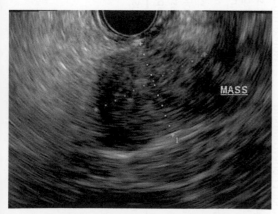

Fig. 9. Hypoechoic mass in the tail of pancreas. EUS-guided biopsy showed neuroendocrine tumor.

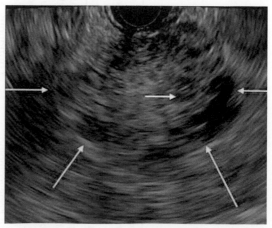

Fig. 11. Serous cystadenoma (*yellow arrows*) of the pancreas showing multiple small cysts (*white arrow*).

Table 3
Consensus-based parenchymal features of chronic pancreatitis

Feature	Definition	Major Criteria	Minor Criteria	Rank	Histologic Correlation
Hyperechoic foci with shadowing	Echogenic structures ≥2 mm in length and width that shadow	Major A		1	Parenchymal-based calcifications
Lobularity	Well-circumscribed, ≥5 mm structures with enhancing rim and relatively echo-poor center			2	Unknown
With honeycombing	Contiguous ≥3 lobules	Major B			
Without honeycombing	Noncontiguous lobules		Yes		
Hyperechoic foci without shadowing	Echogenic structures foci ≥2 mm in both length and width with no shadowing		Yes	3	Unknown
Cysts	Anechoic, rounded/elliptical structures with or without septations		Yes	4	Pseudocyst
Stranding	Hyperechoic lines of ≥3 mm in length in at least two different directions with respect to the imaged plane		Yes	5	Unknown

Data from Catalano MF, Sahai A, Levy M, et al. EUS-based criteria for the diagnosis of chronic pancreatitis: the Rosemont classification. Gastrointest Endosc 2009;69:1251–61.

differentiating between benign and malignant or potentially malignant pancreatic cystic lesions, whereas Frossard and colleagues[57] reported a sensitivity of 97%.

Various tumor markers, such as CEA, CA 19-9, CA 72-4, CA 125, and CA 15-3, have been studied in the aspirated pancreatic cystic fluid. CEA has been found to be the most helpful. A CEA level of less than 5 ng/mL is associated with a sensitivity of 57% to 100% and a specificity of 77% to 86% for serous cystadenomas.[58] A cut-off of more than 400 ng/mL was associated with 100% specificity in differentiating mucinous cystic neoplasms from pseudocysts.[59] Brugge and colleagues[56] did a multicenter collaborative study to determine the most accurate combination of EUS features, cytologic findings, and cyst fluid tumor markers for differentiating mucinous lesions from other types. A total of 341 patients underwent EUS-FNA with measurement of CEA, CA 72-4, CA 125, CA 19-9, and CA 15-3 concentrations. Of these patients, 112 underwent surgical resection. Accuracy of EUS morphology was 51% and cytology was

59%. A CEA concentration above 192 ng/mL was 79% accurate for distinguishing mucinous lesions. No combination of morphologic features, cytology, and tumor markers was better than CEA alone. With regards to amylase levels, a high concentration is found in pseudocysts and IPMN. A level greater than 5000 U/L has a sensitivity and specificity of 61% to 94% and 58% to 74%, respectively, for differentiating pseudocysts from other cystic pancreatic tumors.[57]

CHRONIC PANCREATITIS

The diagnosis of chronic pancreatitis can sometimes be very difficult, especially in early cases of chronic pancreatitis. Different imaging techniques have been used to diagnose this disorder including secretin stimulation test, CT, MRI, magnetic resonance cholangiopancreatography (MRCP), and endoscopic retrograde cholangiopancreatography (ERCP). These imaging modalities specifically look for changes within the pancreatic parenchyma and ducts consistent with chronic

Table 4
Consensus-based ductal features of chronic pancreatitis

Feature	Definition	Major Criteria	Minor Criteria	Rank	Histologic Correlation
MPD calculi	Echogenic structures within MPD with acoustic shadowing	Major A		1	Stones
Irregular MPD contour	Uneven or irregular outline and ecstatic course		Yes	2	Unknown
Dilated side branches	3 or more tubular anechoic structures each measuring ≥1 mm in width, budding from the MPD		Yes	3	Side-branch ectasia
MPD dilation	≥3.5-mm body or >1.5-mm tail		Yes	4	MPD dilation
Hyperechoic MPD margin	Echogenic, distinct structure greater than 50% of entire MPD in body and tail		Yes	5	Ductal fibrosis

Abbreviation: MPD, main pancreatic duct.

Data from Catalano MF, Sahai A, Levy M, et al. EUS-based criteria for the diagnosis of chronic pancreatitis: the Rosemont classification. Gastrointest Endosc 2009;69:1251–61.

pancreatitis. CT can evaluate changes in the main pancreatic duct, presence of cysts, and calcifications. MRCP can examine dilated side branches; however, the resolution of MRCP is poor. The side branches can be better evaluated by ERCP, but this procedure caries the risk of pancreatitis. EUS can evaluate both the changes in the pancreatic parenchyma and the pancreatic duct for the diagnosis of chronic pancreatitis. Smaller cysts, mildly dilated side branches, and calcifications a few millimeters in size can be identified by EUS. Various changes in the pancreatic parenchyma (hyperechoic foci, hyperechoic strands, lobularity, and cysts) and pancreatic ducts (dilation, dilated side branches, main duct irregularity, hyperechoic duct margins, and stones) have been described for the diagnosis of chronic pancreatitis based on EUS.[60] There had been a lack of standardization when EUS was used to diagnose chronic pancreatitis. To address this issue an international consensus conference was held in Rosemont, Illinois, in 2007 and developed the recommendations of the Rosemont classification system for chronic pancreatitis.[61] Changes seen in the pancreatic parenchyma (**Table 3**) and ducts (**Table 4**) were divided into major and minor criteria. Diagnosis of chronic pancreatitis depends on the number of major and minor criteria seen in the pancreas on EUS examination (**Box 1**).

CBD STONES

ERCP has long been used for both diagnosis and removal of CBD stones. It is an invasive procedure, however, with substantial complications in 5% of patients and a mortality rate of 0.1% to 0.2%.[62] Currently, a number of different techniques are available for the diagnosis of CBD stones. Abdominal ultrasound is very specific, but not very sensitive. Helical CT, MRCP, and EUS have improved the diagnosis of CBD stones, avoiding unnecessary ERCP. MRCP is a noninvasive procedure and more accurate than CT, but cannot be performed in patients with permanent pacemakers, cerebral aneurysm clips, or those patients who are extremely claustrophobic. MRCP is also known to miss stones in the periampullary region and has less resolution compared with EUS (1–1.5 mm vs 0.1 mm), and has lower sensitivity in the diagnosis of small stones.[63] Overall, EUS is better than both MRCP and ERCP for detecting small stones.[64] The specificity of EUS in detecting the presence of CBD stones has been noted to be as high as 98% (**Fig. 12**).[65]

SUBMUCOSAL LESIONS

Diagnosis of submucosal lesions of the gastrointestinal tract is one of the main indications for EUS (**Fig. 13**). Submucosal lesions are covered by normal intestinal mucosa, and arise from within the gastrointestinal wall or can be caused by an impression from an adjacent extramural structure. The prevalence of submucosal lesions at routine endoscopy is 0.36%.[66] EUS is the best modality for precise diagnosis of submucosal lesions. Compared with endoscopy, barium contrast radiography, ultrasonography, CT, and MRI, EUS is

---

Box 1
EUS diagnosis of chronic pancreatitis on the basis of consensus criteria[a]

I. Consistent with chronic pancreatitis

A. 1 major A feature (+) ≥3 minor features
B. 1 major A feature (+) major B feature
C. 2 major A features

II. Suggestive of chronic pancreatitis[b]

A. 1 major A feature (+) <3 minor features
B. 1 major B feature (+) ≥3 minor features
C. ≥5 minor features (any)

III. Indeterminate for chronic pancreatitis[b]

A. 3 to 4 minor features, no major features
B. Major B feature alone or with <3 minor features

IV. Normal

≤2 minor[c] features, no major features

[a] EUS diagnosis of CP should be made in the appropriate clinical setting.
[b] Diagnosis requires confirmation by the additional imaging study (ERCP, CT, MRI, or PET).
[c] Excludes cysts, dilated MPD, hyperechoic nonshadowing foci, dilated side branch.
 Data from Catalano MF, Sahai A, Levy M, et al. EUS-based criteria for the diagnosis of chronic pancreatitis: the Rosemont classification. Gastrointest Endosc 2009;69:1251–61.

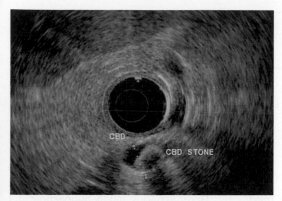

Fig. 12. Gallstone seen within the common bile duct (CBD) with acoustic shadowing.

more accurate in detecting and assessing the size and location of submucosal lesions (**Table 5**).[67] EUS is also able to tell from which layer of the gastrointestinal wall the lesion is originating and allows for tissue sampling by FNA. EUS is more accurate in differentiating between submucosal tumors and extraluminal compression. The accuracy of EUS, ultrasonography, and CT was 100%, 22%, and 28%, respectively, in differentiating submucosal tumors from extraluminal compression.[68]

RECTAL CANCER

As with most malignancies, treatment of rectal cancer depends on the stage of the disease. A number of studies have demonstrated that transrectal EUS is superior to CT and MRI for tumor

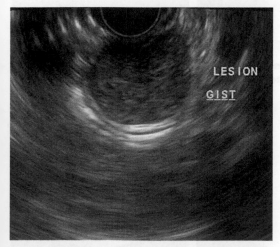

Fig. 13. Hypoechoic lesion arising from muscularis propria. EUS-guided biopsy showed gastrointestinal tumor.

depth and size (T) and nodal (N) staging. The accuracy of transrectal EUS for T staging ranges from 80% to 95%, compared with 65% to 75% for CT, and 75% to 85% for MRI.[69–72] In a meta-analysis of 42 studies the sensitivity and specificity for staging of rectal cancer by EUS for T1 was 88% and 98%, T2 was 81% and 96%, T3 was 96% and 91%, and T4 was 95% and 98%.[73] Based on decision-analysis, Harewood and Wiersema[74] reported that the most cost-effective strategy for evaluation of nonmetastatic rectal cancer was a combination of abdominal CT and transrectal EUS. In a prospective study of 80 patients with nonmetastatic rectal cancer, EUS resulted in the change of management in 31% of the patients.[75]

ANAL SPHINCTERS AND FECAL INCONTINENCE

In patients with fecal incontinence, anal endosonography is used to identify structural defects and tears in the internal and external anal sphincters. This is a relatively simple procedure with a sensitivity of 90% in identifying defects in the anal sphincters. In a study by Deen and colleagues,[76] anal endosonography was 100% sensitive in identifying defects in the internal and external anal sphincters. In another study, endorectal EUS was performed in 28 patients with fecal incontinence before surgery.[77] EUS correctly identified all 25 of the internal anal sphincter defects and all 10 of the external anal sphincter defects. It incorrectly diagnosed external anal sphincter defect in three patients resulting in an overall accuracy of 89%. In a prospective study, the results of endosonography were compared with manometry and electromyography in 12 patients who were scheduled to undergo sphincter repair.[78] Nine of the 12 patients were found to have defects of external anal sphincter at surgery. EUS was superior to other modalities with an accuracy of 100% for detecting sphincter injury, compared with an accuracy of 75% for manometry, 75% for electromyography, and 50% for clinical assessment.

THERAPEUTIC EUS

EUS is now also being used for therapeutic procedures, such as celiac plexus block, stent placement in pancreatic pseudocysts, or failed CBD–pancreatic duct cannulations, and chemotherapy. EUS has been used to perform celiac plexus block or neurolysis in patients with chronic pancreatitis and pancreatic cancer. "Celiac plexus block" is the term used when steroid and local anesthetic is injected in the celiac ganglion. In celiac plexus neurolysis, a neurolytic agent, such

Table 5
EUS characteristics of various submucosal tumors intrinsic to the gastrointestinal wall

Etiology	EUS Layers	Appearance
Gastrointestinal stromal tumors	Fourth	Hypoechoic mass (irregular borders, echogenic foci, anechoic spaces suggest malignancy)
Lipomas	Third	Hyperechoic, often polypoid
Varices	Third	Anechoic, serpiginous structures
Cysts	Third	Anechoic, compressible, round or oval (three- or five- layer walls suggestive of duplication cyst)
Carcinoids	First, second, or third	Homogeneous, mildly hypoechoic mass
Pancreatic rests	Second, third, or fourth	Hypoechoic or mixed echogenicity (ductal structures may be present)
Granular cell tumors	Third	Heterogeneous mass with smooth borders
Metastatic deposits	Any or all	Hypoechoic, heterogeneous mass

Data from Chak A. EUS in submucosal tumors. Gastrointest Endosc 2002;56(Suppl):S43–8.

as alcohol, is injected. In 1996, Wiersma and Wiersma[79] were the first to report on performing celiac plexus neurolysis in patients with pancreatic cancer. EUS-guided celiac plexus neurolysis is a relatively easy procedure. In patients with unresectable pancreatic cancer, EUS-guided celiac plexus neurolysis can be performed at the same time as diagnostic EUS.

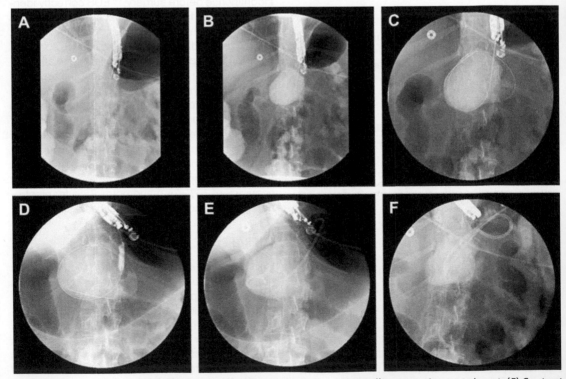

Fig. 14. EUS-guided pseudocyst drainage and catheter placement. (A) Needle puncturing pseudocyst. (B) Contrast injection. (C) Placement of wire. (D) Balloon dilation of tract. (E, F) Pigtail catheter placement.

Pancreatic pseudocysts can be drained by ultrasound or CT guidance. These procedures, however, carry the risk of cutaneous fistula. In 1985, Kozarek and colleagues[80] first reported on endoscopic drainage of pancreatic pseudocysts. With endoscopic drainage there is no risk of cutaneous fistula. Recently, EUS-guided drainage of pseudocysts is more commonly performed. With EUS-guided drainage, vessels present in the gastric, duodenal, or cyst wall can be visualized and avoided. The cyst wall is punctured with a needle under direct vision, reducing the risk of perforation, with subsequent placement of a pigtail catheter (**Fig. 14**).

EUS has been successfully used to perform cholangiography or pancreatography in patients in whom the bile duct or the pancreatic duct cannot be cannulated during ERCP. In a series of 49 patients with failed ERCP, EUS-guided cholangiography and stent placement was performed.[81] The overall success rate was 84% with complication rate of 16% and there were no procedure-related deaths. EUS-guided pancreaticogastrostomy was reported in a series of four patients with strictures secondary to chronic pancreatitis.[82] Gastropancreatic duct stents were placed directly through the gastric wall into the dilated pancreatic ducts. The procedure was successful in all patients with no early complications.

EUS-guided injection of various antitumor agents into unresectable pancreatic cancer has been reported in clinical trials.[83–85] There are case reports describing EUS-guided brachytherapy to malignant perigastric lymph nodes in a patient with recurrent esophageal cancer[86] and EUS-guided injection of 95% ethanol into a gastrointestinal stromal tumor.[87] Injection of paclitaxel after ethanol injection into cystic tumors of the pancreas was reported by Oh and colleagues.[88] Out of 14 patients with cystic tumors of the pancreas, 11 patients had complete resolution, two patients had partial resolution, and in one patient the cyst persisted.

SUMMARY

The convergence of endoscopy and ultrasound has provided an exciting new technology for examination of various anatomic structures and associated diseases. EUS provides a safe procedure with excellent diagnostic capabilities based on both images and tissue diagnosis. As EUS use has expanded, there is now the ability to perform specific therapeutic interventions. Research is ongoing and needs to continue to explore other potential uses, both diagnostic and therapeutic, for this procedure.

REFERENCES

1. Dussik KT, Dussik F, Wyt L. Auf dem Weg zur Hyperphonographie des Gehirnes. Wien Med Wochenschr 1947;97:425–9 [in German].
2. Ludwig GD, Struthers FW. Considerations underlying the use of ultrasound to detect gallstones and foreign bodies in tissue. Naval Medical Research Institute Reports, Project #004 001, Report No. 4, June, 1949.
3. Wild JJ. The use of ultrasonic pulses for the measurement of biological tissue changes. Surgery 1950;27:183–7.
4. Wild JJ, Reid JM. Echographic tissue diagnosis. Proceedings of the 4th Annual Conference of Ultrasonic Therapy. Detroit, August 27, 1955.
5. Wild JJ, Reid JM. Diagnostic use of the ultrasound. Br J Phys Med 1956;19:248–57.
6. Watanabe H, Kato H, Tanaka M, et al. Diagnostic application of ultrasonotomography for the prostate. Jpn J Urol 1968;59:273–7.
7. DiMagno EP, Buxton GL, Regan PT, et al. Ultrasonic endoscopy. Lancet 1980;12:241–4.
8. Strohm WD, Phillip J, Hagenmuller F, et al. Ultrasonic tomography by means of an ultrasonographic fiberendoscope. Endoscopy 1980;12:241–4.
9. Parkin DM, Bray F, Ferlay J, et al. Global cancer statistics, 2002. CA Cancer J Clin 2005;55:74–108.
10. Toloza EM, Harpole L, McCrory DC. Noninvasive staging of non-small cell lung cancer: a review of current evidence. Chest 2003;123(Suppl):137S–46S.
11. Toloza EM, Harpole L, Detterbeck F, et al. Invasive staging of non-small cell lung cancer: a review of current evidence. Chest 2003;123(Suppl):157S–66S.
12. Annema JT, Versteegh MI, Veselic M, et al. Endoscopic ultrasound added to mediastinoscopy for preoperative staging of patients with lung cancer. JAMA 2005;294:931–6.
13. Annema JT, Versteegh MI, Veseleic M, et al. Endoscopic ultrasound-guided fine- needle aspiration in the diagnosis and staging of lung cancer and its impact on surgical staging. J Clin Oncol 2005;23(33):8357–61.
14. Larsen SS, Krasnik M, Vilmann P, et al. Endoscopic ultrasound guided biopsy of mediastinal lesions has a major impact on patient management. Thorax 2002;57:98–103.
15. Mountain CF, Dresler CM. Regional lymph node classification for lung cancer staging. Chest 1997;111:1718–23.
16. Varadarajulu S, Hofman BJ, Hawes RH, et al. EUS-guided FNA of lung masses adjacent to or abutting

the esophagus after unrevealing CT-guided biopsy or bronchoscopy. Gastrointest Endosc 2004;60: 293–7.

17. Annema JT, Veselic M, Rabe KF. EUS-guided FNA of centrally located tumors following a non-diagnostic bronchoscopy. Lung Cancer 2005;48:357–61.

18. Varadarajulu S, Schmulewitz N, Wildi SF, et al. Accuracy of EUS in staging of T4 lung cancer. Gastrointest Endosc 2004;59:345–8.

19. Annema JT. Transesopahgeal ultrasound guided fine needle aspiration in the diagnosis and staging of lung cancer and the assessment of sarcoidosis. PhD Thesis. Leiden; 2005.

20. Wildi SM, Judson MA, Fraig M, et al. Is endosonography guided fine needle aspiration (EUS-FNA) for sarcoidosis as good as we think? Thorax 2004;59: 794–9.

21. Annema JT, Veselic M, Rabe KF. Endoscopic ultrasound-guided fine-needle aspiration for the diagnosis of sarcoidosis. Eur Respir J 2005;25:405–9.

22. Hainaut P, Monthe A, Lesage V, et al. Tuberculous mediastinal lymphadenopathy. Acta Clin Belg 1998;53:114–6.

23. Kramer H, Nieuwenhuis JA, Groen HJ, et al. Pulmonary tuberculosis diagnosed by esophageal endoscopic ultrasound with fine-needle aspiration. Int J Tuberc Lung Dis 2004;8:272–3.

24. Fritscher-Ravens A, Schirrow L, Pothmann W, et al. Critical care transesophageal endosonography and guided fine-needle aspiration for the diagnosis and management of posterior mediastinitis. Crit Care Med 2003;31:126–32.

25. Sriram PVJ, Kaffes AJ, Rajasekhar P, et al. EUS features of mediastinal tuberculosis: a PCR based cytodiagnosis by transesophageal EUS-FNA. Gastrointest Endosc 2004;59:AB216.

26. Wallace MB, Fritscher-Ravens A, Savides TJ. Endoscopic ultrasound for the staging of non-small-cell lung cancer. Endoscopy 2003;35:606–10.

27. Kramer H, Koeter GH, Sleijfer DT, et al. Endoscopic ultrasound-guided fine-needle aspiration in patients with mediastinal abnormalities and previous extrathoracic malignancy. Eur J Cancer 2004;40:559–62.

28. Devereaux BM, LeBlanc JK, Yousif E, et al. Clinical utility of EUS-guided fine-needle aspiration of mediastinal masses in the absence of known pulmonary malignancy. Gastrointest Endosc 2002;56:397–401.

29. Dewitt J, Ghorai S, Kahi C, et al. EUS-FNA of recurrent postoperative extraluminal and metastatic malignancy. Gastrointest Endosc 2003;58:542–8.

30. Ribeiro A, Vazquez-Sequeiros E, Wiersema LM, et al. EUS-guided fine-needle aspiration combined with flow cytometry in the diagnosis of lymphoma. Gastrointest Endosc 2001;53:485–91.

31. Levy MJ, Jondal ML, Clain J, et al. Preliminary experience with an EUS-guided trucut biopsy needle

compared with EUS-guided FNA. Gastrointest Endosc 2003;57:101–6.

32. Faigal DO, Burke A, Ginsberg GG, et al. The role of endoscopic ultrasound in the evaluation and management of foregut duplications. Gastrointest Endosc 1997;45:99–103.

33. Geller A, Wang KK, DiMagno EP. Diagnosis of foregut duplication cysts by endoscopic ultrasonography. Gastroenterology 1995;109:838–42.

34. Kalaheo M, Yoshida C, Kane L, et al. EUS drainage of a mediastinal abscess. Gastrointest Endosc 2004; 60:158–60.

35. Murata Y, Napoleon B, Overgaard S. High-frequency endoscopic ultrasonography in the evaluation of superficial esophageal cancer. Endoscopy 2003;35:429–35.

36. Scotiniotis IA, Kochman ML, Lewis JD, et al. Accuracy of EUS in the evaluation of Barrett's esophagus and high-grade dysplasia or intramucosal carcinoma. Gastrointest Endosc 2001;54:689–96.

37. Tajima Y, Nakanishi Y, Ochiai A, et al. Histopathologic findings predicting lymph node metastasis and prognosis of patients with superficial esophageal carcinoma: analysis of 240 surgically resected tumors. Cancer 2000;88:1285–93.

38. Tio TL. Diagnosis and staging of esophageal carcinoma by endoscopic ultrasonography. Endoscopy 1998;30(Suppl 1):A33–40.

39. Akdamar M, Cerfolio R, Ojha B, et al. A prospective comparison of computerized tomography (CT), 18 fluoro-deoxyglucose positron emission tomography (FDG-PET) and endoscopic ultrasonography (EUS) in the preoperative evaluation of potentially operable esophageal cancer (ECA) patients. Am J Gastroenterol 2005;98:s5.

40. van Westreenen HL, Heeren PA, van Dullermen HM, et al. Positron emission tomography with F-18-fluorodeoxyglucose in a combined staging strategy of esophageal cancer prevents unnecessary surgical explorations. J Gastrointest Surg 2005;9:54–61.

41. Prasad P, Schmulewitz N, Patel A, et al. Detection of occult liver metastases during EUS for staging of malignancies. Gastrointest Endosc 2004;59: 49–53.

42. Legmann P, Vignaux O, Dousset B, et al. Pancreatic tumors: comparison of dual-phase helical CT and endoscopic sonography. Am J Roentgenol 1998; 170:1315–22.

43. Midwinter MJ, Beveridge CJ, Wilsdon JB, et al. Correlation between spiral computed tomography, endoscopic ultrasonography and findings at operation in pancreatic and ampullary tumors. Br J Surg 1999;86:189–93.

44. Mertz HR, Sechopoulos P, Delbeke D, et al. EUS, PET, and CT scanning for evaluation of pancreatic adenocarcinoma. Gastrointest Endosc 2000;52: 367–71.

45. DeWitt J, Devereaux B, Chriswell M, et al. Comparison of endoscopic ultrasound and multidetector computed tomography for the detection and staging of pancreatic cancer. Ann Intern Med 2004;141:753–63.

46. Muller MF, Meyenberger C, Bertschinger P, et al. Pancreatic tumors: evaluation with endoscopic US, CT, and MR imaging. Radiology 1994;190:745–51.

47. Ainsworth AP, Rafaelson SR, Wamberg PA, et al. Is there a difference in diagnostic accuracy and clinical impact between endoscopic ultrasonography and magnetic resonance cholangiopancreatography? Endoscopy 2003;35:1029–32.

48. DeWitt J. EUS on pancreatic neoplasms. In: Hawes RH, Fockens P, editors. Interventional endosonography. London: Elsevier Publishers; 2006. p. 177–203.

49. Rosch T, Braig C, Gain T, et al. Staging of pancreatic and ampullary carcinoma by endosonographic ultrasonography: comparison with conventional sonography, computed tomography, and angiography. Gastroenterology 1992;102:188–99.

50. Sugiyama M, Hagi H, Atomi Y, et al. Diagnosis of portal venous invasion by pancreaticobiliary carcinoma: value of endoscopic ultrasonography. Abdom Imaging 1997;22:434–8.

51. Rosch T, Dittler HJ, Lorenz R, et al. The endosonographic staging of pancreatic cancer. Dtsch Med Wochenschr 1992;117:563–9.

52. Buscai L, Pages P, Berthelemy P, et al. Role of EUS in the management of pancreatic and ampullary carcinoma: a prospective study assessing respectability and prognosis. Gastrointest Endosc 1999;50:34–40.

53. Balthazar EJ, Chacko AC. Computed tomography of pancreatic masses. Am J Gastroenterol 1990;85:343–9.

54. Koito K, Namieno T, Nagakawa T, et al. Solitary cystic tumor of the pancreas: EUS-pathologic correlation. Gastrointest Endosc 1997;45:268–76.

55. Gress F, Gottlieb K, Cummings O, et al. Endoscopic ultrasound characteristics of mucinous cystic neoplasms of the pancreas. Am J Gastroenterol 2000;95:961–5.

56. Brugge WR, Lewandrowski K, Lee-Lewandrowski E, et al. Diagnosis of pancreatic cystic neoplasms: a report of the cooperative pancreatic cyst study. Gastroenterology 2004;126:1330–6.

57. Frossard JL, Amouyal P, Amouyal G, et al. Performance of endosonography-guided fine needle aspiration and biopsy in the diagnosis of pancreatic cystic lesions. Am J Gastroenterol 2003;98:1516–24.

58. Hammel P, Levy P, Voitot H, et al. Preoperative cyst fluid analysis is useful for the differential diagnosis of cystic lesions of the pancreas. Gastroenterology 1995;108:1230–5.

59. Hammel P, Voitot H, Vilgrain V, et al. Diagnostic value CA 72-4 and carcinoembryonic antigen determination in the fluid of pancreatic cystic lesions. Eur J Gastroenterol Hepatol 1998;10:345–8.

60. Sahai AV, Zimmerman M, Aabakken L, et al. Prospective assessment of the ability of endoscopic ultrasound to diagnose, exclude or establish the severity of chronic pancreatitis found by endoscopic retrograde cholangiopancreatography. Gastrointest Endosc 1998;48:18–25.

61. Catalano MF, Sahai A, Levy M, et al. EUS-based criteria for the diagnosis of chronic pancreatitis: the Rosemont classification. Gastrointest Endosc 2009;69:1251–61.

62. Loperfido S, Angelini G, Benedetti G. Major early complications from diagnostic and therapeutic ERCP: a prospective multicenter study. Endoscopy 1999;31:125–30.

63. Lambert R. Clinical outcome of EUS in biliary diseases. Endoscopy 2000;32:558–61.

64. Napoleon B, Dumortier J, Kerivin-Souquet O, et al. Do normal findings at biliary endoscopic ultrasonography obviate the need for endoscopic retrograde cholangiography in patients with suspicion of common bile duct stone? A prospective follow-up of 238 patients. Endoscopy 2003;35:411–5.

65. Liu CL, Lo CM, Chan JK, et al. EUS for detection of occult cholelithiasis in patients with idiopathic pancreatitis. Gastrointest Endosc 2000;51:28–32.

66. Hedenbro JL, Ekelund M, Wetterberg P. Endoscopic diagnosis of submucosal gastric lesions: the results after routine endoscopy. Surg Endosc 1991;5:20–3.

67. Rosch T, Lorenz R, Dancygier H, et al. Endosonographic diagnosis of submucosal upper gastrointestinal tract tumors. Scand J Gastroenterol 1992;27:1–8.

68. Zhang QL, Nian WD. Endoscopic ultrasonography diagnosis in submucosal tumor of the stomach. Endoscopy 1998;30(Suppl 1):A69–71.

69. Kwok H, Bissett IP, Hill GL. Preoperative staging of rectal cancer. Int J Colorectal Dis 2000;15:9–20.

70. Thaler W, Watzka S, Martin F, et al. Preoperative staging of rectal cancer by endoluminal ultrasound vs. magnetic resonance imaging: preliminary results of a prospective, comparative study. Dis Colon Rectum 1994;37:1189–93.

71. Meyemberger C, Huch Boni RA, Bertschinger P, et al. Endoscopic ultrasound and endorectal magnetic resonance imaging: a prospective, comparative study for preoperative staging and follow-up of rectal cancer. Endoscopy 1995;27:469–79.

72. Guinet C, Buy JN, Ghossain MA, et al. Comparison of magnetic resonance imaging and computed tomography in the preoperative staging of rectal cancer. Arch Surg 1990;125:385–8.

73. Puli SR, Bechtold ML, Reddy JB, et al. How good is endoscopic ultrasound in differentiating various T stages of rectal cancer? Meta-analysis and systematic review. Ann Surg Oncol 2009;16:254–64.

74. Harewood GC, Wiersema MJ. Cost-effectiveness of endoscopic ultrasonography in the evaluation of

proximal rectal cancer. Am J Gastroenterol 2002;97: 874–82.

75. Harewood GC, Wiersema MJ, Nelson H, et al. A prospective, blinded assessment of the impact of preoperative staging on the management of rectal cancer. Gastroenterology 2002;123:24–32.

76. Deen KI, Kumar D, Williams JG, et al. Anal sphincter defects: correlation between endoanal ultrasound and surgery. Ann Surg 1993;218:201–5.

77. Meyenberger C, Bertschinger P, Zala GF, et al. Anal sphincter defects in fecal incontinence: correlation between endosonography and surgery. Endoscopy 1996;28:217–24.

78. Sultan AH, Kamm MA, Talbot IC, et al. Anal endosonography for identifying external sphincter defects confirmed histologically. Br J Surg 1994; 81:463–5.

79. Wiersema MJ, Wiersema LM. Endosonography-guided celiac plexus neurolysis. Gastrointest Endosc 1996;44:656–62.

80. Kozarek RA, Brayko CM, Harlan J, et al. Endoscopic drainage of pancreatic pseudocysts. Gastrointest Endosc 1985;31:322–7.

81. Maranki J, Hernandez AJ, Arslan B, et al. Interventional endoscopic ultrasound-guided cholangiography: long term experience of an emerging alternative to percutaneous transhepatic cholangiography. Endoscopy 2009;41:532–8.

82. Francois E, Kahaleh M, Giovannini M, et al. EUS-guided pancreaticogastrostomy. Gastrointest Endosc 2002;56:128–33.

83. Chang KJ, Nguyen PT, Thompson JA, et al. Phase I clinical trial of allogenic mixed lymphocyte culture (cytoimplant) delivered by endoscopic-ultrasound guided fine-needle injection in patients with advanced pancreatic carcinoma. Cancer 2000;88:1325–35.

84. Hecht JR, Bedford R, Abbruzzese JL, et al. A phase I/II trial of intramural endoscopic ultrasound injection of ONYX-015 with intravenous gemcitabine in unresectable pancreatic carcinoma. Clin Cancer Res 2003;9:555–61.

85. Chang KJ, Senzer N, Chung T, et al. A novel gene transfer therapy against pancreatic cancer (TNFerade) delivered by endoscopic ultrasound (EUS) and percutaneously guided fine needle injection (FNI). Digestive Disease Week, oral presentation 2004;59:AB92.

86. Lah JJ, Kuo JV, Chang KJ, et al. EUS-guided brachytherapy. Gastrointest Endosc 2005;62:805–8.

87. Gunter E, Lingenfelser T, Eitelbach F, et al. EUS-guided ethanol injection for treatment of a GI stromal tumor. Gastrointest Endosc 2003;57:113–5.

88. Oh H, Seo DW, Lee TY, et al. New treatment for cystic tumors of pancreas: EUS- guided ethanol lavage with paclitaxel injection. Gastrointest Endosc 2008;67:636–42.

Miniaturization of Ultrasound Scanners

Kai E. Thomenius, PhD, FAIUM

KEYWORDS
- Ultrasound • Scanner • Miniaturization
- Software beamformation

In its nearly 50-year history, ultrasound scanner design has changed dramatically with variations in clinical capability and with the technologies available for achieving that capability. There have been transitions from manual scanning to mechanical and electronic scanning and from bistable black and white images to full gray scale images with electronic scan converters and the migration to digital hardware and to software-based systems. The last decade has seen the increasing conversion of scanner hardware to software, run in either personal computers (PCs) or in digital signal processors. This article reviews most of these developments and tries to anticipate the clinical role of ultrasound scanning in the context of the current trends of development.

Ultrasound scanners are unique among medical imagers in achieving size reduction. This is largely because of the physics involved in data acquisition. With ultrasound scanners, the image data are acquired through an ultrasound transducer whose size is in the range of a few centimeters in any dimension. The rest of the ultrasound scanner is composed of signal processing components of one type or another. This processing can be accomplished with ever smaller electronic components or with software. The contrast with computed tomography, magnetic resonance imaging, positron emission tomography, or radionuclide scanning is stark. All these modalities require large gantries for image data acquisition. All of them have also achieved substantial performance improvement in the last few decades,

although these have not been accompanied by the size and cost reductions achieved in ultrasound scanning. Fortunately for ultrasound instrument manufacturers and users, these reductions have been largely paid for by the semiconductor industry.

STAGES OF ULTRASOUND SCANNER DEVELOPMENT
Early Manual and Mechanical Scanners

Because the early commercial ultrasound scanners were based on investigations of ultrasound technology for medical applications in the 1940s and 1950s, they were more similar to pieces of laboratory equipment than clinical scanners. Invariably, the transducers were low-frequency, single-element devices that were manually positioned and directed. Nonetheless, significant clinical utility was achieved, and the growth of ultrasound scanning achieved a steady double-digit pattern with new users coming in at a rapid rate. Technical progress was rapid, with significant improvements in clinical utility and ease of use.

Phased Array Scanners

During the 1970s, there was rapid development of the multielement arrays that began to replace manual and mechanical scanners. Long linear arrays were initially widely applied for obstetric and abdominal imaging, whereas phased arrays using beam steering were aimed largely at cardiac applications. Some of the digital hardware was replaced

This work was supported in part by United States Army Medical Research Acquisition Activity DAMD17-02-0181 (820 Chandler Street, Fort Detrick, MD 21702-5014, USA) and by the National Institutes of Health (National Institute of Biomedical Imaging and Bioengineering) R01 EB002485, "Low Cost Ultrasound Using Silicon Transduction."
Ultrasound and Biomedical Imaging Technologies Organization, GE Global Research, 1 Research Circle, Niskayuna, NY 12309, USA
E-mail address: thomeniu@crd.ge.com

Ultrasound Clin 4 (2009) 385–389
doi:10.1016/j.cult.2009.10.008
1556-858X/09/$ – see front matter © 2009 Published by Elsevier Inc.

by software run on the newly available microprocessors, and the key here was overall control of image-data acquisition because until this time, ultrasound scanners had no control devices that could strictly be considered computers.

In phased array scanners, the signals from array elements were processed using analog circuitry. For the electronics designer, the achievement of high-quality and robust beamformation with analog components is particularly cumbersome, and they do not permit easy size reduction (eg, it is difficult to construct a scanner with high-quality beamforming delays that will also cover a transducer frequency range from 2 to 10 MHz.) Analog components also have variations associated with temperature changes, which could easily alter intended performance. However, these scanners, with their high frame rates and good image quality, achieved broad clinical application and generated a period of ultrasound growth, which, at times, may have been greater than 20% a year.

Around this time, several semiconductor companies identified medical ultrasound scanning as a growth area and started the development of dedicated circuitry for this industry segment. The earliest time-gain compensation (TGC) amplifiers in articulated arm scanners often occupied a small circuit board; today as many as 8 of them can be on a single chip.

Digital Beamformation

With the development of high-speed integrated circuits for the conversion of analog signals to digital form, a development similar to the conversion from vinyl analog records to compact discs, digital beamformers began to replace the analog beamformers in ultrasound scanners. With this development, ultrasound scanners were able to take advantage of the size reductions and the increased stability and reliability of each new generation of integrated circuits.

This miniaturization characteristic of electronic circuitry is sometimes referred to as Moore law,[1] which argues that integrated circuits will halve in size and double in their speed approximately every 2 years. This has been the trend for almost the last 30 years, although it seems to be slowing down. However, in the 1980s and 1990s, ultrasound scanners directly benefited from Moore law, particularly with the reduction of the size of the electronic components required for beamforming electronics (Fig. 1). The earliest digital beamformers had feature sizes in the order of 1 μm, whereas today those dimensions are often less than 100 nm. Such tenfold size reductions (accompanied by speed and power consumption

improvements) dramatically reduced the space requirements for ultrasound scanners.

Displays

The earliest displays on articulated arm scanners were cathode ray tubes; several manufacturers used the displays available in the oscilloscopes marketed by Tektronix Inc (Beaverton, OR, USA) or Hewlett-Packard (Palo Alto, CA, USA). The need for superior displays and more convenient storage of the displayed information pushed for the development of scan converter technologies for the faster video scanning systems. These became widely available in the 1980s. With the increasing use of liquid crystal displays and the change in the video display industry, this migration occurred for ultrasound scanners.

Migration of Functionality to Software

The earliest articulated arm scanners had no discernible computer controller simply because none were available at the time. This situation changed rapidly when microprocessors arrived in the late 1970s and early 1980s in several forms. Microprocessors became the logical master controller device for ultrasound scanners. Various operating systems, including UNIX, were used in ultrasound scanning systems. Today some version of Microsoft Windows is commonly used in the larger scanners. Along with these operating systems came convenient user interfaces, display capabilities (often driven by the video game industry), and electronic communication and storage. These improvements rapidly enhanced the overall capabilities of the scanners. The drivers behind much of this technology were the PC industry and Moore law.

With the availability of superior processors, some of the functionalities of the scanners were transferred to them. This migration is illustrated in **Fig. 1**, which shows a typical block diagram of a scanner and the technologies being used to implement them. In many cases, the first function to be moved was scan conversion. Specific capabilities in the newer processors allowed Doppler and image processing to be moved over during the late 1990s and early 2000s. As seen in **Fig. 1**, the line between software and hardware has been steadily drifting toward the transducer end during the last 2 decades. It has been debated whether the receive beamformer itself could be executed in software. This processing block includes some very high-speed electronics technology, and the logical choice has been their implementation in dedicated hardware. However, there are several developments that suggest that

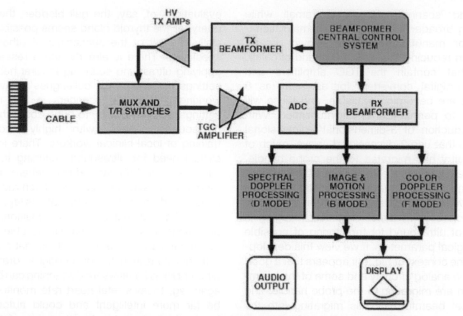

Fig. 1. A typical ultrasound scanner. The blue boxes indicate system functionality that has already been implemented in software, that is, in a PC or a digital processor. The yellow boxes show processing steps that are commonly performed in digital application-specific integrated circuits. Of these, the receive beamformer (RX beamformer) is starting to be moved to the software column. The remaining blocks contain analog signal processing components; some of this is actually moving into the probe itself. The net result is the hollowing out of the ultrasound console.

even this functionality can shift to the software side (eg, a patent application[2] proposes a scheme of pixel-based processing in which the determination of the gray level of a pixel is determined by a matrix multiplication of the raw data). The major challenges in conversion to software may not be processor speed; rather they are in the area of data transfer from frontend electronics to the processing unit. There are analog methods of beamformation that can be implemented as highly miniaturized integrated circuits.[3] These are referred to as charge-coupled devices, and their operation is termed charge domain processing.

IMPLICATIONS OF MIGRATION TO SOFTWARE BEAMFORMATION

With multiple advances in frontend electronics and the introduction of software beamformation, it is apparent that ultrasound scanners are becoming simply a combination of an analog frontend unit and a computing unit. With appropriate packaging, an additional round of size reductions will become possible. More importantly, new beamformation strategies will become available. Hardware implementation of the beamformation function tended to favor the conventional delay-and-sum architecture. This is not the case with software beamformers, and many new strategies can be contemplated. In contemplating the future of medical ultrasound technology, this may be the most exciting stage for further development, offering superior image reconstruction and possible solutions for image reconstruction errors due to variations in the speed of sound in different tissues.

Many machines will still retain their console format, more for user convenience rather than for the actual space requirements of the scanner. The need for large displays in clinical diagnosis will establish the limit for size reductions; such displays are the easiest to use with small consoles. There are other applications for which a handheld device may be the most appropriate. The migration of ultrasound scanners from the hospital to the offices of primary care physicians and even to earlier health care providers is a likely outcome.

It is interesting to contemplate how small ultrasound scanners might develop, given the current miniaturization trends. Moore's law seems to have run its course, although new semiconductor fabrication technologies are continuously being developed and one of these might extend the run of this law. Most of the processors being sold today come in multicore versions, and these allow an increased number of parallel operations and hence greater speed without much of an increase in the size of the devices. Based on these developments, it appears that the back ends of the ultrasound scanner will remain small while achieving broader functionality. The major semiconductor manufacturers have shown greater interest in reducing the size of frontend circuitry. Chips that contain the TGC amplifiers and analog-to-digital converters for as many as 8 channels are becoming available, and these will continue to permit further miniaturization. With the introduction of 3-dimensional/4-dimensional scanners that use 2-dimensional arrays, much of this circuitry has migrated to the probe handle. These developments permit more size and cost reduction, and high-quality diagnostic handheld devices will become available. Another interesting application beyond direct diagnostic imaging is the use of ultrasound for monitoring of possible physiological parameters. If we view this development in the context of **Fig. 1**, it appears that a good part of the analog circuitry and some of the beamformation are migrating to the probe handle, and the digital beamformation is migrating into the system processor. When complete, this process will end with a complete hollowing of the ultrasound scanner, which will consist of the probe and a system processor. The size of each will be determined by the degree of miniaturization achievable with the analog electronics in the probe and the nature of the system processor.

APPLICATIONS OF MINIATURIZED SCANNERS

Several companies have introduced laptop-sized scanners, and these have found many uses with the early adopters. Laptop scanners are highly mobile and can readily be moved around the hospital. Some common applications include use in the emergency department,[4] in intervention guidance, in placement of peripherally inserted central catheters,[5] and in nerve block guidance for regional anesthesia. Each of these applications introduces its own technical challenges, but the utility of the information is of sufficient value to sustain further use and acquisition of additional scanners. As the systems migrate from the hands of trained and highly experienced users, there will be a greater emphasis on maintaining high image quality. Some approaches toward miniaturization trade off cost and size for image quality; this has significant application risks. Further, the need for automated features such as gain adjustment is far greater. This is partially because of the reduced size of instruments that may not allow the existence of slide pots for TGC controls.

With the improvements in handheld scanners, it is likely that their role will expand into point-of-care applications. The ability of a primary care physician to perform rapid first-order imaging

evaluations of, say, the gall bladder, the carotid artery, or the thyroid gland seems possible, especially in view of the successes of other clinical specialists. There is already active research into applying ultrasound scanning in rural health care settings.[6] Garra and colleagues[7] have been working with laptop scanners in low resource settings, such as Belize, to bring about the use of ultrasound scanning with highly accelerated training of local clinical workers. There is a clear clinical need for ultrasound scanning in regions such as sub-Saharan Africa, where maternal mortality ratios remain very high. Even rudimentary skills in performing fetal examinations (eg, determination of gestational age, breech position, multiple gestations, placenta previa) will be able to bring about substantial improvements in that ratio.

If miniaturization trends continue, dramatically different roles for ultrasound scanning can be envisaged, eg, today's fetal heart rate monitors could be far more intelligent and could automatically locate the atrioventricular plane in a fetus even

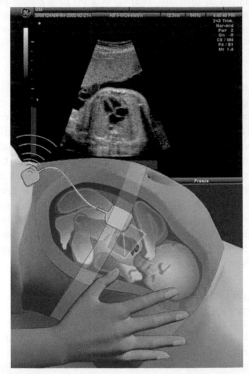

Fig. 2. Concept of fetal monitoring with highly miniaturized ultrasound scanner. In this example, the array locates the atrioventricular plane of the fetal heart by determining the location of the strongest Doppler echoes corresponding to fetal heart motion. With subsequent possible maternal or fetal motion, the ultrasound scanner can relocate the fetal heart and continue with monitoring. If fetal heart rate anomalies occur, the system can scan and transmit the image data to a central station for further analysis.

with maternal or fetal motion (**Fig. 2**).[8] The concept of patient monitoring can be extended beyond fetal heart rate to include the measurement and monitoring of other physiologic parameters, such as vascular properties.[9–11] Whereas research into determinants of vascular compliance remains to be completed, ultrasound monitoring of blood pressure without a cuff is a real possibility. Concepts such as using a handheld ultrasound scanner to guide the placement of an intravenous needle have been proposed for battlefield settings.

In 2004, the American Institute of Ultrasound in Medicine organized a workshop to review the implications of small scanners.[12] This issue had already been discussed in publications that generated extended sets of responses.[13,14] The implications of small scanners are numerous. Clearly, such devices would be used more in point-of-care settings rather than in referral settings. The regulatory agencies will have to define new requirements, such as whether the output display standard should apply, for scanners operated by personnel without extended training in ultrasonic safety and the ALARA (As Low As Reasonably Achievable) concept. New reimbursement rules may have to be defined and the question of quality assurance considered. Ultrasound system manufacturers will have to identify new formats for marketing and servicing these devices. Many of these issues remain unaddressed.

SUMMARY

This article discusses the development of ultrasound scanners toward miniaturization. This development is a continuous interplay between clinical needs and the application of novel technologies to bring about superior solutions. Far more than the other imaging modalities, ultrasound imaging has been a major beneficiary of emerging technologies, especially in the areas of electronic hardware and software. Much of this achievement is simply associated with the nature of the ultrasound scanner that is largely composed of processing electronic components.

The exciting aspect is the evolution of the scanner into an ultrasound probe containing an analog frontend attached to a processing unit and a display. Such devices open up a host of possibilities and allow interesting possibilities for improvements in the delivery of medical care. With further improvements and developments, ultrasound scanning will migrate even further from the hospital and the imaging center to specific point-of-care settings.

However, this need not be the only future for ultrasound scanners. The handheld scanner is not attractive for a detailed imaging examination, and the likelihood of a console display being developed is high. Further, as our understanding of ultrasound interaction and propagation in tissue improves, there will be a need for a larger console size to deal with the increased complexity of ultrasound data. New concepts such as ring arrays for breast imaging with high element counts and large computing needs will retain the requirement for larger consoles.

REFERENCES

1. Moore GE. Cramming more components onto integrated circuits. Electronics Magazine; 1965. p. 4.
2. Daigle RE. Ultrasound imaging system with pixel oriented processing. Patent Application WO 2006/113445 A1.
3. Wong W, et al. Modular portable ultrasound systems. Patent no. WO 2005/053664 A2, 2005.
4. Jain AR, Stead L, Decker W. Ultrasound in emergency medicine: a colorful future in black. Int J Emerg Med 2008;1:251–2.
5. Falkowski A. Improving the PICC insertion process. Nursing 2006;36:26–7.
6. Harris RD, Marks WM. Compact ultrasound for improving maternal and perinatal care in low-resource settings. J Ultrasound Med 2009;28: 1067–76, 0278–4297.
7. Garra BS, et al. Scan protocols for use by nonmedical personnel in developing countries: organ visibility and reproducibility evaluation. J Ultrasound Med 2008;27:S16.
8. Hoctor RT, Thomenius KE. Method and apparatus for noninvasive ultrasonic fetal heart rate monitoring. US Patent no. 7, 470232 B2, 2008.
9. Hoctor RT, Dentinger AM, Thomenius KE. Signal processing for ultrasound-based arterial pulse wave velocity estimation. Proc IEEE Ultrasonics Symposium; 2004. p.1492–96.
10. Hoctor RT, Dentinger AM, Thomenius KE. Array signal processing for local arterial pulse wave velocity measurement using ultrasound. IEEE UFFC Trans 2007;54:1018–27.
11. Hoctor RT, Thomenius KE, Dentinger AM. Method and apparatus for ultrasonic continuous, noninvasive blood pressure monitoring. US Patent no. 7,425,199 B2, 2008.
12. Greenbaum LD, Benson CB, Nelson LH 3rd, et al. Proceedings of the compact ultrasound conference sponsored by the American Institute of Ultrasound in Medicine. J Ultrasound Med 2004;23:1249–54.
13. Greenbaum LD. It is time for the sonoscope. J Ultrasound Med 2003;22:321–2.
14. Filly RA. Is it time for the sonoscope? If so, then let's do it right! J Ultrasound Med 2003;22:323–5.

Ultrasound Imaging and Advances in System Features

Mary C. Whitsett, AS, BA, RT(R, T), RVT, RDMS

KEYWORDS

- Ultrasound • Auto-optimization • 3-D imaging
- 4-D imaging • Digital technology • Fusion imaging

Ultrasound physics is the basis of all ultrasound imaging and is a complex subject. All diagnostic ultrasound images are created using an ultrasound machine and an ultrasound transducer. An electric current is applied to a piezoelectric crystal, which produces an ultrasound beam. The returning signal from that ultrasound beam is then processed by a beam transformer and displayed on a monitor to be viewed as an ultrasound image. This is a simplified description of how an ultrasound image is created. The purpose of this article is to introduce readers to newer technologies used in diagnostic ultrasound imaging, not to provide readers with detailed information in the science of ultrasound physics and image creation. Trained operators of any piece of ultrasound equipment should know these basic principles in order to understand how their equipment works and to understand the basics of ultrasound imaging and image acquisition. The basics of ultrasound physics will never change. What has changed is the use of newer digital technologies and innovative engineering ideas that are used in the development and manufacturing of ultrasound machines and transducers today. These new technologies are changing the way basic physical principles are used in the applications of ultrasound. It would not matter how much technology a piece of equipment has if an operator of the equipment did not have basic knowledge in the principles of ultrasound physics. It is this knowledge that allows operators to maximize each system's features to acquire images, differentiate between what is real and what is artifact, and image the area of interest adequately for diagnostic interpretation

by a qualified professional. This is an exciting time in ultrasound imaging because newer applications in the use of ultrasound in imaging for the diagnosis of disease are developed every day. Using a combination of powerful new engineering tools, an ultrasound beam and the miniaturization of transducers and machines have made the imaging possibilities in ultrasound limitless. This article reviews basic system features and provides an overview of advances in ultrasound technology.

BASIC EQUIPMENT FEATURES AND 2-D REAL-TIME ULTRASOUND IMAGING

All ultrasound machines operate on these basic principles: electrical generation of a sound wave and ultrasound beam; reception of the returning echoes; and processing of the returning signal for display. The standard gray-scale real-time image is referred to as 2-D real-time (live) imaging. 2-D real-time imaging consists of two spatial coordinates plotted against time for the returning ultrasound echo. Each detected echo is determined by a scan line using the echo range principle and the speed of sound through tissue (average velocity of sound through tissue is 1540 cm/s). The sound wave produced must have an ultrasound frequency that is greater than 20 kHz and is of uniform intensity with good spatial resolution.[1] Beam formation is accomplished through a combination of internal system components, applied transducer technology, and transducer construction. Manufacturers strive to provide innovative transducer technology that results in the highest-quality axial and lateral resolution with improved

St Luke's Hospital and Health Network, Ultrasound Department, 801 Ostrum Street, Bethlehem, PA 18015, USA
E-mail address: whitsem@slhn.org

Ultrasound Clin 4 (2009) 391–401
doi:10.1016/j.cult.2009.11.005

depth penetration. Axial resolution and lateral resolution are determined by the number of transducer elements and the number of channels. Axial resolution and lateral resolution are the two key ultrasound requirements that must be present to provide high-resolution, quality ultrasound images. Axial resolution is the ultrasound system's ability to see the smallest detectable object along the perpendicular axis of the beam. Lateral resolution is the ultrasound system's ability to distinguish two objects adjacent to each other that are oriented perpendicular to the ultrasound beam.[1] Transducer frequency is another important factor in image quality. Higher-frequency transducers provide higher-quality images with excellent axial and lateral resolution. Today's ultrasound transducers are multifrequency transducers that image for detail at higher frequencies and use lower frequencies for better depth penetration. Multifrequency transducers allow operators to image with improved axial and lateral resolution without the need to use multiple transducers during the performance of an examination.

Basic system features, such as overall gain (transmit power in decibels), time gain compensation, dynamic range (in decibels), field of view (or depth), and focal zones (region of minimum beam width), comprise the basic tools to producing an ultrasound image.[1] Because newer systems have enhanced technology to improve the speed of image acquisition, it is possible to add multiple focal zones to an image without compromising frame rate. Manufacturers have improved equipments' ability to scan with more than two focal zones on, scan at much deeper depths, and maintain fast frame rates. The ability to scan with the entire region of interest in focus and at deeper depths is critical to aiding an operator's ability to find and image normal anatomy and pathology within these areas.

Some new features used to enhance old technology are the addition of auto-optimization buttons or automatic system image adjustments, which allow operators to adjust the sound beam for the organ-specific region of interest. The auto-optimization feature adjusts the image for differences in the speed of sound in varying types of organ tissues and enhances the ability to see these tissue differences. A simple explanation of auto-optimization is to describe it as an automatic adjustment to the image quality that otherwise would have to be adjusted by an operator. Auto-optimization assists in bringing out some of the ultrasound image detail, or contrast differences, that might not have been seen before its application.[2] It is useful for imaging anechoic areas adjacent to soft tissue and subtle masses in an organ

and for bringing out details that require higher than normal levels of contrast. Some systems automatically adjust to these changes as the transducer is moved whereas others require an operator to turn auto-optimization on or off as needed. Some manufacturers program this feature to automatically adjust the time gain compensation and overall gain controls with movement of the transducer or as auto-optimization is applied.[2]

ADVANCES IN ULTRASOUND TECHNOLOGY: BUILDING A SMALLER ULTRASOUND UNIT

The past decade has seen some dramatic changes in ultrasound imaging. Each year researchers have developed new digital ultrasound technology that aids in the diagnosis and treatment of disease processes without the use of ionizing radiation. Digital computerized technology and microprocessors have made it possible for manufacturers to develop powerful equipment and allow them package it in smaller, lightweight, mobile units. Some of the newest generations of ultrasound units are small enough to place in a laboratory coat pocket and light enough to take anywhere. These newer units offer the ability to obtain exceptional quality images at a fraction of the cost of a full-sized unit. The laptop-sized machines have made it possible to perform diagnostic high-quality images that are equivalent in quality to those from higher-end pieces of equipment. These smaller units have also made it possible to take them to locations and perform ultrasound examinations where they has not been able to be done before. Emergency departments across the United States have integrated these small units for use in trauma assessments, or quick scans, and for easy access to vessels for central line placements. Most emergency department training programs for physicians now include training in the use of ultrasound in an emergency department setting. These units have also become popular within the sports medicine field and are routinely used during athletic events for instant diagnosis of sports injuries. These compact units are also battery operated, an added feature to their compact size and portability. These smaller ultrasound units have also become attractive to the veterinary medicine field where they are portable enough to take directly to an animal to use as an assessment tool for diagnostic purposes. Medical professionals can bring the equipment to patients and diagnose disease in a much shorter period of time than previously. Use of compact, portable ultrasound technology for diagnostic purposes has helped lower cost of care to patients and provide earlier diagnoses of diseases.

3-D AND 4-D TECHNOLOGY

3-D, or easy 3-D, is created by using real-time 2-D imaging to acquire a volume of images through an area of interest. On-board ultrasound system software reproduces the image in three orthogonal planes: sagittal, transverse, and coronal. Mechanical and freehand scanning methods may be used to acquire the volume or data set of images. Volume image acquisition requires appropriate transducer movement and speed and frame rates in order to acquire enough image frames for quality reconstruction.[1] Another use of 3-D volume imaging is sometimes referred to as a cine loop or real-time image clip, which can be reviewed after being captured in real time and after digital storage.[1] The volume data set can be acquired in the sagittal or transverse plane and reconstructed through digital data acquisition. The digital data set collected in either plane is what gives users the ability to reconstruct the coronal plane to be viewed. Image acquisition in CT and MRI easily provides the ability to reconstruct the coronal plane because the data sets in these two modalities are large and can be easily completed with reconstruction software. The coronal plane is the one dimension in ultrasound that has not previously been able to be imaged prior to 3-D and 4-D technology (**Figs. 1** and **2**).

Several different scan methods may be used to acquire a 3-D data set. These include linear motion, tilt motion, rotational motion, and freehand with or without a positional sensing device. In order to get the rotational and dimensional information from the 3-D scan, a positional sensing device must be used and is attached to the transducer with a remote magnetic sensor placed near the patient. This enables the machine to plot transducer position in the volume of images, which can then be used to reconstruct a 3-D polyhedron image cube. It allows a viewer to move the plane of reference in or out and rotated to any orientation. Without the sensors, there is no ability to calculate distance within the volume of images.[1]

There are several 3-D–rendering methods using computer graphics, including multiplanar formatting, surface rendering, and volume rendering. Multiplanar formatting consists of a volume set called a voxel (volume of image boxes).[1] The image volumes, or voxel, contain huge amounts of ultrasound information. When frame rates and scan speeds are maximized, these volumes may contain 200 image frames or more in a single image data set. The combination of the multiple image frames make up the layers of the voxel.[1] A voxel[1] data set has an appearance similar to a Rubik's Cube, where each cube, when used as a unit, allows users to view a single plane in the 3-D image volume (**Fig. 3**).

Another use of a 3-D volume set is to depict the surface of organs or structures for display, called volume rendering. Rendering allows color and imaging opacity factors to be adjusted to depict anatomic structures in the image.[1] This technique is frequently used in fetal and vascular imaging. 3-D rendering of fetal anatomy does not have the degree of dramatic depth perception that a 4-D image has but it can be used as a less expensive method of dimensional imaging because it can be performed with a standard transducer and volume acquisition methods and software. 3-D imaging is most useful in imaging of vascular structures, gynecology, and obstetrics. It is a useful tool for reconstructing the coronal plane for diagnosing uterine anomalies, locating gestational sacs in a uterus with a uterine anomaly, and for imaging of the endometrial lining in sonohysterography.

4-D imaging[1] has become one of the newest diagnostic tools used in ultrasound imaging. Its application in fetal imaging has changed the way fetal anomalies are diagnosed and has allowed prospective parents the first opportunity to see their baby before birth. Although 4-D imaging has been controversial in its use for entertainment

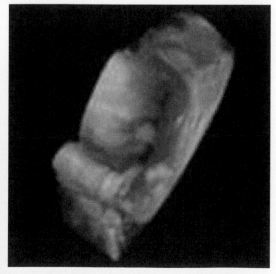

Fig. 1. Easy 3-D representation of fetal face and surface rendering. (*Courtesy of* GE Medical Systems, Wauwatosa, WI; with permission.)

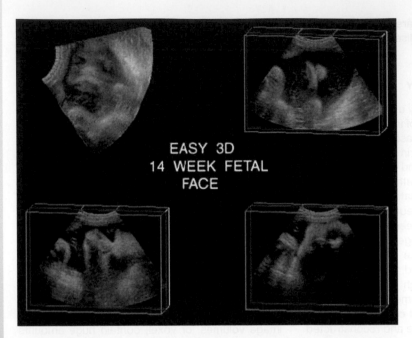

EASY 3D
14 WEEK FETAL
FACE

Fig. 2. Easy 3-D surface rendering obtained from the volume data set. The boxes represent the different planes in which the images can be viewed for surface-rendering purposes. (*Courtesy of* GE Medical Systems, Wauwatosa, WI; with permission.)

purposes and for keepsake photos of the fetus, 4-D imaging has given perinatologists and sonographers another tool for imaging a fetus and has aided in their ability to detect and diagnose life-altering fetal abnormalities. It has proved useful in detecting facial and cranial anomalies and limb abnormalities, imaging documentation of multiple pregnancies, and fetal heart assessment through special cardiac software. Research studies are being conducted to develop additional usefulness of the technology of 4-D imaging in ultrasound (**Figs. 4** and **5**).

4-D imaging requires a transducer that can scan simultaneously in three planes with the fourth dimension of time combined with volumetric sampling to produce the 4-D and surface image. A mechanical transducer is constructed with multiple rows of crystal array encased in fluid to allow enhanced energy transmission into tissue. The crystal array allows the electronic steering of the beam to create an arc of scan lines, which are then converted to a 4-D image. The data set acquired allows an operator to change or modify the 4-D view needed by adjusting the X, Y, and Z

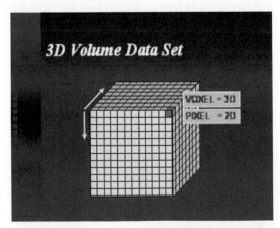

3D Volume Data Set

VOXEL = 3D
PIXEL = 2D

Fig. 3. A voxel is a volume of images that can be used to reformat images or reconstruct for 3-D and 4-D imaging. (*Courtesy of* J.P. Moreland, RT(R), (CT), (ARRT), RDMS, RVS, Kaiser Customer Relationship/VIP Manager, GE Healthcare Ultrasound; with permission.)

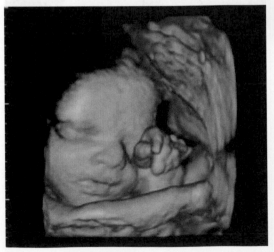

Fig. 4. 4-D surface rendering of a fetal face, arm, and hand. (*Courtesy of* GE Medical Systems, Wauwatosa, WI; with permission.)

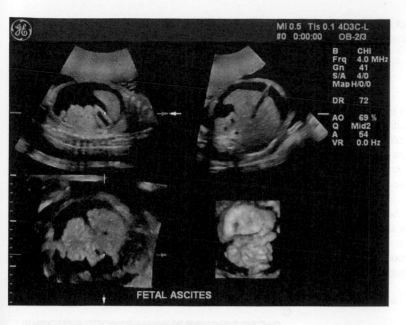

Fig. 5. Use of 4-D imaging of and evaluation of fetal ascites and other fetal abnormalities. (*Courtesy of* GE Medical Systems, Wauwatosa, WI; with permission.)

planes of the volume of images. These X, Y, and Z planes are adjusted by using the system instrumentation, which is specified by the manufacturer.[1] The quality of 4-D imaging depends on the overall 2-D image quality, motion within the field of view, frame rates, region of interest or scan width of the 4-D acquisition area, and line density. Initial 4-D transducers were large, heavy, and cumbersome because the transducer had to contain the mechanics to scan all four planes.[1] According to John Fitzpatrick, Ultrasound Account Executive for GE Healthcare, "new developments in 4-D technology are allowing manufacturers to incorporate solid-state electronic technology in the creation of 4-D imaging transducers which will eliminate the need for mechanical moving parts in the acquisition of 4-D images. Solid-state transducers send scan lines based on a 10 × 10 matrix crystal arrangement. This technology is currently used in cardiac and esophageal transducer construction with research under way to extend the technology to other imaging transducers" (**Fig. 6**). Eventually, this solid-state transducer technology will result in smaller,

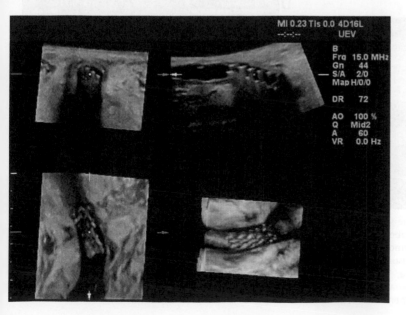

Fig. 6. Other applications of 4-D imaging in location and evaluation of an intraluminal stent. (*Courtesy of* GE Medical Systems, Wauwatosa, WI; with permission.)

high-definition imaging transducers, which will enable their use in 2-D and more sophisticated 4-D image acquisition.

HARMONIC IMAGING

Although 3- and 4-D imaging is expanding the use of ultrasound technology in ultrasound imaging, there are other new tools in ultrasound imaging that are helping in the diagnosis of diseases.

Harmonic imaging, also known as coded harmonics or tissue harmonic imaging, is not a new technology in ultrasound.[1] It is now routinely used in ultrasound imaging, however, and has become an integral part of any ultrasound examination. Harmonic waves are generated from nonlinear distortion of an acoustic signal as an ultrasound wave passes through tissues of the body. In simplified terms, the harmonic frequency is higher on its return to the transducer, which aids in improved axial and lateral resolution and reduces the effect of side lobe artifacts.[3] The returning echoes or harmonic frequency is double the original frequency sent into the body. The harmonic imaging improves resolution but because the harmonic frequency is higher, the trade-off to imaging is decreased penetration. Decreased penetration with harmonic imaging may not be useful in large patients for abdominal and pelvic imaging because the returning harmonic frequency decreases a transducer's ability to penetrate and limits its use in organs deep in the body.[3] New advances in engineering techniques have allowed harmonic frequencies to be applied in most applications with little or no effect in penetration. Most systems manufactured

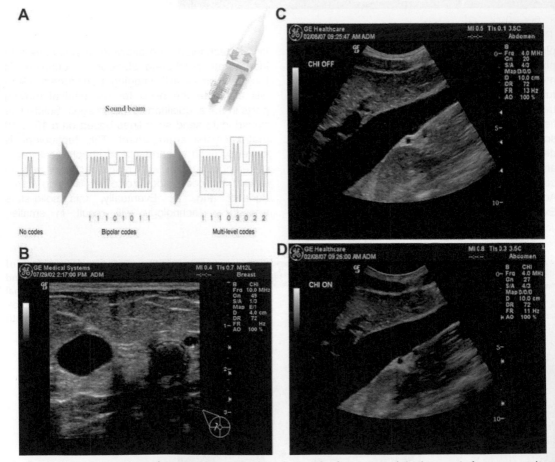

Fig. 7. (*A*) Illustration of how the sound beam changes during the formation of the harmonic frequency as it returns back to the ultrasound probe. (*Reprinted from* GE Medical Systems, 9900 Innovation Drive, Wauwatosa, WI 53226; with permission.) (*B*) Harmonic imaging used to visualized cystic and solid nodules in breast tissue. Use of harmonics is most effective in visualization of both types of lesions in breast tissue. (*Reprinted from* GE Medical Systems, 9900 Innovation Drive, Wauwatosa, WI 53226; with permission.) (*C*) Abdominal imaging without harmonic imaging applied in image. (*D*) Harmonics imaging applied to the image. (*Courtesy of* GE Medical Systems, Wauwatosa, WI; with permission.)

today have these engineering technologies and enhancements and allow users of ultrasound systems to scan and to penetrate the area of interest even with harmonics turned on (**Fig. 7**).

Harmonic imaging is useful in 2-D real-time imaging in the detection of cystic or fluid-filled structures or solid masses within an area of interest, and it also provides improved contrast resolution of the ultrasound image.[1] It has become a useful tool in breast imaging in the detection of small lesions and cysts. Breast tissue is typically gray in ultrasound and is inherently filled with beam noise artifacts and scatter. Use of harmonics improves image contrast in breast tissue and allows easier detection of small cystic structures. The breast lends itself perfectly to the use of harmonics because there are few restrictions to depth penetration in breast tissue.

Harmonic imaging is standard in most equipment sold today. Harmonics is used in almost every application of ultrasound imaging and has become routine for use in the diagnosis of lesions or cystic structures in most organs. Because the harmonic frequency limits penetration, it is not a good tool to use in morbidly obese patients.[3]

EXTENDED FIELD-OF-VIEW IMAGING

In the early days of ultrasound, static imaging was the primary method of ultrasound image acquisition. Static images were made by moving a transducer attached to an articulated arm. As the transducer was moved over a patient, the returning echoes were plotted on X and Y axes and an image was produced on a monitor.[1] Static imaging was the foundation for real-time imaging and in its day was exciting. It was the first nonradiation imaging technique for fetal imaging. Static imaging technique eventually led to the creation of real-time mechanical transducers and the rest is history. Static imaging was the foundation for the ultrasound imaging used today. A need to return to the ability to acquire a larger area of interest for ultrasound eventually led manufacturers to develop a new style of static imaging using real-time techniques. Although manufacturers have coined their own phrases for the technique, the new version of static imaging that emerged is referred to as extended field of view. This feature works in much the same fashion as static imaging, except a hand-held real-time transducer is moved along a plane, which is then plotted internally, and a panoramic (large) image is displayed. Early versions did not allow measurements from extended field-of-view images but the newer versions do. Uses of extended field of view can include imaging of large masses, large subcutaneous fluid collections of abscess, or large areas that cannot be imaged in normal, conventional fields of view. This scan technique requires that the transducer travel or be moved along a straight line along a relatively straight path.[1] Movement of the transducer face during extended field-of-view imaging must be steady in order to avoid overlap of the scan beam and distortion of the area of interest. For this reason, it is not effectively used on curved or bumpy surfaces. Measurements can be made of much larger areas when extended field of view is used in imaging. Sector scans are typically not large enough to include larger than normal areas. This software allows the measurement of larger volumes of tissue. Using extended field of view is useful when ultrasound imaging is required of a large area of interest, such as a leg, arm, neck, or torso (**Fig. 8**).

COMPOUND IMAGING

Compound imaging, or real-time transmit spatial compound imaging, uses electronic beam steering to produce multiple overlapping scan lines that originate at different angles from the transducer crystal. Overlapping multiple scan lines improve the ability to see tissue boundaries and reduce

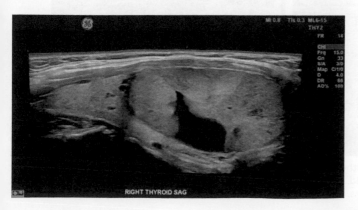

Fig. 8. Extended field-of-view image of a right lobe of the thyroid. The use of this feature provides the capability to include large areas of interest. (*Courtesy of* GE Medical Systems, Wauwatosa, WI; with permission.)

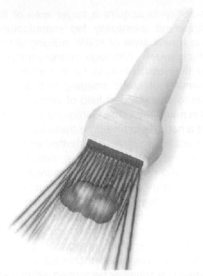

Fig. 9. Illustration of a transducer that is applying a compounded ultrasound beam to a round object. Note how the beam hitting the surface at multiple angles allows for increased visualization of the borders of this type of lesion. (*Courtesy of* GE Medical Systems, Wauwatosa, WI; with permission.)

noise variations in the image.[1] Compound imaging is used most effectively in rounded surfaces and is useful in imaging of calcifications, the cortex of the kidney, ovaries, fibroids, thyroid nodules, and masses within most organs. Because compound imaging uses multiple scan line angles, it is also useful in vascular imaging for plaque characterization as it provides a clear image of plaque arising from vessel walls.[4] Because there is some reduction in image noise and scatter, compound imaging may also improve contrast resolution and tissue differentiation (**Figs. 9** and **10**).

SPECKLE REDUCTION IMAGING ALGORITHM

Imaging of the body with ultrasound can be easy with patients who have perfect anatomy, minimal body fat, and great acoustic windows to scan through. Needless to say, ultrasound operators are not always presented with ideal patients to scan. One commonly occurring artifact in most ultrasound examinations was once referred to as noise or scatter.[5] Now referred to as a speckle artifact,[6,7] it is often difficult to eliminate or reduce even when an operator changes transducers or frequencies. Ultrasound product engineers have discovered an algorithm found to reduce the image degradation effect of this speckle artifact.[5] Applying this algorithm reduces the speckle artifact effect on the image, improving spatial and contrast resolution, which often obscures the underlying anatomy. Speckle reduction improves overall image contrast by increasing the signal-to-noise ratio while retaining all information, so diagnostic quality is maintained.[5] This reduction allows operators to detect differences in tissue planes by defining the differences between tissue types. Levels of speckle reduction applied can be variable and are operator dependent; in other words, operators can change the effect depending on what effect is desired. The application of speckle reduction to an image is sometimes difficult for the eye to adapt to and sonographers using this tool may need a period of adjustment to what they see when first applying speckle reduction to their images. This is especially true when first moving from standard imaging with noise to the application of the speckle reduction algorithm to the same image. Speckle reductions can be adjusted to apply low, medium, and high levels to an image depending on the application and

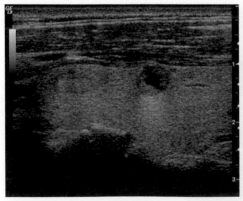
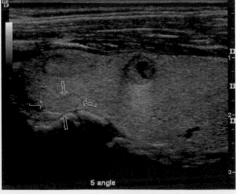

Fig. 10. Thyroid imaging on the left without compounding applied. The image on the right is the same thyroid nodule with compounding applied. Note the distinct difference in visualization of the thyroid nodule (*arrows*). (*Courtesy of* GE Medical Systems, Wauwatosa, WI; with permission.)

may be applied during live scanning or as a post-processing tool (**Fig. 11**).[5]

Speckle reduction is useful in all applications of ultrasound imaging, although it may be more useful in abdominal and pelvic applications because of the higher incidence of noise artifact in those areas. Use of speckle reduction aids in improving contrast and is especially useful in imaging of fluid-filled structures.

ELASTOGRAPHY

The use of elastography ultrasound imaging in diagnosis of disease processes is currently in the early stages of research and development. This technology uses sound wave and pressure readings to determine the degree of stiffness seen in an organ as the sound beam passes through it. The ultrasound pressure can be applied by an operator with external transducer compression or by the equipment software. Tissues that contain tumors or cells that are suspicious for cancer are stiffer than the normal tissue that surrounds the abnormal area. When abnormal tissues are compressed as the sound wave is applied, they are less responsive to pressure than is normal tissue surrounding the area of abnormality. Tissue

stiffness is displayed in hues of color. Areas of abnormality are displayed as darker hues of color in the image. Elastography may be most useful for the diagnosis of breast cancer lesions in which sonographic findings are indeterminate and may lead to unnecessary biopsy and anxiety for patients.[8] Other applications for elastography under investigation include its use in imaging of the prostate, thyroid, colorectal area, and liver fibrosis and in the characterization of arterial plaque. It remains to be seen how it will be used in the diagnosis and treatment of cancer and other disease processes. Research studies are currently under investigation to determine the usefulness of this technology for patients in the future.

FUSION IMAGING

Fusion imaging is a new ultrasound technology that fuses images from CT or MRI with an ultrasound image and allows scan operators to determine the location and correlation of pathologic findings in the two blended modalities.[7] The ability to fuse images is made possible through the use of global positioning system technology and sensors placed in close proximity to the patient. As the global positioning system sensor marks the

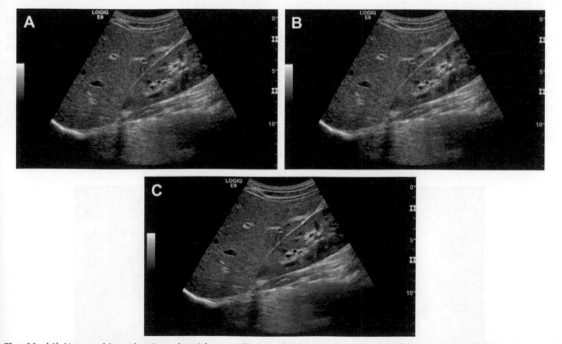

Fig. 11. (*A*) No speckle reduction algorithm applied in this image. Note mottled appearance of this image and loss of tissue differentiation. (*Reprinted from* GE Medical Systems, 9900 Innovation Drive, Wauwatosa, WI 53226; with permission.) (*B*) Low level of speckle reduction algorithm is applied to the same image. Note reduction of speckle in echoes and some moderate smoothing of the overall image. (*C*) Maximum speckle reduction algorithm is applied to the same image. Note improved contrast resolution and tissue plane differentiation compared to the original image without speckle reduction. (*Courtesy of* GE Medical Systems, Wauwatosa, WI; with permission.)

starting location of the transducer, it is possible to match, or synchronize, the anatomy in the ultrasound image to the same anatomic position on the downloaded CT or MRI image (**Fig. 12**).

The images from both modalities can be used as an overlay (one on top of the other simultaneously) or as a side-by-side function in which the ultrasound image location on one side of the image is compared with the matching anatomy from CT or MRI scan on the other side of the monitor.[9] The ability to merge these two different types of examinations gives operators the ability to correlate findings on the CT or MRI with almost pinpoint accuracy. There are, however, some limitations in this technology, such as patient body habitus, whether or not patients can hold still and hold their breath adequately, and a lack of adequate sonographic windows, which can hamper fusion of the ultrasound beam to the CT or MRI. Health care changes in the United States and concerns over rising costs in health care may make fusion ultrasound technology an attractive alternative to the much higher cost of using CT or MRI for biopsy procedures. Because ultrasound is so operator dependent, fusion imaging may also be useful in locating small, indeterminate lesions that have been detected on CT or MRI imaging. Fusion imaging is emerging in the field of ultrasound and its future uses are yet to be seen.

SCAN ASSISTANT SOFTWARE

A final new software feature marketed to ultrasound operators allows them to scan and follow the required image sequence or protocol as the machine automatically labels the images and guides users to the next required image. This scan assistant theoretically helps eliminate mislabeling and inconsistencies in producing the required images for a specific department protocol.[10] The software guides sonographers through an examination by automatically moving to the next required image while automatically labeling the image on screen. The ultrasound scan protocol can be followed exactly without need of a written reference or memorization of written protocols. The scan assistant may also be capable of improving study throughput and help reduce musculoskeletal injuries by reducing repetitive motions of the hand and arm during an examination. It can also automatically apply color Doppler and pulsed-wave Doppler to an image and change the color box direction, as each required image is obtained during the examination. This application can be especially useful in vascular examinations because most vascular examinations require a standard scan protocol with minimal variation in image sequence. It can be used as a teaching tool for entry-level sonographers by illustrating correct scan sequence and protocols for any examination. The scan assistant can be stopped during an examination if additional views must be added. Some of these programs can be written and modified offline and then downloaded to the ultrasound machine as protocols or needs change.[10]

The use of more advanced software and computer-based systems is changing the way systems are developed. Off-system image viewing and manipulation or mini–patient archiving communication systems are also allowing ultrasound operators to view their studies offline, remeasure, reannotate, and prepare their preliminary reports for interpretation, eliminating extra time that patients might need to remain on the equipment.

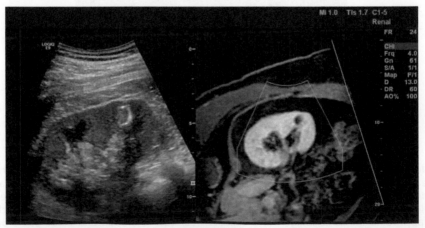

Fig. 12. Fusion imaging in the side-by-side format. The CT image of a renal mass is fused to locate the same lesion seen on the ultrasound image on the left. (*Courtesy of* GE Medical Systems, Wauwatosa, WI; with permission.)

Digital technology has made imaging advances in ultrasound software possible. The future of digital technology in ultrasound is limitless and it will be exciting to see what the future brings to the field of ultrasound.

SUMMARY

The information obtained from ultrasound imaging largely depends on beam characteristics, frequency, operator experience, technique, and many other factors affecting an image. Many of the new advances in ultrasound technology have been developed because skilled ultrasound operators are always looking for ways to improve disease diagnosis through ultrasound imaging. The future of ultrasound may see elastography and fusion imaging become commonly used tools for imaging. The development of increasingly smaller ultrasound machines and transducers and the adoption of wireless technology also are on the horizon. The possibilities are endless and the future of ultrasound is promising.

REFERENCES

1. Hedrick W, Hykes D, Starchman D. Ultrasound physics and instrumentation. 4th edition. St. Louis (MO): Elsevier Mosby; 2005.
2. Jag J, Anderson M. Patent title: automatic ultrasound scanning initiated by protocol stage. Patentdocs. com. Available at: http://www.faqs.org/patents/app/20080306385. Accessed September 12, 2009.
3. Choudhry S, Gorman B, Charboneau W, et al. Comparison of tissue harmonic imaging with conventional US in abdominal disease [Electronic version]. Radiographics 2000;20:1127–35. Available at: http://radiographics.rsna.org/content/20/4/1127.full. Accessed September 12, 2009.
4. Entreken R, Porter B, Sillesen H, et al. Real-time spatial compound imaging: application to breast, vascular and musculoskeletal ultrasound. Semin Ultrasound CT MR 2001;22(1):50–64. Available at: http://www.ncbi.nlm.nih.gov/pubmed/11300587. Accessed September 12, 2009.
5. Milkowski A, Li Y, Becker D, et al. Speckle reduction imaging-white paper [Electronic version]. Available at: http://www.gehealthcare.com/euen/ultrasound/docs/education/whitepapers/whitepaper_SRI.pdf. Accessed September 12, 2009.
6. Crawford D, Cosgrove D, Tohno E, et al. Visual impact of adaptive speckle reduction on US B-mode images. Radiology 1992;183:555–61. Available at: http://radiologyrsna.org/content/183/2/555.abstract. Accessed September 12, 2009.
7. Imaging Economics. GE launches ultrasound fusion. Available at: http://www.imagingeconomics.com/news/2008-09-04_01.asp. Accessed September 19, 2009.
8. Hayes E. Elastography stretches horizons of breast ultrasound. DiagnosticImaging.com. June 3, 2006. Available at: http://www.diagnosticimagingcom/display/article/113619/1191987?verify=0. Accessed October 24, 2009.
9. Healthimaging, New Products. GE releases ultrasound scanner with fusion, GPS, capabilities. Available at: http://www.healthimaging.com/index.php?option=com_articles&view=article&id=12015:ge-releases-ultrasound-scanner-with-fusion-gps-capabilities. Accessed September 19, 2009.
10. GE Heathcare Scan Assistant. Available at: http://www.gehealthcare.com/euen/ultrasound/products/general-imaging/logiq-e9/scanassistant.html. Accessed October 24, 2009.

Basics and Clinical Applications of Photoacoustic Imaging

Keerthi S. Valluru, MS[a],*, Bhargava K. Chinni, MS[a],
Navalgund A. Rao, PhD[b], Shweta Bhatt, MD[a],
Vikram S. Dogra, MD[a]

KEYWORDS

- Photoacoustic imaging • Medical imaging
- Cancer detection

In medical imaging, radiography, ultrasound (US), X-ray computed tomography (CT), magnetic resonance imaging (MRI), positron emission tomography (PET), and single photon emission computed tomography are some of the current clinically established modalities. Photoacoustic (PA) imaging is a new modality that has matured from its research stage in the last decade and is now making a transition into the clinical arena. The purpose of this article is to introduce the basics of PA imaging and then present a short review of the developments to date. The review consists of a description of various technologies used by different groups, including the authors' group. The article puts the future in perspective by illustrating clinical areas in which the authors believe progress is taking place.

BASICS OF PA IMAGING
What is PA Effect?

PA effect refers to a phenomenon in which acoustic waves are produced by absorbing points or objects of a medium, such as soft tissue, that is exposed to a beam of low-energy nanosecond (ns) pulse of laser light in the near-infrared (NIR) region, usually defined for wavelengths from 600 nanometers (nm) to 1100 nm. The absorption of an optical pulse of a few nanoseconds causes localized heating and rapid thermal expansion, which generates thermoelastic stress waves (US waves). These waves are referred to as the "PA signal." The waves are generated instantaneously and simultaneously everywhere in the three-dimensional (3D) tissue volume exposed by the laser beam (**Fig. 1**). These waves propagate and spread away from the source point as spherical waves. The imaging task is to record this signal with 1 or more US sensors, located on the surface of the object being imaged, and then use this information to predict or image the location of the sources. The signal amplitude at the source point can be represented by some calibrated grayscale value in the image. This signal amplitude is proportional to the absorbed light energy at that point. Therefore, imaging based on PA effect is sensitive to the optical absorption property of the object being imaged.

Why PA Imaging?

There are several reasons. First, every imaging modality noninvasively depicts some specific tissue property that results from tissue-radiation interaction inherent in that modality. For example, X-ray CT depicts the attenuation of X-rays, US

[a] Department of Imaging Sciences, University of Rochester, 601 Elmwood Avenue, Box 648, Rochester, NY 14642, USA
[b] Center for Imaging Sciences, Rochester Institute of Technology, 54 Lomb Memorial Drive, Rochester, NY 14623, USA
* Corresponding author.
E-mail address: keerthi_valluru@urmc.rochester.edu (K.S. Valluru).

Ultrasound Clin 4 (2009) 403–429
doi:10.1016/j.cult.2009.11.007
1556-858X/09/$ – see front matter

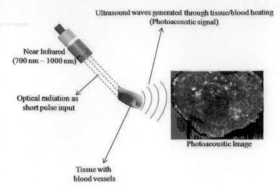

Fig. 1. PA image formation process.

depicts one of the mechanical properties (reflectivity or acoustic impedance difference) of the tissue, and PET depicts the concentration of injected radio nucleotide in the body. Similarly, PA imaging depicts the tissue optical absorption at the wavelength of interrogating laser light. Therefore this is a completely new, henceforth unexplored modality in medical imaging. It may be argued that pure optical imaging[1] can also provide a map of this tissue property, which introduces the second point that differentiates PA imaging from US and pure optical imaging. PA is neither purely acoustical nor purely optical in nature, but a hybrid of the two. It uses light as the input source for tissue excitation, but detection and image formation are achieved using the US waves generated by light absorption in the tissue. Thus it keeps the best of the optical and acoustical counterparts. For example, image contrast comes from the difference in optical absorption of the incident light. As discussed later, evidence for high contrast with PA imaging is strong. Furthermore, unlike pure optical tissue imaging, PA imaging does not depend on the backscattered optical radiation. Because of excessive scattering of light in turbid media, pure optical imaging suffers from depth penetration and poor resolution. Instead, in PA imaging the excited US waves are used for imaging and localization. Good resolution in PA imaging is because US does not scatter, refract or attenuate so much in tissue, it can be focused easily, and speed of propagation does not deviate much from ~1500 m/s so that the wave arrival time can provide the depth information. The third point is that the tissue and its major constituents (eg, water, blood, lipid, fat, melanin, collagen) have widely varying absorption spectra in the NIR that not only promises abundant contrast mechanism, they also allow PA imaging based spectroscopy, noninvasive tissue characterization, and functional imaging. On the other hand, inherent contrast in US imaging has already

been fully exploited. Yet there are many clinical scenarios, such as US imaging of prostate, where tumor contrast in pure US imaging is inadequate for diagnosis and biopsy.

Contrast and Penetration in PA Imaging

Fig. 2 shows the absorption coefficient μ_a of various tissue constituents in NIR.[2] Absorption coefficient of blood is sensitive to hemoglobin concentration, oxy and deoxy state, and the wavelength of light. For a given laser light exposure, the PA signal from any specific location in the tissue is proportional to absorption coefficient μ_a value at that location.[3] Although μ_a values for specific tissues are not known, they are usually significantly lower than blood in the NIR. On this basis significant contrast between blood vessel and surrounding tissue is possible for most wavelengths in the NIR. It is this aspect that most researchers have exploited to image blood vessels in small animals and humans at shallow depths. There is a disadvantage to imaging through high absorption medium. Scattering of light, quantified by the parameter called reduced scattering coefficient μ'_s, dominates in tissue. As a result, in the diffusion limit, the effective attenuation parameter $\mu_{eff}=\sqrt{3\mu_a(\mu_a+\mu'_s)}$ determines the effective penetration depth $l_{eff}=\mu_{eff}^{-1}$ of laser light in tissue.[3] If because of high absorption or scattering or both, effective attenuation is high in the tissue, then the penetration of laser light will be low, limiting the depth for practical PA imaging. For example, for prostate, $l_{eff}\approx 0.24$ cm and 0.42 cm at 1064 nm and 800 nm, respectively.[4,5] Choice of the wavelength often is a compromise between penetration depth and contrast. To increase penetration the laser pulse energy could be increased

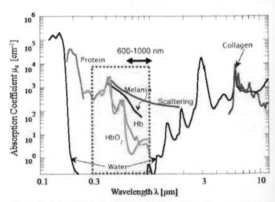

Fig. 2. Absorption coefficient of various tissue constituents as a function of wavelength. (*From* Vogel A, Venugopalan V. Mechanisms of pulsed laser ablation of biologic tissues. Chem Rev 2003;103(2):577–644; with permission.)

but not indefinitely. Limits are set by American National Standards Institute (ANSI) safety guidelines.[6] For example, at 1064 nm the limit for safe laser exposure is 100 mJ/cm^2. The present review indicates feasibility of PA imaging up to a depth of 3 to 4 cm, while keeping the light intensity below the ANSI limits.

PA Signal Generation and Detection

There are several important factors that affect the temporal and frequency spectra of PA signal. Theoretic estimation of the temporal shape of the PA signal indicates that at the point of origin the short temporal US wavelet has an "N" shape (compression followed by rarefaction pressure) for a spherical absorber.[7] The temporal pulse width of this PA signal is directly proportional to the absorber diameter. Therefore small absorbers generate a short pulse that is rich in high frequencies. The second factor that affects the temporal pulse width is caused by the laser pulse duration. Ideally this tissue heating time should be short enough that heat does not diffuse out of the region of interest (ROI) and simultaneously the generated US PA signal does not have time to travel out of the ROI.[3] With 1- to 10-ns laser pulses, it is easy to satisfy this "confined stress condition." If longer (eg, >100 ns) laser pulses are used, the PA signal frequency content is filtered to lower frequencies.[8] The third effect is caused by wave propagation. The PA pulse undergoes frequency-dependent attenuation in tissue, typically 0.5 dB/cm/MHz, on its way toward the US transducer.[8] Consequently, the frequency content shifts toward lower frequencies because higher frequencies are preferentially absorbed. Finally, the US transducer imposes another filter because its frequency response is usually band-limited. The major difference from US imaging is that the PA signal is generated by absorbers in the tissue ROI and its frequency content at the transducer, generally not known a priori, can be estimated based only on the assumptions described earlier. Therefore choice of transducer (or sensor) is an important system design parameter. The best approach is to match the center frequency to the anticipated PA signal frequency and choose the largest possible bandwidth.

Image Formation or Reconstruction

Fig. 3 illustrates all the major PA image formation methodologies used by researchers. In general, the laser source and the sensors may be on the same side or at an angle to each other. An overlap between laser beam and the sensor directivity pattern must exist. The CT-like reconstruction

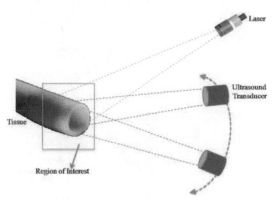

Fig. 3. Diffraction tomography.

method is known as diffraction tomography.[9] The sensor may be a single-element transducer that rotates around the tissue ROI[10,11] or may consist of multiple stationary elements of an array around the ROI.[12–15] It is normally assumed that the US PA signals travel with a constant speed of approximately 1500 m/s in the tissue. The sensors usually have a wide-angle directivity pattern (shown in red). PA signal arriving at each sensor is filtered back-projected along circular arcs in the spatial domain, and then all the back-projections are summed up to construct the final image that approximately represents the spatial distribution of light absorption in the ROI. An alternative method, commonly referred to as "delay and sum", is more efficient.[14,16] The PA signal travel time from a given point source in the ROI to each sensor element location can be calculated exactly for a fixed geometry. To reconstruct an image value at each spatial location in the ROI, 1 contribution from each sensor PA signal at a precalculated delay time is summed up and the process is repeated for all points in the ROI. This method has been scaled up to 3D image reconstruction.[15,17]

The second method is identical to B-scan 2-dimensional (2D) medical US imaging[8,18] as shown in **Fig. 4**. The sensor is usually a focused circular disk transducer that has a thin linelike receiving beam or directivity pattern that is scanned mechanically in a direction perpendicular to the beam axis, or in a radial sectorlike format.[19,20] At each scanning step, PA time signal is recorded and the time is converted into distance along the beam axis using 1-way travel time in tissue, as opposed to 2-way, which is used in pulse echo medical US. Alternatively, a linear array of multiple transducer elements can be used to focus, steer, or scan the beam electronically with a synthesized aperture without mechanical motion.[8,18] This concept has been used by several researchers to

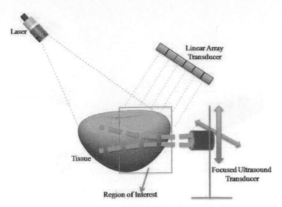

Fig. 4. Alternative reconstruction technique.

modify the existing US scanners to perform PA imaging.[21,22]

While most researchers have selected one of the many available US sensors made of material such as lead zirconate titanate (PZT), polyvinyl difluoride (PVDF), or composites, Beard and colleagues[15] have invented a Fabry-Perot (FP) polymer film sensor that uses interferometric technique. The Stanford group has developed 2D Capacitive Micro-machined Ultrasonic Transducer arrays and used them for PA and US imaging.[23] Ashkanazi and colleagues[24] have also used optical detection of US in PA imaging. The authors introduce a lens-based focusing of PA signal and their experience in building an imaging prototype is discussed later.

Image Resolution

Regardless of the image formation method, the best resolution that can be obtained is ultimately diffraction limited because of focusing of US waves. If the US detection system has full 360° angular access surrounding the object, then the theoretic resolution limit on the order of γ is possible for the tomographically reconstructed image; γ stands for the wavelength of PA US signal in the tissue. In vivo imaging is practical only for small animal imaging and imaging of human breast. Otherwise for most practical purposes, a limited angle or restricted aperture imaging has to be used. The resolution value can be estimated from $\gamma f_{\#}$, where $f_{\#}$ is (focal length)/(aperture or diameter) of the focusing system. Unlike US imaging in which the backscattered signal wavelength γ is determined by the choice of transmitting US source, in PA imaging it is determined mostly by the absorber size and the nanosecond pulse width of the laser source, but most importantly by the sensor frequency response.[8,18] The sensor finite size also affects resolution. Smaller pointlike sensors (size $<< \gamma$) are better, while larger

sensors produce more spatial smoothing effect on the reconstructed image and therefore lower the resolution. However, there is a trade-off between sensor signal-to-noise ratio (SNR) and the resolution that needs to be considered. Generally with other factors notwithstanding, the observed resolution will approximately scale with γ. There are differences among different research groups in details of imaging geometry, sensor size and sensor frequency response, the reconstruction methodology, and even the way resolution is defined. In view of the comments made earlier, differences in resolution are expected. A general idea is provided by a few representative examples of systems in which resolution values have been reported. Kruger and colleagues[25] have developed a small animal system in which data acquisition has full 360° access with a 5-MHz, 128-element linear array transducer, with element size in the imaging plane ~ 2 mm, and a well-designed back-projection algorithm. The measured resolution is about 0.2 mm, close to the theoretic limit. In another clinical breast imaging system developed by Manohar and colleagues[26] the US sensor frequency is around 1 MHz. The sensor is a 2D planar array of 90 mm diameter with 590 sensor elements each of size ~ 2 mm $\times$ 2 mm, but the sensor plane does not rotate around the breast. The observed resolution is between 3 and 4 mm. Another group[27] has designed a breast imaging system that uses a wider bandwidth PVDF-film-based curved sensor array that covers approximately 180° around the breast and have claimed to achieve 0.5 mm resolution with additional signal processing of PA signal. At the other extreme there are examples of laboratory systems that have achieved resolution of less than 50 μ for PA microscopy in which imaging is limited to superficial depths ($<$ a few millimeters).[28] This was achieved by scanning the object with a 50-MHz focused US sensor (f-number ~ 0.44).

EXAMPLES OF PA IMAGES

A few high quality examples of PA images generated by different groups are provided to show the capability of this imaging modality. In most cases correlation with histology has been depicted. The group at Washington University in St Louis, Missouri, USA, has studied in vivo PA imaging of mouse brain extensively. **Fig. 5** shows images from their small animal scanner depicting the brain anatomy in 2 axial planes, 1 mm and 5 mm below the skin surface.[29] Major veins and arteries are resolved and appear as high contrast against the surrounding tissue background because of the difference in light absorption of

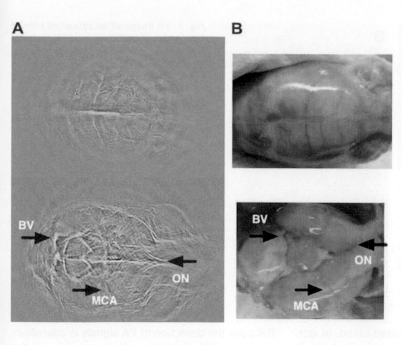

Fig. 5. (*A*) PA images at 1 and 5 mm below skin surface. (*B*) Open-skull photographs of top and basal surfaces of brain. Basalar vein (BV), mid-cerebral artery (MCA), optic nerve (ON) are shown in the image. (*From* Gamelin J, Maurudis A, Aguirre A, et al. A fast 512-element ring array photoacoustic imaging system for small animals. Proc SPIE 2009;7177: 1–10; with permission.)

blood from surrounding tissue in the 710- to 900-nm window.

Fig. 6 provides an example of coregistered US and PA images of ex vivo swine ovary.[30] The imaging system has a 1.75D transducer array that can steer the beam in the sector scan plane and change image plane in elevation direction electronically without moving the transducer. Antral follicles usually show up with low signal value (dark) in US and PA images. Increased blood in theca stands out around the follicle in the PA image. **Fig. 7** is an example of an ex vivo PA image of a late-stage polycystic kidney in a rodent model.[31] Such a kidney contains hemoglobin as a dominant absorber in the NIR, whereas normal parenchyma and cyst contain fluid with Na^+ and Cl^- are expected to absorb less. Correlation of the cysts (dark regions in the PA image) with histology is evident. Vascular structures appear as brighter regions, usually distributed as the outer layer of the kidney. Less evident are the mid-gray level bands around the cyst that represent normal parenchyma.

From the absorption spectra of blood in **Fig. 2** significant amplitude differences can be expected between PA signal from blood that is saturated

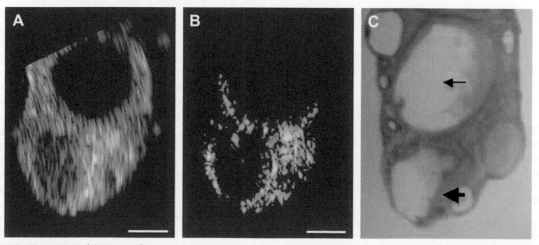

Fig. 6. Coregistered images of ex vivo swine ovary. (*A*) US pulse-echo image. (*B*) PA image. (*C*) Histologic slide. (*From* Aguirre A, Gamelin J, Guo P, et al. Photoacoustic characterization of ovarian tissue. Proc SPIE 2009;7177:1–9; with permission.)

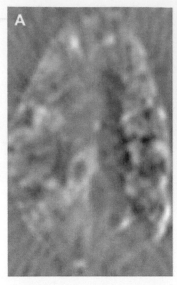
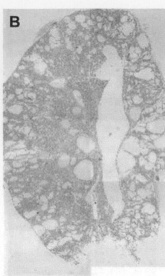

Fig. 7. PA image of an extracted kidney from a late-stage PCY mouse (*A*) and corresponding histology photograph (*B*). (*From* Liu B, Gattone VH, Kruger R, et al. Assessment of photoacoustic computed tomography to classify tissue in a polycystic kidney disease mouse model. Proc SPIE 2006;6086:54–61; with permission.)

with oxygen and the deoxygenated blood. In fact oxygen saturation fraction can be calculated if PA signal amplitude values are known at 2 different wavelengths.[32] This is the simplest application of PA spectroscopy. An example is taken from group that has developed a small animal scanner as shown in **Fig. 8**. An axial slice of PA image through a tumor in a rat model is shown.[32] **Fig. 9** is a 2D PA image of a portion of palm from the skin down to a depth of 4 mm below the skin.[33] This imaging system uses the technology developed by a group at University College, London. This group has also carried out work on PA spectroscopy. **Fig. 10** shows the richness of information that is contained in spectroscopic evaluation of PA imaging data.[34]

RECENT ADVANCES IN PA IMAGING

To date, only a few researchers have had success in developing a complete PA imaging system that can be used in a proper clinical setting, and most others are still either in the research phase, conducting preliminary experiments to prove the concepts, or in the transformation phase from benchtop to bedside. This section presents a brief review of technological advances in PA imaging, categorized into 3 major sections: (1) PA imaging at breadboard level, (2) preclinical imaging using small animals, and (3) PA imaging in the clinical setting.

PA Imaging at Breadboard Level

It has only been a decade or so since researchers have started using photoacoustics in medicine and hence most of the work is still experimental.

Because the detection of PA signals is essentially similar to US detection, the resolution of the system depends mostly on the optical absorption and scattering properties of the tissue being investigated. If there is a priori information about the absorbers in a specific tissue, proper selection of the laser wavelength is all that is needed to perform PA imaging, making sure that the thermal confinement conditions are met. The ease of performing PA imaging and its noninvasive nature have led many researchers to investigate its potential in clinical diagnostics. Systems that have showed promise in addressing a specific clinical issue or those are currently under development are reviewed in this section.

Characterization of atherosclerotic plaques using PA imaging was illustrated by many researchers.[34–36] Allen and Beard[34] conducted an experimental study to discriminate between normal and atheromatous (lipid-rich plaques) arterial tissue using PA imaging. For this purpose, formalin-fixed human aortas were used as tissue samples. These investigators have used a fiber-coupled optical parametric oscillator (OPO) based laser system that can generate laser pulses of diameter 4 to 6 mm at the tissue surface with pulse energy less than 20 mJ over the wavelength range of 740 to 1800 nm in steps of 20 nm. The experiment was set up in forward mode by using a custom-built 25-MHz circular focused PVDF transducer on the opposite side of the tissue sample. The tissue sample was placed on a translation stage and was scanned mechanically in the focal plane of the detector so that the PA signals are acquired at different spatial points. The PA signals obtained were compared with spatially

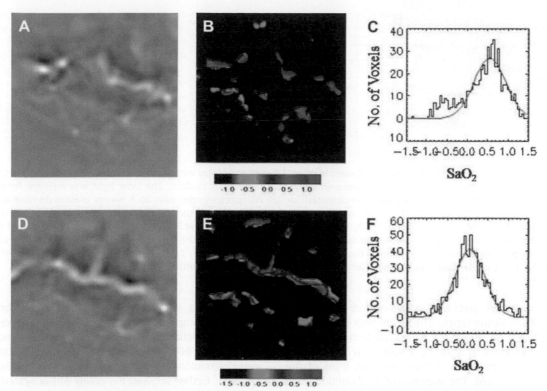

Fig. 8. An axial slice of PA image through a tumor in a rat model. Grayscale images (*A, D*) shows the vasculature through the tumor, Images (*A, B, C*) are taken when rat was alive and the images (*D, E, F*) are taken 1 hour after it was killed. Color plots (*B, E*) depict oxygen saturation value at each pixel. A statistically significant difference can be seen in the oxygen saturation after death. (*From* Stantz KM, Liu B, Cao M, et al. Photoacoustic spectroscopic imaging of intra-tumor heterogeneity and molecular identification. Proc SPIE 2006;6086:36–47; with permission.)

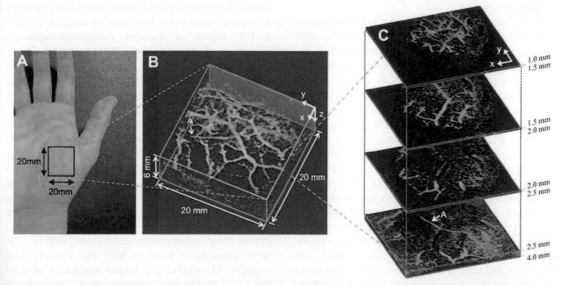

Fig. 9. PA image of vasculature in the palm in vivo at 670 nm. (*A*) The imaged region, (*B*) volume rendered image, (*C*) lateral slices at different depths. Deepest visible vessel (*arrow A*) is located 4 mm beneath the surface of the skin. (*From* Zhang EZ, Laufer JG, Pedley RB. In vivo high-resolution 3D photoacoustic imaging of superficial vascular anatomy. Phys Med Biol 2009;54:1035–46; with permission.)

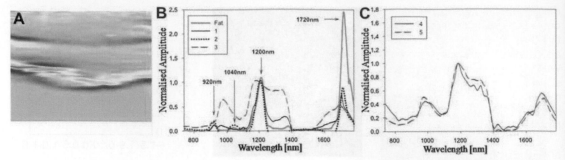

Fig. 10. Ex vivo study of human arterial sample using a B-scan geometry with a single-element transducer. (*A*) PA image at 1200 nm. Wall structure of approximately 2.8 mm vessel is evident. The laser light was incident from below and optical attenuation was compensated for. (*B*) PA spectroscopic data at 3 mainly plaque dominated regions labeled 1, 2, and 3 in the vessel image. It shows normalized amplitude of the PA signal for laser excitation varying from 700 nm to 1800 nm. The spectrum most resembles that of fat. (*C*) Spectrum at 2 locations labeled 4 and 5 where the tissue is expected to be normal. Between 800 and 1200 nm, this spectrum resembles that of water because about 70% of arterial tissue content is water. (*From* Allen TJ, Beard PC. Photoacoustic characterization of vascular tissue at NIR wavelengths. Proc SPIE 2009;7177:1–9; with permission).

resolved PA spectra of ex vivo normal and atheromatous tissue types. The study was extended to assess the capability of the system to perform PA imaging in vivo by inserting a 4-mm-thick cuvette filled with human blood in front of the tissue sample. The experiment was conducted in a similar fashion except that the 25-MHz PVDF detector was replaced by a 15-MHz focused PZT detector. The results of this study indicate that the PA spectroscopy was successful in distinguishing normal and lipid-rich plaques in the NIR wavelength range. Also, the study suggests that the blood has minimal effect on the ability to distinguish between different tissue types based on spectral properties.

Similar studies were conducted by Sokolov and Emelianov[36,37] to address the atherosclerotic plaques in the arteries. They developed an intravascular PA (IVPA) imaging system with a tunable laser source that can generate 7-ns laser pulses at an energy fluence of 11 mJ/cm^2 over a 680- to 950-nm spectral range. The system comprises a 40-MHz intravascular US (IVUS) imaging catheter that is capable of detecting the PA signals and US signals through a pulse echo technique. This catheter allows for spatial coregistration of IVPA and IVUS images for a single cross section of the vessel. To acquire the images, the sample is rotated 360°, and the IVUS catheter and the laser beam remain stationary. The feasibility of using gold nanoparticles as contrast agents for IVPA imaging of macrophages was studied. The IVPA imaging was performed at a wavelength of 680 nm on PVA-based arterial-mimicking phantoms that contain mouse microphages loaded with different concentrations of gold nanoparticles, and was successful in detecting the

macrophages with gold nanoparticle detection sensitivity comparable to the ferromagnetic nanoparticle detection limit of MRI.[36] Spectroscopic studies (700–900 nm) conducted on similar blood vessel mimicking phantoms using an IVPA imaging system[37] further showed the ability of the system to detect tissue constituents that have unique absorption spectra.

Wang and colleagues[20] have shown the potential of PA imaging of neonatal brains through infant skull operated in reflection mode. A 50-μm-diameter blood vessel phantom was constructed using soft transparent tube filled with canine blood and was embedded in a canine brain at different depths to perform transcranial PA imaging through a piece of newborn infant skull ex vivo. To induce a PA effect, a tunable neodymium:yttrium-aluminum-garnet (Nd:YAG) laser pumped OPO-based laser system was used that can generate 5.5-ns pulses at a pulse repetition frequency (PRF) of 10 Hz over a spectral range of 680 to 950 nm. A wideband focused US transducer was raster scanned along the skull surface to reconstruct a 3D volumetric image from the acquired PA data with the vessel placed in the focal plane of the transducer. Wang and colleagues reported use of 2 transducers (5 MHz and 10 MHz). The system was able to detect the vessel at a depth of up to 21 mm beneath the skull when operated at a wavelength of 850 nm with a 5-MHz transducer. The experiments conducted with a 10-MHz transducer suggest that the system was capable of achieving a lateral resolution of 420 μm. That study also involved an in vivo rat tail model to monitor the blood oxygenation level in the main artery of the rat tail, which is placed beneath the infant skull. The obtained PA measurements agreed well with recordings read out by a pulse oximeter, suggesting a good sensitivity for the system to monitor the blood oxygenation level in the brain through the infant skull. Wang and colleagues have also shown PA C-scan imaging by performing a point-by-point 2D raster scan over the skull surface, but the the scan took more than 4 hours, which is significantly high for a clinical setting.

Aguirre and colleagues[38,39] have developed a 3D US and PA imaging system based on a custom-designed 1280-channel 1.75D PZT US phased array that can scan a 3D volume and provide coregistered PA and US images. The system uses a tunable (700- to 1000-nm) Ti:sapphire laser that can output 10-ns laser pulses with a maximum energy of 50 mJ/pulse at a PRF of 15 Hz, which are expanded to a diameter of 20 mm to induce the PA effect in the tissue. The 1.75D US array consists of 128 elements in an azimuthal plane with a pitch of 0.27 mm and 10 elements in the elevation plane with a pitch of 1 mm and a mechanical elevation focal depth of 40 mm. The array is capable of performing $\pm40°$ sector scans in azimuth and $\pm10°$ sector scans in elevation directions with measured azimuth, elevation, and axial resolutions at the elevation focus depth of 40 mm being 0.785°, 2.75°, 0.77 mm for pulse echo and 0.75°, 2.875°, 0.41 mm for PA modes, respectively.[38] A custom-designed electronics circuitry is used that multiplexes, amplifies, and digitizes the acquired RF data, which are subsequently stored on a computer for further beam forming. The system has an ability to perform either traditional pulse echo US imaging or PA imaging, which allows for coregistration of the acquired US and PA images. The 3D PA and US images are reconstructed using a standard delay-and-sum algorithm. Initial studies conducted with tumor-mimicking phantoms reported the advantage of PA and US image coregistration.[39] The clinical potential of the system was shown by performing PA and US imaging on ex vivo porcine ovarian tissue samples immersed in 0.9% saline solution at a wavelength of 740 nm while the laser fluence was maintained at less than 8 mJ/cm^2.[30] The ovarian samples were placed at the elevation focus of the transducer during imaging and the acquired US and PA images were coregistered and compared with corresponding histologic sections. The study indicates that highly vascularized ovarian tissue structures that were not seen in US images were clearly observed in PA images and histologic slices, which shows the potential of PA imaging.

Germer and colleagues[40] have developed a PA detection system based on PA spectroscopy for asthma diagnostics that exploits the absorption properties of nitric oxide (NO) in the exhaled air. It is assumed that a strong correlation exists between asthma and level of exhaled NO concentration. Their system uses a quantum cascade laser, with repetition frequency and pulse width variable up to 2 MHz and 100 ns, respectively, which generates tunable pulses in the spectral range of 5.269 to 5.275 μm by changing its operational temperature. To show the clinical ability of the system, an experimental setup consisting of a flow chamber filled with a calibrated mixture of 100 ppm NO in nitrogen is employed. A microphone connected to a phase-sensitive lock-in amplifier is used to detect PA signals. The PA spectroscopic measurements recorded by varying the laser pulse width from 17.5 ns to 30 ns over a temperature range of −25°C to −18°C indicate an increase in absolute value of the measured PA signal and the spectral resolution with shorter pulse width. A gas blending system was later used with the flow chamber to yield 20-ppm to 1-ppm concentrations of NO in nitrogen, and PA measurements were performed at a wavelength of 5.2715 μm, which resulted in an average PA signal of 17.8 μV with a detection sensitivity of 70 ppb. Germer and colleagues' study suggests that this detection sensitivity is sufficient to distinguish asthmatic patients from healthy patients.

Ren and colleagues[41] have reported the use of PA technique for noninvasive monitoring of blood glucose concentration. Their system uses a fiber-coupled Nd:YAG laser to generate 3-ns laser pulses of wavelength 532 nm to irradiate the sample. The setup consists of a cuvette with a diameter of 4 cm to hold the test sample. A 3- to 12-MHz PVDF ultrasonic transducer array orthogonal to the laser beam is used to detect the PA signals from the sample, which are amplified and digitized before transferring to a computer for subsequent data processing. These investigators have conducted in vitro studies to show the ability of their system to track blood glucose levels. The system was preheated for about an hour, after which the cuvette was filled with 100 mL of aqueous glucose solution. PA measurements were then recorded by adding 0.5 g of glucose powder to the solution at specific time intervals for 2 hours. As the glucose concentration was increased, an increase in the PA signal amplitude was observed. With an additional signal processing on the recorded PA data, Ren and colleagues were able to minimize the noise associated with the PA glucose spectrum, with a considerable improvement in SNR.

Another application of photoacoustics is diagnosis of burn wounds based on the contrast in optical properties of burnt and healthy tissue as investigated by Talbert and colleagues.[42] These investigators have shown the potential of PA technique in differentiating noncoagulated blood from thermally coagulated blood to assess the depth of burn injuries. Their system exploits the spectral differences in optical absorption of thermally coagulated blood and noncoagulated blood at 543- and 633-nm wavelengths. Their study indicates that a strong difference exists in the spectral absorption ratios of coagulated and noncoagulated blood samples. They collected blood samples from 18 swine and performed spectroscopic analysis to determine the spectral absorption ratio values ($\mu a_{543}/\mu a_{633}$) for coagulated and noncoagulated blood samples, which are then compared with experimentally determined PA ratio values. PA measurements were recorded by placing the blood samples in polyacrylamide cylinders. An OPO laser was used to generate the laser pulses of 5-ns pulse width at a PRF of 10 Hz, which illuminate the blood samples from the top via an optical fiber. The generated PA transients were detected by a high frequency ($\approx$40 MHz) PVDF transducer placed beneath the cylinder (transmission mode). The results suggest that the PA ratios calculated from the obtained pressure waveforms agree well with the spectroscopic absorption ratios and hence it was possible to differentiate coagulated and noncoagulated blood samples using this dual wavelength technique. A polyacrylamide gel phantom that consists of 2 vessels filled with coagulated and noncoagulated blood samples separated by a small distance at a depth of 1.75 mm was inserted in intralipid medium to mimic burn wound. The transducer and the optical fiber were fixed to a single scan arm, and 2D raster scanning of the phantom was performed in reflection mode. The acquired data were then used to compute the spectroscopic ratio values at each pixel location, yielding a 2D PA image that showed strong discrimination between noncoagulated and coagulated blood vessels.

To induce PA transients in a sample, a pulsed laser source capable of producing short ns pulses is required. Most of the PA excitation sources that are being used are high-energy Q-switched lasers that operate at a few tens of Hertz. The use of these laser sources in a clinical setting is often limited by their high cost, large, and cooling requirements. Allen and Beard[43] have shown PA effect in vivo using an alternative excitation source consisting of pulsed laser diodes. They have developed a fiber-coupled pulsed laser diode system that comprises 12 high peak power laser diodes, 6 of them being able to generate laser pulses at wavelength of 850 nm and the other 6 at 905 nm wavelength, with variable pulse widths ranging from 50 ns to 500 ns at PRFs of 100 to 5 kHz. The output of each laser diode is coupled to an optical fiber, thus forming a fiber bundle to deliver the laser pulses onto the tissue. The tip of the middle finger was illuminated with the excitation source with a PRF set to 1 kHz. The pulse energy at the output of the bundle was measured to be 80 μJ and 120 μJ for wavelengths 850 nm and 905 nm, respectively, at a pulse width of 200 ns. A cylindrically focused PZT US sensor was used with the excitation source in backward mode to detect PA A-line signals. More experimental details can be found elsewhere.[43] The results of Allen and Beard's study suggest that the setup using the high-power pulsed laser diode excitation source mentioned earlier was capable of generating detectable PA signals in superficial vasculature to monitor the changes in blood oxygenation and volume during arterial and venous occlusions of the forearm. To illustrate the 2D imaging capabilities of the system, they have conducted phantom studies using a cylindrical scanner that rotates a 3.5-MHz PZT detector through 306°.[43] At each angular increment, the detected signal is amplified, averaged, and downloaded on to a computer, until the entire scan is completed. The acquired data are then used to reconstruct a 2D image using a modified backprojection algorithm.

Another active research area that has drawn much attention recently is the detection of circulating metastatic tumor cells (CTCs) using photoacoustics.[44–49] Viator and colleagues[44–46] have developed a PA flowmetry system to detect individual circulating melanoma cells in human blood samples. Most of the melanoma cells contain melanin, which is a broadband optical absorber and can generate strong PA signals on laser illumination.[46] Their system consists of an OPO laser that can generate 5-ns pulses of wavelength 450 nm at 10 Hz to irradiate the sample. The performance of the system was assessed by circulating saline solution suspended with varying concentrations of cultured human melanoma cells through a flow cell by means of a peristaltic pump at a predefined rate.[44,45] The laser pulses of spot size 1.1 mm are delivered on to the sample via an optical fiber, whereas a 100-μm PVDF sensor sealed along the lateral surface of the flow cell is used to detect the PA signals generated from the melanoma cells.[44] To show the clinical potential of their system, Viator and colleagues collected blood samples from a healthy human volunteer and a patient with stage IV melanoma, and performed an investigation.[46] The collected blood samples were centrifuged to separate white blood cells along with melanoma cells from the rest of the blood constituents, and the resultant sample was circulated through the flow cell. Their system was able to detect as few as 5 melanoma cells in the laser beam path with a detection threshold of 1 single melanoma cell suspended in saline solution.[45,46] Further improvement in SNR is promised by using additional signal processing and denoising techniques.[45]

In an in vivo study conducted by Galanzha and colleagues,[49] detection sensitivity of 1 CTC in the presence of approximately 1000 red blood cells (RBCs) is reported. To detect CTCs, these investigators have developed a PA flow cytometry (PAFC) system using a tunable OPO laser that can produce 8-ns laser pulses of 15 μm spot size at 10 to 50 Hz or a 905-nm diode laser that can generate 15-ns pulses at a repetition rate of 10 kHz. They have performed an in vivo mouse study by injecting melanoma cells suspended in saline solution into the mouse circulatory system through a tail vein. Diode laser based PA monitoring of the melanoma CTCs was conducted at a different anatomic site (50-μm-diameter ear vein) to verify the detection sensitivity of the system using a 3.5-MHz US transducer or a 20-MHz focused cylindrical transducer. A tumor progression study conducted on ear and skin tumor mouse models using a 15-μm OPO laser beam suggested that the chance of detecting metastatic processes is higher in the vicinity of the primary tumor than in the systemic circulation at early stages. The study also reports the possibility of spontaneous metastatic cell damage at higher laser exposure levels, illustrating the therapeutic ability of their system. To explore the sensitivity of the PAFC system in detecting melanoma cells in a background with high RBC count, in vitro studies were conducted on whole blood samples drawn from normal mice. A focused laser beam (≈ 10 μm) was scanned over the glass tubes filled with these blood samples after adding mouse melanoma cells to the blood, which resulted in an occasionally strong PA signal appearance against lower PA signals from RBCs.[49] A similar study conducted on healthy human blood samples doped with cultured human melanoma cells revealed a detection limit of 1 melanoma cell in the laser beam path of 50 μm at an SNR of 2. Overall, this study suggests that a 10-minute PA monitoring of a large blood vessel results in an improvement in CTC detection sensitivity by 10^2- to 10^3-fold compared with existing assays.[49]

Preclinical Imaging Using Small Animals

Wang and colleagues[50,51] developed a PA imaging system for small animal in vivo imaging that uses a diffraction tomography technique (which they call PA tomography [PAT]) to reconstruct the PA images. A tunable Ti:sapphire laser pumped by a Q-switched Nd:YAG laser that can provide 8- to 12-ns laser pulses with pulse energy less than 15 mJ/cm^2 at a PRF of 15 Hz over a wavelength range of 700 to 950 nm was used as an excitation source for PA generation. The laser beam was expanded to a diameter of about 50 mm and was homogenized to achieve a uniform illumination over the sample. A 128-element, 90° curved US array with a 5-MHz center frequency and 80% bandwidth was employed to detect the generated PA signals from the sample in the plane orthogonal to the illuminated laser beam. The elements are 0.208 mm × 10 mm in size and are focused in the elevation direction to produce an arc-shaped beam at 19 mm from the transducer surface. The sample is mounted on a rotation stage which is positioned at the center of the detector curvature and turned 3 times in increments of 90° to acquire the PA data over 360°, which are amplified, digitized, and transferred onto a computer, in which the images are reconstructed using a delay-and-sum algorithm. More recently, the use of a 512-element ring transducer array constructed from 4 128-element units whose elements are arranged along the inner curvature of a circular aperture was reported.[29] Along with some improvement in receiver electronics, it enabled the system to achieve a complete 2D tomographic PA imaging in less than 1 second and display the images in real time. The backprojection algorithm was used to reconstruct the 2D PA images from the acquired data. The PA imaging was performed in a rat brain ex vivo and the system was able to discriminate the anatomic features in the brain clearly with a resolution better than 200 μm up to depths of 6 mm. To facilitate in vivo imaging, a flexible clear plastic bag with water was used between the sample and the transducer array to achieve good acoustic coupling along with a breathing bag and a provision for delivering anesthesia to the patient. In vivo spectroscopic imaging was also shown using this system with mice as subjects, the brain being the area of interest.[29] The PA experiments were conducted over the wavelengths 710 to 900 nm to obtain real-time spectroscopic images during a time interval of 30 seconds. The study suggests that the presence of the bag and the breathing apparatus has resulted in lower resolution images; nevertheless, the potential of the PAT system in obtaining real-time functional images was shown.

Yang and Wang[52,53] have shown that the PAT system is also capable of large animal brain cortex imaging by conducting experiments on monkey brains with intact scalp and skull ex vivo. The experiments were conducted using a 1064-nm Nd:YAG laser operating at 10 Hz PRF with an energy fluence of 50 mJ/cm^2 and a 1-MHz single-element unfocused US transducer of diameter 12 mm that can be scanned circularly around the monkey brain to acquire the generated PA signals. Formalin-fixed head samples of a young rhesus monkey and an old pigtail monkey were imaged with and without skull bones and the images of the exposed brain were compared with the skull intact brain. The PAT system was capable of detecting PA signals from the brain cortex even in the presence of a thick skull bone. The acquired signals were used to reconstruct a 2D image using a back-projection algorithm. Song and Wang[54,55] developed a PA imaging system to image deeper structures (up to 38 mm) in biologic tissue. They adopted a dark-field ring-shaped illumination technique that employs a spherical conical lens followed by an optical condenser to improve the penetration of the laser light into the tissue with reduced surface reflections. This geometry allows reflection-mode imaging, making the system usable with otherwise inaccessible areas. The study involved the use of a single-element spherically focused US transducer that can be raster scanned to detect the PA transients. PA imaging performed on a rat using this system revealed the structures in the thoracic cavity and information about vasculature in the cervical area.[55] The study has also demonstrated the performance of the system in visualizing the abdominal structures, including interlobar arteries and spinal cord in situ and the rat kidney vasculature up to depths of 15 mm in vivo. The reflection-mode dark-field illumination technique was further adopted in realizing a PA microscopy (PAM) system, which is capable of performing B-scan imaging at 50 Hz and 3D imaging at 1 Hz.[56,57] The higher rates were achieved by means of a custom-designed light delivery system in conjunction with custom-designed back end electronics. To induce PA signals in vivo, an Nd:YLF laser pumped tunable dye laser that can generate 7-ns pulses with 12 mJ energy at a high PRF of 1 kHz was used. A specially fabricated 48-element, 30-MHz high-frequency US linear array was used in the system to detect the generated PA transients. The array was linearly translated by a motorized actuator for 3D imaging. At a wavelength of 584 nm, an in vivo rat study was conducted using the PAM system, which was able to resolve the subcutaneous blood vessels of diameter 70 to 300 μm that lie within 1 to 2 mm beneath the skin surface.[57] PAM studies conducted by Stein and colleagues[58,59] further

suggest that the system is capable of imaging blood oxygenation dynamics in mouse brain using endogenous hemoglobin contrast with a resolution of 70 μm and 54 μm in lateral and axial dimensions, respectively. Fang and colleagues[60] have developed an M-mode PA flow imaging system that combines PAM with a flow setup including a syringe pump. A spherically focused US transducer with center frequency 22 MHz was used in the system to detect the generated PA signals. Blood flow was simulated using a diluted carbon powder suspension in a Tygon tube (Saint-Gobain Performance Plastics, Akron, OH) oriented perpendicular to the ultrasonic axis, and M-mode PA flow images were obtained at 3 different flow speeds of 1.1 mm/s, 2.2 mm/s, and 4.4 mm/s.

Another application of PA imaging is the endoscopic PAM system as shown by Wang and colleagues.[61] A stainless steel endoscopic probe of about 4 mm in diameter was developed that is capable of obtaining radial B-scan images over a 250° angular field of view at a sampling rate of 200 MHz. Each B-scan image consisted of 254 A-lines, with angular increment of 1.42° between successive A-lines. The imaging ability of the system was demonstrated by conducting rat studies at 570 nm wavelength and the laser energy fluence being 17.6 mJ/cm^2. In situ imaging performed on rat's abdominal tissues show the capability of the endoscopic PAM system in visualizing the blood vessels that are at a depth of up to 1.8 mm. PA imaging was also performed by inserting the endoscopic probe into the rat's large intestinal tract ex vivo, which displayed the ability of the system to visualize the morphology of the intestine.

Kruger and colleagues[25,31,62–65] developed a 3D PA scanning system for small animal imaging that uses a tunable OPO laser source that can generate laser pulses over 680 to 1064 nm wavelength range at a rate of 10 Hz and a 128-element transducer array whose elements (1.8 × 2.0 mm with a center frequency of 2.5 MHz) are lined along a cylindrical surface of radius 40 mm to detect PA signals. This system, the Photoacoustic CT (PCT), in principle, is similar to the PAT system developed by Wang and colleagues in that both employ rotating scanning geometry to acquire PA signals. However, unlike the PAT system, in which the transducer array is rotated around a fixed sample, in the PCT system, the sample is rotated about the vertical axis although the transducer array remains stationary. The PCT system consists of a water tank in which the sample holder (made of a transparent thin-walled plastic tube affixed to a computer-controlled rotary stage) is submerged. The holder has a diameter of about

25 mm and has a provision for supplying air for the subject to keep it alive during the test procedure. The holder is in turn connected to a linear stage to allow the vertical alignment of the sample. Once the sample is aligned, the laser pulses are delivered on to the sample through the plastic wall via 4 fiber-optic bundles that are positioned around the sample holder. The PA imaging is performed by rotating the sample holder 64 times about its vertical axis, spanning 360°. At each scanning angle, the PA data acquired by each element of the transducer array are signal averaged, amplified, digitized, and downloaded to a computer, resulting in a total acquisition time of about 2 minutes for the entire 3D volume.[63] The acquired data are later used to reconstruct a 3D volume by means of a custom-developed filtered back-projection algorithm.[62]

To show the potential of the PCT system, in vivo studies were conducted on mice at wavelengths of 800 nm and 1064 nm. The resulting PA images showed differences in the appearance of anatomic features with a spatial resolution of less than 350 µm. At the 1064-nm wavelength, brain, trachea, scapulae, heart, and lungs of the mice were clearly visualized, whereas at 800 nm, the vascular anatomy along with the 2 kidneys and the abdominal aorta were identified.[63] The clinical ability of the PCT system was further evaluated by conducting ex vivo studies on 4 mice with late-stage polycystic kidney disease and 1 normal mouse.[31] Kidneys were excised from each of the freshly killed mice and were imaged using the PCT scanner over the spectral range of 680 to 940 nm at increments of 20 nm. At each wavelength, the sample holder with the kidney was rotated 96 times, accounting for an acquisition time of approximately 4.5 minutes to complete a scan. The obtained PCT images and the histology images when compared show that both the images are in good correspondence in identifying the cysts (see Fig. 7). The diameter of the smallest cyst visible on the PCT image was reported as 0.4 mm. The ability of the PCT scanner to perform small animal imaging was further shown by conducting studies on ex vivo tissue samples and in vivo mouse models to track tumor hypoxia and angiogenesis. For this purpose, breast cancer or ovarian cancer cells were grown in immune-deficient mice on which PA spectroscopic studies were performed using the PCT scanner.[32] The study also reports the potential of the PCT scanner in monitoring the distribution of indocyanine green (ICG), an exogenous contrast agent that binds to plasma proteins when injected into the blood stream, commonly used to determine liver and cardiac function. In vivo measurements of hemoglobin concentration and oxygen saturation levels were also reported by imaging mice tails using the PCT scanner. To determine the hemoglobin concentration values obtained from the PCT images more accurately, these investigators have developed and implemented a reconstruction correction technique that yielded the values that are in good correspondence with actual CO-oximeter measurements.[64] To reduce the data acquisition time, they have proposed using a new back-projection technique called HYPR (HighlY constrained back PRojection) by means of which the images can be reconstructed by data taken in fewer projections.[65] Recently, development of a new 128-element US detector with its elements (3 mm diameter with 5 MHz center frequency) laid on a hemispherical surface, to be used with the PCT scanner was reported.[65] The detector array can be depicted as a hemispherical cup with elements arranged on the inner surface uniformly with a clear aperture at the bottom for laser delivery. To perform PCT, the small animal is placed above the detector array, which is filled with water to achieve good acoustic coupling. The detector can then be rotated about its vertical axis to acquire additional interleaved projections. The use of this detector array in conjunction with the HYPR technique is expected to yield PA images with high resolution at a faster rate.

PA Imaging in Clinical Setting

The laser optoacoustic imaging system (LOIS) developed by Oraevsky and colleagues[7,12,27,66,67] is a clinical prototype that was developed to diagnose breast malignancies. The setup consists of an examination table on which the patient lies with the breast suspended down through a circular opening (Fig. 11). To induce the PA effect, a pulsed NIR laser source with wavelength 757 nm consisting of a compact Q-switched Alexandrite laser is employed that can generate laser pulses at a repetition rate of 10 Hz and pulse width of 75 ns. The system operates in forward (transmission) mode (ie, the excitation source [laser] and the detector are on the opposite side of the tissue). The laser beam is delivered through a 1-mm-diameter optical fiber and is expanded to 70 mm to achieve a uniform illumination on the breast surface with a maximum fluence of 10 mJ/cm^2. The PA signals generated from the breast tissue are detected by 64 rectangular ultrasonic transducers that are arranged in an arc-shaped array beneath the circular vent of the examination table, orthogonal to the laser beam.[27] Each ultrasonic transducer is fabricated using PVDF and has dimensions of $20 \times 3 \times 0.11$ mm with a center frequency around

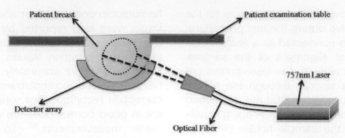

Fig. 11. Laser optoacoustic imaging system.

1 MHz and bandwidth of 2.5 MHz. The PA signals detected are amplified, digitized, and processed to yield a PA image in the plane of the array orthogonal to the incident laser beam. This system was able to reconstruct the PA images using a radial back-projection algorithm representing 2D slices of the breast with a resolution of around 0.5 mm with additional signal processing. With the help of a dedicated computational environment, the LOIS system was able to perform real-time PA imaging, yielding 256 × 256 pixel images at a frame rate of 10 Hz or 512 × 512 pixel images at a frame rate of 1 Hz.

The Twente photoacoustic mammoscope developed by Manohar and colleagues[16,17,26,68,69] is another example of a forward-mode PA imaging clinical prototype that was intended for breast imaging. The setup comprises a patient examination table with provision for suspension of the patient's breast. The suspended breast is mildly compressed between a glass plate and a flat US detector array that consists of 590 elements arranged in a circular grid of 90 mm diameter (**Fig. 12**). The system employs a 1064-nm Q-switched Nd:YAG laser with pulse width of 5 ns and pulse repetition rate of 10 Hz as the excitation source to generate PA signals inside the breast tissue. The laser beam is coupled into a custom-developed light delivery system, the output of which can be translated into 2 dimensions by a scanning system to facilitate localized breast tissue illumination. The laser beam is delivered onto the breast through the glass plate and the

generated PA transients that propagate in the forward direction are received by the 2D detector array. Each detector array element is fabricated using PVDF of thickness 110 μm and has a size of 2 mm × 2 mm, with interelement spacing (pitch) of 3.175 mm. The center frequency of the detector elements is 1 MHz with −6 dB bandwidth range of 450 kHz to 1.78 MHz. The PA images are reconstructed using a delay-and-sum beam focusing algorithm with a measured lateral resolution of 2.3 mm to 3.9 mm and an axial resolution of 2.5 mm to 3.3 mm for depths between 15 mm and 60 mm.[17] Tests conducted on healthy human volunteers with this system suggest an approximate scan time of 45 minutes to acquire PA data over an area of 52 × 52 mm with a signal averaging of 100,[68] 30 minutes being the average scan time.[17]

Petrov and colleagues[70] have developed a high-sensitivity reflection-mode PA system to monitor cerebral venous oxygenation noninvasively in patients with traumatic brain injury and cardiac surgery. Their system probes the ocular tissue at low energy levels to monitor the blood oxygenation levels in superior sagittal sinus (SSS). A compact tunable OPO-based laser system that can generate 10-ns laser pulses at a PRF of 20 Hz with pulse energy of 1 to 2 mJ over a spectral range of 680 to 2400 nm was used to induce PA signals in the SSS. The laser beam was delivered to the ocular tissue via an optical fiber that attenuates the energy to 60 μJ to achieve safe levels of exposure. A 3-MHz broadband US sensor

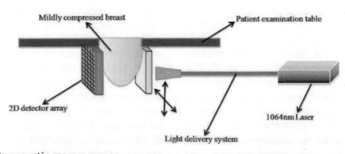

Fig. 12. Twente photoacoustic mammoscope.

was used to detect the PA A-line signals. In vivo experiments were conducted on sheep and healthy human volunteers with their system within 700 nm to 1064 nm and the results show the potential of the system to accurately measure the cerebral blood oxygenation at wavelengths of 700, 760, 800, and 1064 nm. These investigators have conducted similar studies using this system on healthy human volunteers by performing PA measurements on the neck area superficial to the internal jugular vein (IJV) with laser fluence less than 4 mJ/cm^2.[71] The system was capable of probing the IJV, which is 6 to 12 mm deep within the neck with high SNR and high resolution, thus providing noninvasive accurate measurements of cerebral blood oxygenation. Noninvasive multispectral in vivo PA measurements of external jugular vein conducted on sheep (which is anatomically similar to the IJV in humans) were also reported[72] to have a strong correlation, with invasive blood oxygenation measurements taken from the same location measured by CO-oximeter.

Petrova and colleagues[73] have developed a portable laser diode based PA system for noninvasive monitoring of total hemoglobin concentration (THb). The diode laser is operated at a wavelength of 905 nm and generates 100 ns laser pulses with pulse energy of 18 μJ at a repetition rate of 100 Hz, which are delivered on to the radial artery through a 1-mm fiber-optic cable. The generated PA signals are detected by a broadband single-element PVDF transducer of center frequency 10 MHz and are transferred on to a laptop for acquisition and real-time processing after suitable amplification and digitization. Clinical studies were conducted on the radial arteries of 4 normal and 2 anemic human volunteers using this system, and the PA measurements obtained, after signal averaging, were used to predict THb values, which are compared with the actual THb concentrations determined from blood samples of each volunteer analyzed with a clinical CO-oximeter. During the trials, each volunteer's wrist was held stationary using a holder and the PA probe was translated over the radial artery using a linear stage. Statistical analysis was also performed on the data, which suggested that the predicted PA measurements of THb concentrations agreed well with the actual THb measurements, thereby showing the potential of PA technique in monitoring THb concentrations noninvasively.

Beard and colleagues[33,34,43,74–79] developed a high-resolution NIR PA imaging system that is capable of performing multiwavelength studies to characterize the tissue at depths less than 1 cm based on an optical detection system. The system is designed to work in backward (reflection) mode,

in which the laser and the detector are on the same side of the tissue. The system comprises a frequency tripled Q-switched Nd:YAG laser pumped tunable (410–2100 nm) fiber-coupled OPO-based laser system that can generate 8-ns optical pulses at a PRF of 10 Hz with energies ranging from 12 to 36 mJ/pulse.[77] As mentioned earlier, these investigators have used an optical interferometry based detector FP polymer film sensor. The FP sensor head is transparent in the NIR wavelength range 650 to 1200 nm, with a high reflectivity in the 1500- to 1700-nm wavelength range. The NIR laser pulses from the tunable laser are illuminated on to the FP sensor head and are transmitted through it into the underlying tissue, and are eventually absorbed and generate PA signals inside the tissue. The generated PA waves that propagate back to the FP sensor head induce modulation of the optical thickness of the FP film, thereby changing the reflectivity by producing a small phase shift that is linearly converted to reflected optical power modulation that corresponds to the 2D distribution of PA waves incident on the sensor.[74,77] To read out the modulated reflectivity pattern, a continuous-wave 1550-nm focused laser interrogating beam of spot size 64 μm is raster scanned two-dimensionally over the FP film surface with a step size of 10 μm. The reflected laser beam at each scanning location is detected using a photodiode, which converts it into a time-varying electrical signal (PA waveform) that is digitized and stored on to a computer, thus yielding a 3D data array that can be used to reconstruct a 3D image using k-space or Fourier transform based reconstruction algorithm[74,80] once the entire 2D raster scan is completed. These investigators have reported the use of FP sensors of thicknesses 22 μm and 38 μm. The lateral spatial resolution was experimentally observed as 40 μm for 22-μm-thick polymer film, whereas the vertical spatial resolution of the system was estimated to be 20 μm for 22-μm-thick film and 30 μm for 38-μm-thick film, respectively.[33,77] The frequency response of the sensor depends on the polymer film thickness and the backing material. The −3-dB bandwidth of the sensor was reported as 38 MHz for 22-μm-thick FP film and 22.2 MHz for 38-μm film.

The performance of the system was initially assessed by conducting experiments with tissue-mimicking phantoms: dye-filled tubes and artificial blood vessels at multiple wavelengths.[75–77] The PA imaging on a human middle finger in vivo was reported with 1.5-cm-diameter laser pulses at a maximum fluence of 17 mJ/cm^2 over a wavelength range of 740 to 980 nm in steps of 20 nm.[76] Three blood vessels located at depths 1 to

2 mm were clearly distinguished in the images and were analyzed to determine intravascular oxy- and deoxyhemoglobin concentrations and blood oxygen saturation levels. The usefulness of the system was further shown through the experiments conducted by Zhang and colleagues,[33,77] in which the PA imaging was performed using a 38-μm sensor on a human palm in vivo and a mouse abdominal skin ex vivo to visualize subcutaneous vasculature, with 670-nm and 590-nm excitation wavelengths, respectively. Results indicate higher penetration depth in human palm (maximum depth of 4 mm) than in the mouse (maximum depth of 2 mm) because of the high optical attenuation by blood at 590 nm. The study also reports PA imaging on nude mice with implanted tumors. The thickness of the FP sensor film was 22 μm in this case. Two human colorectal tumors with different but known pathophysiologic conditions were grown in 2 separate mice and were imaged at visible wavelengths (650 nm and 630 nm). One of the mice had tumor covering a larger area of approximately 20 mm × 20 mm, whereas the other had a tumor grown to a size approximately 8 mm × 8 mm. Results indicate that the system is capable of characterizing tumor vasculature in small animal models besides being able to visualize superficial vascular networks to assess soft-tissue abnormalities, including burns, wounds, and lesions.[33]

PA IMAGING OF PROSTATE

Unlike breast, skin, or small animal imaging, the imaging of prostate poses certain challenges for developing a PA imaging system because of its anatomic origin. Because the prostate lies close to the rectal wall, a probe that can fit into the rectum similar to a transrectal US (TRUS) probe to perform PA imaging would be an ideal choice. Yet, in this configuration, only backward (reflection) PA imaging can be performed. Hence, the major limitation lies in the delivery of light to the prostate to induce the PA effect. However, if it is necessary to develop such a system, the next most obvious problem lies in detecting the generated PA transients. Because the acoustic transients must be detected on the same side from which the optical pulses are propagated, the placement of the US transducer becomes challenging relative to the light delivery mechanism such as a fiber-optic cable.

A dog study was conducted by Oraevsky and colleagues[81] to show the feasibility of PA imaging in a surgically exposed prostate. A custom-designed transrectal probe with a 128-element convex PZT US transducer array whose elements are aligned over a 154° arc was used to detect the PA signals, whereas an optical fiber of diameter 1 mm was attached to the probe through the biopsy needle channel to deliver the laser pulses on to the prostate. Each transducer element has dimensions of 6 mm (elevation) × 0.23 mm (width) × 0.25 mm (thickness), with a pitch of 0.25 mm and an upper frequency limit of 6.7 MHz. The detected PA transients are used to reconstruct 2D images using a radial back-projection algorithm. In vitro studies on prostate-mimicking phantoms were conducted with the system and the measured lateral resolution was found to be approximately 1 mm, whereas the axial resolution was 0.8 mm. The probe was used to perform PA imaging of canine prostate in vivo.[81] For this study, small lesions were mechanically created in the dog's prostate, which was surgically exposed to perform PA imaging. The laser light was delivered from the top on to the prostate by means of a beam expander, and the transrectal probe in the absence of the optical fiber was pressed against the prostate to acquire the PA signals. The obtained PA images showed the blood-containing lesion with high contrast. In vitro experiments conducted by Oraevsky and colleagues[82,83] also showed the potential of PA imaging in detecting prostate malignancies.

PA imaging of prostate with a commercially available TRUS probe was reported.[84] A Q-switched Nd:YAG laser that can generate 1064-nm laser pulses with a pulse width of 6 ns at a PRF of 10 Hz was coupled to an optical fiber to deliver the laser beam on to the tissue. The potential of the imaging system in detecting PA signals was shown by conducting in vitro experiments with tissue-mimicking phantoms. 2D images were reconstructed from the obtained PA signals using a directivity-weighted filtered radial back-projection algorithm. The study suggests that a PA imaging system using an alternative method of delivering laser pulses on to the prostate by inserting an optical fiber in the urethra is under development. The laser pulses will emerge from the center of the prostate through the urethra, and the generated PA signals will be detected by the US transducer array housed in the TRUS probe, which can be used to reconstruct 2D images.

Prostate cancer is the most common malignancy in men and the leading cause of death from cancer in the United States (source: American Cancer Society, 2009). Current screening protocols for prostate cancer include the prostate specific antigen test and digital rectal examination, which have low positive predictive values. TRUS guided biopsy is the only diagnostic modality being currently used. TRUS, however, is not reliable because of its low sensitivity and specificity, often missing cancer in more than 30% of cases. There is a great need for an improved imaging modality in definitive diagnosis of prostate cancer, which motivated the authors to develop a novel method and a device for prostate imaging, C-Scan Photoacoustic Imaging of the Prostate (CSPIP). The authors have developed a PA imaging probe to detect prostate malignancies in vivo that will overcome most of the limitations mentioned earlier. To show the potential of the system, the authors have conducted feasibility studies using a breadboard setup and then designed a prototype that can perform PA imaging in vivo. The design parameters along with experimental observations are presented in the following sections.

ACOUSTIC LENS-BASED C-SCAN PA IMAGING

C-scans are 2D images produced by spatially sampling the US signal amplitude at a fixed time while the interrogating sensor is scanned over some surface. In contrast to a US or PA B-scan imaging system, real time C-scan image formation is possible only by means of a 2D sensor. **Fig. 13** highlights the B-scan and C-scan image formation processes. The size and number of elements in a 2D sensor depend on the area being investigated. The larger the area, the greater the number of elements needed to perform imaging with a good resolution. To form a 3D image, the time resolved A-line signal acquired by each sensor element has to be amplified, digitized, and then transferred onto a computer. A 2D sensor with a large number of elements requires a significantly large set of communication channels or cables running down from the back of the sensor array, thus presenting a bottleneck for the sensor designers. Moreover, to achieve high SNR and high-resolution images, focusing of the transducer is required, making the design more cumbersome. As opposed to software-based focusing or filtered back-projection algorithms used by many researchers, in our design, focusing of the transducer is performed by an acoustic lens.

Consider a nanosecond laser beam that irradiates the object at time t=0. Let there be 2 optical point absorbers (color coded in red and blue) in plane A and B, respectively. The PA US wave is shown diverging from the 2 points. The proposed idea is to achieve focusing of the PA waves with an acoustic lens system, much like optical image formation (**Fig. 14**). An appropriately designed lens will converge the wave front from the red point in plane A to the red point in plane A* and the blue point in plane B to the blue point in plane B*, respectively. A detector array located in plane A* will capture this energy as a focused image in the form of a C-scan.

PA C-Scan Imaging Breadboard Setup

A single-element acoustic lens was designed with 25 mm diameter and 27.5 mm focal length to perform C-scan imaging. The authors have adopted the 4f acoustic lens imaging technology[85] to obtain high-contrast PA images that exactly resemble the optical absorption distribution in

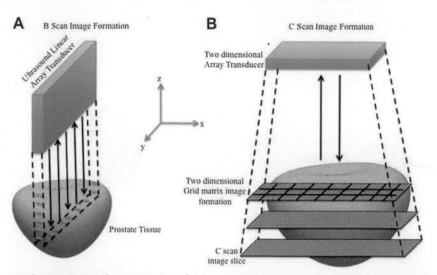

Fig. 13. B-scan and C-scan image formation. Set of A-lines in (*A*) taken by each sensor element of 1D array constitutes a B-scan image and set of A-lines in (*B*) taken by each sensor element of 2D array forms a 3D image. Signal arrival time encodes the depth direction z.

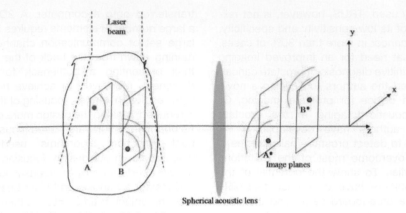

Fig. 14. Concept of lens based C-scan PA imaging.

the tissue. Initial in vitro experiments were performed with a breadboard setup shown in **Fig. 15.** An Nd:YAG laser with 1064 nm wavelength, 10 ns pulse width and 1 to 10 Hz PRF has been used as an excitation source. A 0.2-mm-diameter lead pencil placed in the object plane was illuminated by a 2-mm laser beam with the help of a fiber-optic cable terminated into a collimator. To simulate the experimental conditions in vivo, the energy was maintained less than 5 mJ, which is well within the ANSI laser safety limits for skin exposure.[6]

The authors have used needle hydrophones that are excellent sensors in US field mapping, with pinpoint access and good spatial resolution. The US detector was a 1.5-mm-diameter needle hydrophone with a wide bandwidth to detect US signals from 0 to 10 MHz. The hydrophone was raster scanned in the image plane, shown as a grid matrix. At each grid point (pixel location), a time-resolved A-line signal was acquired, amplified, and then digitized at a sampling rate of 100 MHz. The target (lead pencil) acts as a 2-mm point source which is located in an "object plane-O," generating PA waves that are focused and can be detected on the other side of the lens in any "image plane" by appropriate time-gating of A-line signal (**Fig. 16**).

Fig. 17 shows a series of C-scans. Object distance-O was 55 mm and image distance-I was varied from 49 mm to 59 mm from the acoustic lens. According to physical optics,[86] focused image should form at image distance of 55 mm from the acoustic lens, which is confirmed in **Fig. 17** because the image spot size is the smallest (in focus) for image distance of 55 mm. **Fig. 18**A shows a PA object formed of the letters "AAIT" written with 0.7-mm lines of black tape.

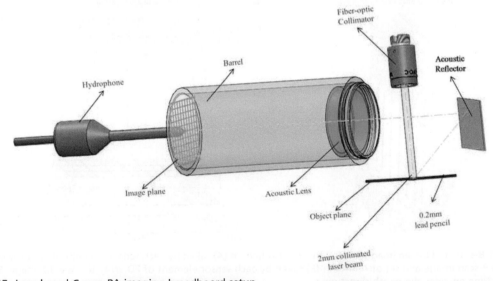

Fig. 15. Lens-based C-scan PA imaging breadboard setup.

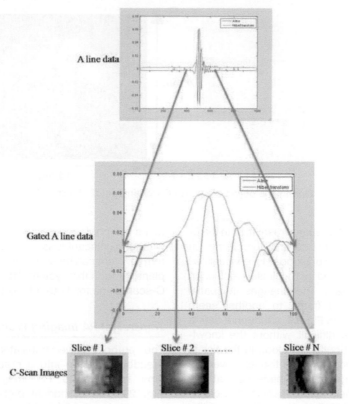

A line data

Gated A line data

Slice # 1   Slice # 2 ....   Slice # N

C-Scan Images

Fig. 16. PA C-scan image formation.

Its focused C-scan PA image is shown in **Fig. 18**.B.

Neonatal Mouse Imaging

A sequence of C-scan images from the thigh region of a dead neonatal mouse with prominent superficial vessels are shown in **Fig. 19**. Each C-scan represents the same 6-mm × 6-mm ROI in the region indicated by the arrow in the photograph in the upper left image. The time increment to select different slices was 0.05 μs, corresponding to slice spacing in object of 0.075 mm. The total range of distances covered by the slices

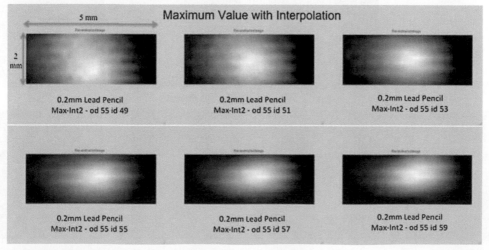

Fig. 17. C-scan images of lead pencil exposed by 2-mm laser beam.

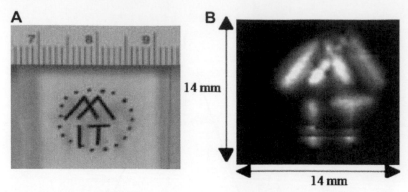

Fig. 18. (*A*) Letters in black tape in the object plane. (*B*) C-scan image of object in (*A*).

was about 0.75 mm. The spatial resolution in the 6-mm × 6-mm depicted planes is around 2 mm. In brightness the presence of blood pool is visualized in the tissue in 3D blurred by the limited resolution of the imaging system. The changes in spatial image pattern from 1 frame to another seem consistent, as shown in **Fig. 19**, although a definitive interpretation is difficult without the knowledge of spatial distribution of blood in the tissue or absorption coefficient of the tissue. Nevertheless, these results generate confidence that it is possible to image field inhomogeneity of biologic systems with our CSPIP method. The feasibility of C-scan PA imaging technique to visualize biologic tissues has been validated using our laboratory breadboard setup. These experiments helped us gain practical knowledge in selecting the appropriate lens materials that will work best to

focus the photoacoustically generated US waves without significant loss. A spatial resolution of 0.5 mm to 1 mm can be achieved in the C-scan image plane through this system. The resolution between C-scan plane for 1- to 5-MHz PA signals is 100 μ.

Transrectal PA Imaging Probe

The authors have translated their laboratory breadboard setup into a practical probe prototype for prostate PA imaging, presented in **Fig. 20**. The cylindrical probe has a diameter between 1 and 1.25 inches, and a length approximately 3 inches. The probe is divided into optical and acoustic chambers that are separate and sealed. The acoustic chamber contains water as the US propagation medium. The laser pulses are delivered via a high quality fiber-optic cable,

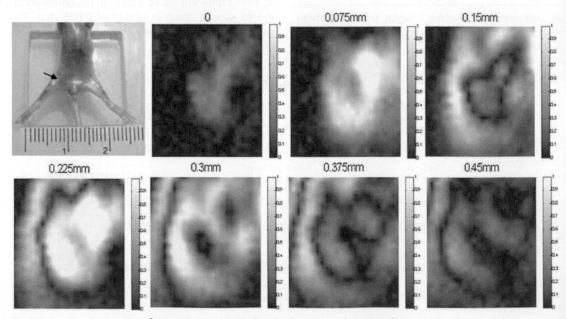

Fig. 19. C-scan planar slices from a 6 × 6 mm region in the thigh of neonatal mouse.

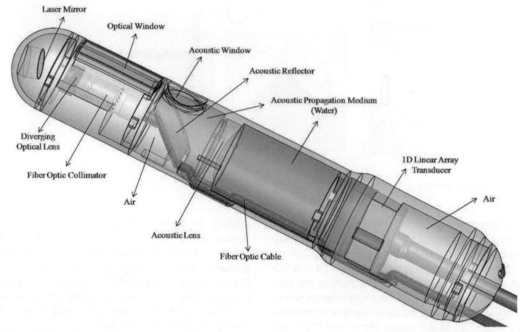

Fig. 20. CSPIP probe design.

which are expanded to a desired beam diameter over the tissue at the object plane. This laser beam emerges from an optical window at a grazing angle to illuminate the tissue. The acoustic window is aligned in front of the prostate when inserted into the rectum. With the help of acoustic coupling gel, the PA waves generated in the prostate enter through the acoustic window and are guided toward the linear array transducer by means of an acoustic reflector.

From our experience, we have designed a custom acoustic lens that is placed in the acoustic chamber that achieves improved image quality with high SNR. A custom-designed 32-element linear (1D) US transducer array is placed in the image plane for detecting the PA transients. Data acquisition by the array is performed at every trigger of laser exposure to the tissue for each line scan. The present configuration allows acquisition and display of only B-scan images because of the mechanical limitations posed by the array inside the probe. A probe that can perform PA C-scan prostate imaging is under development. To acquire real-time C-scan images, the transducer array will have to be moved perpendicularly to the line scan direction to a different location for another line scan. Likewise, 32 to 64 line scans will constitute 1 C-scan image data acquisition sequence. Dedicated back end electronics will time-gate and process the signals to produce an image on a monitor.

PA C-Scan Imaging with 1D Linear Array Transducer

To demonstrate the ability of our system to perform C-scan imaging, a biplanar sample was constructed and imaged. The sample was made using a black tape (PA absorber) with "□" on 1 plane and "Λ" on the other plane. The distance between the 2 planes is 5.79 mm. The dimensions are shown in **Fig. 21**. The experimental setup is shown in **Fig. 22**. To illustrate the C-scan imaging ability, the probe with the 1D array was immersed in a water bath without the optical chamber. The experiments were performed in forward propagation mode in which the laser beam was illuminated from the opposite side of the sample, as shown in **Fig. 22**. A beam expander was used to expand the laser beam to 10 mm at the object plane. The entire probe was translated in 1 direction in increments of 200 µm to acquire the PA signals generated from the sample until a series of PA B-scan images were obtained. The present data acquisition rate with linear array transducer is 1 B-scan image per second at 100-MHz sampling rate. Once the scan is completed, the PA B-scan images obtained were used to reconstruct a 3D volumetric data from which C-scan images can be readily constructed, as shown in **Fig. 23**. Strength of the PA signal is represented on a scale corresponding to the normalized pixel value obtained by linear array transducer.

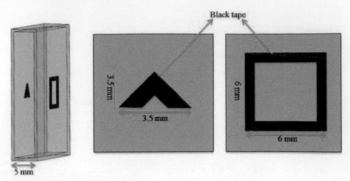

Fig. 21. Biplanar sample with "Λ" and "□" planes.

The size of the reconstructed image is 7 mm × 14 mm with a pixel size of 200 μm × 700 μm, as defined by the scan increment and the pitch of the transducer array, respectively. **Fig. 24** is a 3D volume reconstructed by postprocessing the obtained B-scan images with the experimental setup described earlier. The biplanar sample is investigated with "Λ" in the object plane and "□" out of focus and vice versa The volumetric data obtained are presented in **Fig. 24**A and B, respectively. The features of "Λ" have been visualized clearly in **Fig. 24**A compared with **Fig. 24**B because it was in the focus (object) plane. Diffraction limited C-scan slice thickness is approximately 620 μm.

C-scan PA imaging was shown by acquiring and postprocessing B-scans at defined intervals, yet the total time taken to perform a complete scan with this system was at least 70 seconds. The

authors are currently designing a probe with a 2D sensor array that can produce real-time PA C-scan images. Because the system employs acoustic lens imaging technology to acquire C-scan images, the need for electronic focusing is completely eliminated and the computational overhead involved in sampling and storing the data is effectively minimized.

Merits of the Approach

Our methodology will produce C-scan planar images, depicting the prostate in sequential coronal planes with distances ranging from close to the rectal wall to the far edge of the prostate gland. Lens focusing is expected to produce a 10- to 20-fold improvement in the SNR of the PA signal at each sensor pixel, compared with existing methodologies. Because of the lens

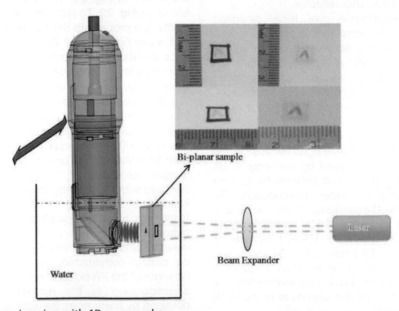

Fig. 22. PA C-scan imaging with 1D array probe.

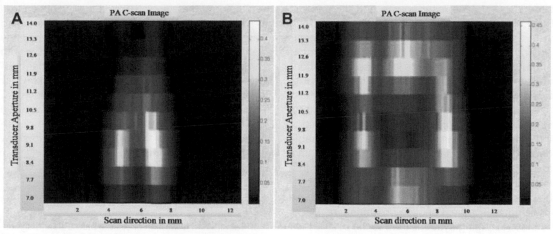

Fig. 23. (A) PA C-scan image when "Λ" is in focus, (B) PA C-scan image when "□" is in focus.

focusing, there is no computational overhead in the system, which gives room for an image display at 2 to 10 Hz, making it suitable for biopsy guidance. This novel C-scan imaging technology makes it possible to locate the lesion spatially with all 3 coordinates, providing accurate information about its position in length, width, and depth directions of the lesion. Once the spatial coordinates of the lesion are obtained, they can be used to operate a mechanical (robotic) arm to perform diagnostic, therapeutic, and other interventions accurately.

DEVELOPMENT OF PA IMAGING SYSTEMS FOR CLINICAL USE

The authors believe the state-of-the-art for PA imaging has reached a stage at which transition from bench to bedside is possible. With appropriate choice of the wavelength of laser light in NIR, tissue penetration and imaging up to 3 to 4

cm deep are feasible. There are a few challenges. Achieving good SNR, while maintaining the intensity of laser light within the ANSI limit,[6] is difficult. Therefore initial efforts might focus on imaging at shallow depths such as skin and superficial veins. The rationale for introducing PA imaging into any existing modality will remain connected to presence of blood, any other appropriate chromophore, or exogenous absorbers such as ICG and nanoparticles, unless in vivo spectroscopic data on different tissue types become available to indicate any other reasons. Ideally, access to the imaged organ from all directions (4π radians) is impossible, but this is not a serious impediment. Image reconstruction of sufficient quality has been shown even for limited angle reception by the sensors. Systems to image organs such as breast, in which there is flexibility to choose the direction from which the incident light exposure occurs and the location of the sensors, will be easy to design and fabricate. In contrast,

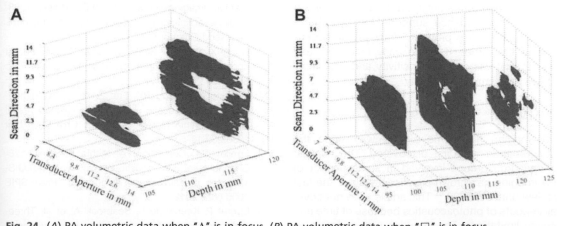

Fig. 24. (A) PA volumetric data when "Λ" is in focus. (B) PA volumetric data when "□" is in focus.

situations in which laser source and the sensors have to be on the same side, such as prostate, skin, or thyroid, will be technologically more challenging. For a given desired resolution, the number of required sensor elements increases proportionately to the area of the final reconstructed image. Designing large sensor arrays and the associated dedicated hardware is another challenge. Finally, the data acquisition and image reconstruction time must be short. How short is acceptable depends on many factors, but the time will have to be reduced for many benchtop systems that currently take several tens of minutes. The authors believe progress has been made to meet these challenges. The next section presents a review of all the PA imaging systems that, to the best of their knowledge, have been developed for use in a clinical setting.

Twente University group[16,17] has developed a PA breast imaging system and showed its usefulness as an adjunct to mammography. The system has resolution ~3 to 4 mm but the 3D image acquisition time is long at ~40 minutes. However, in a compressed breast it can provide 2D planar PA images in planes parallel to the compression plates. The group at Fairway Medical Technologies has also developed a breast imaging system and used it for clinical trials.[27] The technology they use has been described earlier. It works on a vertically hanging breast, in which mammography can be performed simultaneously in mediolateral configuration for comparison. The expected resolution is ~1 mm in plane. The dedicated hardware can produce planar images in a few seconds.

There are no other large-scale clinical trials using PA technology that the authors are aware of. Both the breast imaging technologies mentioned earlier have shown in their initial clinical trials that a strong PA signal is coming from an area where a suspect lesion could be seen on the mammogram, confirmed to be cancer on biopsy. This evidence supports the hypothesis that PA imaging is probably detecting angiogenesis in the tumor. It is too early to expect any results that will explain sensitivity and specificity of this new imaging modality.

SUMMARY

PA imaging has come a long way since the phenomenon was first discovered. The number of research groups involved in some aspect of PA imaging has grown significantly since the last review paper in 2006.[87] This article does not cover all aspects of photoacoustics because of time and space limitations. The intention was to focus on

technology that is relevant to clinical system development. The authors believe that PA imaging has great promise for medical imaging in early detection of cancer, guiding biopsy, imaging with targeted nanoparticles, application of spectroscopy, and blood oxygen level determination, for example. It is a safe and noninvasive, or at worst, minimally invasive, modality. The authors believe clinical PA imaging systems will be further developed, and more clinical trials will be able to show the potential of PA imaging.

REFERENCES

1. Tuchin VV. Handbook of optical biomedical diagnostics. Bellingham (WA): SPIE press; 2002.
2. Vogel A, Venugopalan V. Mechanisms of pulsed laser ablation of biological tissues. Chem Rev 2003;103(2):577–644.
3. Oraevsky AA, Jacques SL, Tittel FKK. Determination of tissue optical properties by piezoelectric detection of laser-induced stress waves. Proc SPIE 1993;1882:86–101.
4. Nau WH, Roselli RJ, Milam DF. Measurement of thermal effects on the optical properties of prostate tissue at wavelengths of 1064 and 633 nm. Lasers Surg Med 1999;24:38–47.
5. Levy DA, Schwartz Jon, Ostermeyer Martin, et al. Transurethral in vivo optical properties of the human prostate gland. Proc SPIE 1996;2671:329–34.
6. American National Standard for Safe Use of Lasers. Laser Institute of America. New York: ANSI Z136.1;2000.
7. Andreev VG, Karabutov AA, Oraevsky AA. Detection of ultrawide-band ultrasound pulses in optoacoustic tomography. IEEE Trans Ultrason Ferroelectr Freq Control 2003;50:1383–90.
8. Szabo TL. Diagnostic ultrasound imaging: inside out. Burlington (MA): Elsevier; 2004.
9. Kak AC, Slaney M. Principles of computerized tomographic imaging. New York: IEEE Press; 1988. Availabe at: http://www.slaney.org/pct/pct-toc.html. Accessed October 5, 2009.
10. Wang X, Pang Y, Stoica G, et al. Laser-induced photo-acoustic tomography for small animals. Proc SPIE 2003;4960:40–4.
11. Yi-Xiong SU, Wang RK, Fan Z, et al. Two-dimensional photoacoustic imaging of blood vessel networks within biological tissues. Chin Phys Lett 2006;23:512–5.
12. Ermilov SA, Conjusteau A, Mehta K, et al. 128-Channel laser optoacoustic imaging system (LOIS-128) for breast cancer diagnostics. Proc SPIE 2006;6086:1–12.
13. Ephrat P, Keenliside L, Seabrook A, et al. Three-dimensional photoacoustic imaging by sparse-array

detection and iterative image reconstruction. J Biomed Opt 2008;13(5):1–12.

14. Yang DW, Xing D, Yang SH, et al. Fast full-view photoacoustic imaging by combined scanning with a linear transducer array. Optic Express 2007;15:15566–75.

15. Laufer J, Elwell C, Delpy D, et al. In vitro measurements of absolute blood oxygen saturation using pulsed near-infrared photoacoustic spectroscopy: accuracy and resolution. Phys Med Biol 2005;50:4409–28.

16. Vaartjes SE, van Hespen JC, Klaase JM, et al. First clinical trials of the Twente photoacoustic mammoscope (PAM). Proc SPIE 2007;6629:1–12.

17. Manohar S, Vaartjes SE, van Hespen JC, et al. Initial results of in vivo non-invasive cancer imaging in the human breast using near-infrared photoacoustics. Optic Express 2007;15:12277–85.

18. Rao NAHK. Ultrasound imaging. In: Hornak JP, editor. Encyclopedia of imaging science & technology. New York: John Wiley & Sons Inc; 2002. p. 1412–35.

19. Karpiouk AB, Wang Bo, Emelianov SY. Development of catheters for combined intravascular ultrasound and photoacoustic imaging. Proc SPIE 2007;7177:1–7.

20. Wang X, Chamberland DL, Xi G. Noninvasive reflection mode photoacoustic imaging through infant skull toward imaging of neonatal brains. J Neurosci Methods 2008;168:412–21.

21. Park S, Aglyamov SR, Emelianov SY. Beamforming for photoacoustic imaging using linear array transducer. IEEE Ultrasonics Symposium 2007;856–9.

22. Agarwal A, Huang SW, O'Donnell M, et al. Targeted gold nanorod contrast agent for prostate cancer detection by photoacoustic imaging. J Appl Phys 2007;102:1–4.

23. Vaithilingam S, Wygant IO, Kuo PS, et al. Capacitive micromachined ultrasonic transducers (CMUTs) for photoacoustic imaging. Proc SPIE 2006;6086:1–11.

24. Ashkenazi S, Hou Y, Buma T, et al. Optoacoustic imaging using thin polymer etalon. Appl Phys Lett 2005;86:1–3.

25. Kruger RA, Kiser WL Jr, Reinecke DR, et al. Thermoacoustic computed tomography using a conventional linear transducer array. Med Phys 2003;30(5):856–60.

26. Manohar S, Kharine A, Molenaar R, et al. Characterization of a clinical prototype for photoacoustic mammography and some phantom studies. Proc SPIE 2005;5697:27–34.

27. Ermilov SA, Khamapirad T, Conjusteau A, et al. Laser optoacoustic imaging system for detection of breast cancer. J Biomed Opt 2009;14(2):1–14.

28. Li ML, Wang JC, Schwartz JA, et al. In-vivo photoacoustic microscopy of nanoshell extravasation from solid tumor vasculature. J Biomed Opt 2009;14(1):1–3.

29. Gamelin J, Maurudis A, Aguirre A, et al. A fast 512-element ring array photoacoustic imaging system for small animals. Proc SPIE 2009;7177:1–10.

30. Aguirre A, Gamelin J, Guo P, et al. Photoacoustic characterization of ovarian tissue. Proc SPIE 2009;7177:1–9.

31. Liu Bo, Gattone VH, Kruger R, et al. Assessment of photoacoustic computed tomography to classify tissue in a polycystic-kidney disease mouse model. Proc SPIE 2006;6086:54–61.

32. Stantz KM, Liu Bo, Cao M, et al. Photoacoustic spectroscopic imaging of intra-tumor heterogeneity and molecular identification. Proc SPIE 2006;6086:36–47.

33. Zhang EZ, Laufer JG, Pedley RB. In vivo high-resolution 3D photoacoustic imaging of superficial vascular anatomy. Phys Med Biol 2009;54:1035–46.

34. Allen TJ, Beard PC. Photoacoustic characterisation of vascular tissue at NIR wavelengths. Proc SPIE 2009;7177:1–9.

35. Henrichs PM, Meador JW, Fuqua JM, et al. Atherosclerotic plaque characterization with optoacoustic imaging. Proc SPIE 2005;5697:217–23.

36. Wang B, Yantsen E, Sokolov K, et al. High sensitivity intravascular photoacoustic imaging of macrophages. Proc SPIE 2009;7177:1–6.

37. Su JL, Wang Bo, Emelianov SY. Spectroscopic intravascular photoacoustic imaging of neovasculature: phantom studies. Proc SPIE 2009;7177:1–7.

38. Guo P, Gamelin J, Yan S, et al. Co-registered 3-D ultrasound and photoacoustic imaging using a 1.75D 1280-channel ultrasound system. Proc SPIE 2007;6437:1–11.

39. Aguirre A, Gamelin J, Guo P, et al. Feasibility study of three-dimensional co-registered ultrasound and photoacoustic imaging for cancer detection and visualization. Proc SPIE 2008;6856:1–10.

40. Germer M, Wolff M, Harde H. Photoacoustic NO detection for asthma diagnostics. Proc SPIE – OSA Biomed Opt 2009;7371:1–6.

41. Ren Z, Liu G, Huang Z, et al. Laser-induced photoacoustic glucose spectrum denoise using an improved wavelet threshold translation-invariant algorithm. Proc SPIE 2009;7382:1–8.

42. Talbert RJ, Holan SH, Viator JA. Photoacoustic discrimination of viable and thermally coagulated blood using a two-wavelength method for burn injury monitoring. Phys Med Biol 2007;52:1815–29.

43. Allen TJ, Beard PC. Dual wavelength laser diode excitation source for 2D photoacoustic imaging. Proc SPIE 2007;6437:1–9.

44. Weight RM, Viator JA, Dale PS, et al. Photoacoustic detection of metastatic melanoma cells in the human circulatory system. Opt Lett 2006;31(20):2998–3000.

45. Holan SH, Viator JA. Automated wavelet denoising of photoacoustic signals for circulating melanoma

cell detection and burn image reconstruction. Phys Med Biol 2008;53:N227–36.

46. Viator J. Photoacoustic detection of circulating melanoma cells in human blood. SPIE Newsroom 2009. Available at: http://spie.org/documents/Newsroom/Imported/1630/1630_5734_0_2009-04-21.pdf. Accessed November 1, 2009.

47. Gupta SK, Katti K, Viator JA. Photoacoustic detection of gold nanorods tagged prostate cancer cells in-vitro. Proc SPIE 2009;7177:1–6.

48. Galanzha EI, Shashkov EV, Tuchin VV, et al. In vivo multispectral photoacoustic lymph flow cytometry with natural cell focusing and multicolor nanoparticle probes. Cytometry A 2008;73(10):884–94.

49. Galanzha EI, Shaskov EV, Spring PM. In vivo, noninvasive, label-free detection and eradication of circulating metastatic melanoma cells using two-color photoacoustic flow cytometry with a diode laser. Cancer Res 2009;69(20):7926–34.

50. Gamelin J, Aguirre A, Maurudis A, et al. Curved array photoacoustic tomographic system for small animal imaging. J Biomed Opt 2008;13(2):1–10.

51. Yang X, Wang LV. Three-dimensional photoacoustic tomography of small animal brain with a curved array transducer. Proc SPIE 2009;7177:1–9.

52. Yang X, Wang LV. Monkey brain cortex imaging by photoacoustic tomography. J Biomed Opt 2008;13(4):1–5.

53. Yang X, Wang LV. Monkey brain cortex imaging by use of photoacoustic tomography. Proc SPIE 2008;6856:1–10.

54. Song KH, Wang LV. Deep reflection-mode photoacoustic imaging of biological tissue. J Biomed Opt 2007;12(6):1–3.

55. Song KH, Wang LV. Deep reflection-mode photoacoustic imaging of internal organs. Proc SPIE 2008;6856:1–8.

56. Song L, Maslov K, Bitton R, et al. Fast 3-D dark-field reflection-mode photoacoustic microscopy in vivo with a 30-MHz ultrasound linear array. J Biomed Opt 2008;13(5):1–5.

57. Song L, Maslov K, Bitton R, et al. Fast 3-D photoacoustic imaging in vivo with a high frequency ultrasound array towards clinical applications. Proc SPIE 2009;7177:1–9.

58. Stein EW, Maslov K, Wang LV. Noninvasive, in vivo imaging of blood-oxygenation dynamics within the mouse brain using photoacoustic microscopy. J Biomed Opt 2009;14(2):1–3.

59. Stein EW, Maslov K, Wang LV. Noninvasive, in vivo imaging of the mouse brain using photoacoustic microscopy. J Appl Phys 2009;105:1–5.

60. Fang Hui, Maslov K, Wang LV. M-mode photoacoustic flow imaging. Proc SPIE 2009;7177:1–8.

61. Yang J-M, Maslov K, Yang H-C, et al. Endoscopic photoacoustic microscopy. Proc SPIE 2009;7177:1–9.

62. Kruger RA, Kiser WL Jr, Miller KD, et al. Thermoacoustic CT: imaging principles. Proc SPIE 2000;3916:150–9.

63. Kruger RA, Kiser WL Jr, Reinecke DR, et al. Thermoacoustic optical molecular imaging of small animals. Mol Imaging 2003;2(2):113–23.

64. Liu Bo, Reinecke D, Kruger RA, et al. Phantom and in vivo measurements of hemoglobin concentration and oxygen saturation using PCT-S small animal scanner. Proc SPIE 2007;6437:1–9.

65. Kruger RA, Reinecke D, Kruger G, et al. HYPR-spectral photoacoustic CT for preclinical imaging. Proc SPIE 2009;7177:1–10.

66. Oraevsky AA, Savateeva EV, Solomatin SV, et al. Optoacoustic imaging of blood for visualization and diagnostics of breast cancer. Proc SPIE 2002;4618:81–94.

67. Khamapirad T, Henrichs PM, Mehta K, et al. Diagnostic imaging of breast cancer with LOIS: clinical feasibility. Proc SPIE 2005;5697:35–44.

68. Manohar S, Kharine A, van Hespen JC, et al. The Twente photoacoustic mammoscope: system overview and performance. Phys Med Biol 2005;50:2543–57.

69. Manohar S, Vaartjes SE, van Hespen JC, et al. Region-of-interest breast studies using the Twente photoacoustic mammoscope (PAM). Proc SPIE 2007;6437:1–9.

70. Petrov YY, Petrova IY, Esenaliev RO, et al. Clinical tests of noninvasive, optoacoustic, cerebral venous oxygenation monitoring system. Proc SPIE 2009;7177:1–5.

71. Petrov YY, Petrova IY, Patrikeev IA. Multiwavelength optoacoustic system for noninvasive monitoring of cerebral venous oxygenation: a pilot clinical test in the internal jugular vein. Opt Lett 2006;31(12):1827–9.

72. Brecht HP, Prough DS, Petrov YY, et al. In vivo monitoring of blood oxygenation in large veins with a triple-wavelength optoacoustic system. Optic Express 2007;15(24):16261–9.

73. Petrova IY, Petrov YY, Prough DS, et al. Clinical tests of highly portable, 2-lb, laser diode-based, noninvasive, optoacoustic hemoglobin monitor. Proc SPIE 2009;7177:1–6.

74. Beard PC, Zhang EZ, Cox BT. Transparent Fabry Perot polymer film ultrasound array for backward-mode photoacoustic imaging. Proc SPIE 2004;5320:230–7.

75. Zhang EZ, Beard P. 2D backward-mode photoacoustic imaging system for NIR (650–1200nm) spectroscopic biomedical applications. Proc SPIE 2006;6086:1–8.

76. Laufer J, Zhang E, Beard P. Quantitative in vivo measurements of blood oxygen saturation using multiwavelength photoacoustic imaging. Proc SPIE 2007;6437:1–9.

77. Zhang ED, Laufer J, Beard P. Backward-mode multiwavelength photoacoustic scanner using a planar Fabry–Perot polymer film ultrasound sensor for high-resolution three-dimensional imaging of biological tissues. J Appl Opt 2008;47(4):561–77.

78. Laufer J, Zhang ED, Raivich G, et al. Three-dimensional noninvasive imaging of the vasculature in the mouse brain using a high resolution photoacoustic scanner. J Appl Opt 2009;48(10):D299–306.

79. Cox BT, Arridge SR, Beard PC. Estimating chromophore distributions from multiwavelength photoacoustic images. J Opt Soc Am 2009;26(2):443–55.

80. Köstli KP, Beard PC. Two-dimensional photoacoustic imaging by use of Fourier-transform image reconstruction and a detector with an anisotropic response. J Appl Opt 2003;42(10):1899–908.

81. Oraevsky A, Ermilov S, Mehta K, et al. In vivo testing of laser optoacoustic system for image-guided biopsy of prostate. Proc SPIE 2006;6086:1–11.

82. Andreev VG, Ponomaryov AE, Henrichs PM, et al. Detection of prostate cancer with optoacoustic tomography: feasibility and modeling. Proc SPIE 2003;4960:45–57.

83. Spirou GM, Vitkin IA, Wilson BC, et al. Development and testing of an optoacoustic imaging system for monitoring and guiding prostate cancer therapies. Proc SPIE 2004;5320:44–56.

84. Yaseen MA, Brecht HP-F, Ermilov SA, et al. Hybrid optoacoustic and ultrasonic imaging system for detection of prostate malignancies. Proc SPIE 2008;6856:1–11.

85. Chen Z, Tang Z, Wan W. Photoacoustic tomography imaging based on a 4f acoustic lens imaging system. Optic Express 2007;15(8):4966–76.

86. Hecht E. Optics. San Francisco (CA): Addison Wesley; 2002.

87. Xu M, Wang LV. Photoacoustic imaging in biomedicine. Rev Sci Instrum 2006;77:1–22.

Index

Note: Page numbers of article titles are in **boldface** type.

Ultrasound Clin 4 (2009) 431–438
doi:10.1016/S1556-858X(10)00016-2

Printed and bound by CPI Group (UK) Ltd, Croydon, CR0 4YY
03/10/2024
01040353-0007